CELL BIOLOGY RESEARCH PROGRESS

THE STELLATE CELL (VITAMIN A-STORING CELL) SYSTEM

Cell Biology Research Progress

Additional books in this series can be found on Nova's website under the Series tab.

Additional e-books in this series can be found on Nova's website under the e-book tab.

CELL BIOLOGY RESEARCH PROGRESS

THE STELLATE CELL (VITAMIN A-STORING CELL) SYSTEM

HARUKI SENOO

NOVA BIOMEDICAL

New York

For permission to use material from this book please contact us:
Telephone 631-231-7269; Fax 631-231-8175
Web Site: http://www.novapublishers.com

Library of Congress Cataloging-in-Publication Data

ISBN: 978-1-62808-516-7

LCCN: 2013947628

Published by Nova Science Publishers, Inc. † New York

Contents

Preface		**vii**
Chapter 1	Introduction	**1**
Chapter 2	Morphology of HSC	**11**
Chapter 3	Functions of HSCs	**33**
Chapter 4	Relation with other Cells in the Liver	**99**
Chapter 5	Extrahepatic Stellate Cells	**105**
Chapter 6	Aging and HSCs	**117**
Chapter 7	Roles of HSCs during Liver Regeneration	**119**
Chapter 8	Hepatic Diseases and HSCs	**121**
Chapter 9	Immunity and HSCs	**147**
Chapter 10	Epigenetics of HSCs	**153**
Chapter 11	Artificial Organs and HSCs	**155**
Chapter 12	Global Climate Change and HSCs	**161**
Chapter 13	Conclusion	**165**
Acknowledgment		**167**
References		**169**
Index		**231**

Preface

Past, present, and future of the research of hepatic stellate cells (HSCs; also called vitamin A-storing cells, lipocytes, interstitial cells, fat-storing cells, Ito cells) are summarized and discussed in this review. Kupffer discovered black-stained cells in the liver by gold chloride method and named the cells the stellate cells (Sternzellen in German) in 1876. Wake re-discovered the cells in 1971 using the same gold chloride method and various modern histological techniques including electron microscopy. Between the discovery and re-discovery, the HSCs disappeared from the research history. Identification, establishment of cell isolation and culture methods, the development of cellular and molecular biological techniques have promoted the HSC research after the re-discovery of the cell. The research is entering new era, namely, the golden age after the dark ages. In mammals, HSCs exist in the space between liver parenchymal cells or hepatocytes (PCs) and liver sinusoidal endothelial cells (LSECs) of the hepatic lobule, and store 50-80 % of vitamin A in the whole body as retinyl ester in lipid droplets in the cytoplasm. HSCs also exist in extrahepatic organs such as pancreas, lung, and kidney. Hepatic (HSCs) and extrahepatic stellate cells (EHSCs) form the stellate cell (SC) system or SC family; the main storage site of vitamin A in the body is the HSC in the liver. In physiological conditions, HSCs and EHSCs play pivotal roles in the regulation of vitamin A homeostasis; they take up, store, and release retinol. HSCs play an important role in the liver regeneration. In pathological conditions such as liver fibrosis, HSCs lose vitamin A, and synthesize a large amount of extracellular matrix (ECM) components including collagen, proteoglycan, glycosaminoglycan, and adhesive glycoproteins. The morphology of these cells also changes from the star-shaped HSCs to that of fibroblasts or myofibroblasts. The three-dimensional structure of ECM components regulates reversibly the morphology, proliferation, and functions of the HSCs. Molecular mechanisms in the reversible regulation of the HSCs by ECM imply cell surface integrin-binding to ECM components followed by signal transduction processes and then cytoskeleton assembly. The distribution of HSCs, EHSCs, and retinoid-storing cells differs between non-mammalian vertebrates and mammals, suggesting that the SC system has appeared in lamprey, and vitamin A-storing site has shifted from whole body to the liver during vertebrate evolution. The relationship between HSCs and biodiversity has been proposed. HSCs are now to be a target of the treatment and therapy of hepatic fibrosis and liver cirrhosis. In the future, the research of HSCs will develop more into not only the clinical field but also into the basic research fields. In this monograph we would like to describe the past, present, and future of the HSC research.

Chapter 1

Introduction

The research of hepatic stellate cells (HSCs) has re-started when the cells was re-discovered by Wake (Wake 1971; reviewed by Wake 1980a). Establishment of cell isolation and culture methods of HSCs and standardization of the nomenclature, namely, hepatic stellate cells (HSCs), have promoted the development the HSC research (reviewed by Friedamn 2008b, Senoo et al. 2010, 2011a, 2011b). Not only physiological roles but also roles in pathogenesis of diseases are now under investigation in many laboratories in the world. Under such circumstances, the authors would like to summarize the past and present and try to describe the future of the HSC research. Excellent and new reviews on HSCs have been already published (Blomhoff and Wake 1991; Friedman 2008b; Li and Friedman 2001; Sato et al. 2003; Senoo 2004; Senoo et al. 1997, 2010, 2011a, 2011b; Smedsrød et al. 2009; Wake 1980, 1998), but we would like to describe this review emphasizing pioneer works, basic research, and important but not well-known studies.

The hepatic lobule consists of liver parenchymal cells or hepatocytes (PCs) and non-parenchymal cells (NPCs) associated with the liver sinusoids: liver sinusoidal endothelial cells (LSECs), Kupffer cells (KCs), pit cells, dendritic cells, and hepatic stellate cells (HSCs) (Bloom and Fawcett, 1994; Wake, 1971, 1980) (Fig. 1). LSECs (Wisse 1970, 1972; Brouwer et al. 1988b) express lymphocyte co-stimulatory molecules (Kojima et al. 2001) and form the greater part of the extremely thin lining of the sinusoids, which are larger than ordinary and more irregular in shape.

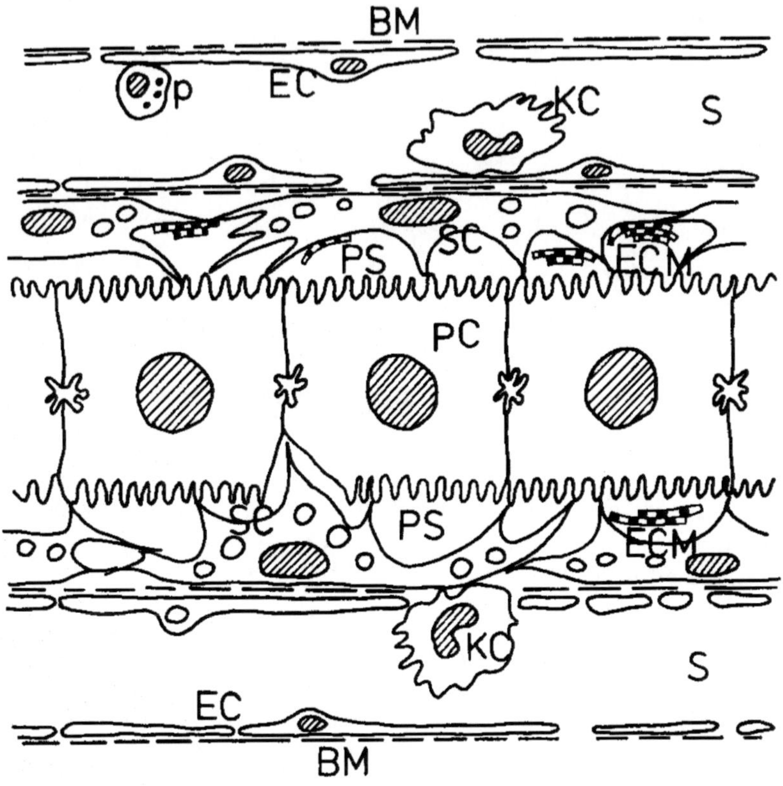

Figure 1. Structure of hepatic lobule. Hepatic cords of the lobule consist of parenchymal cells or hepatocytes (PC). Endothelial cells (EC) form the thin lining of the sinusoids (S). Kupffer cells (KC) are tissue macrophages and belong to the monocyte-macrophage cell lineage. Pit cells (p) have natural killer activity. Stellate cells (SC) lie in the space between parenchymal cells and endothelial cells, and store 50-80 % of retinoids of the whole body as retinyl palmitate in the lipid droplets in the cytoplasm. The classical definition of the perisinusoidal space (space of Disse) was the space between PCs and ECs. Whereas the new concept of the perisinusoidal space (PS) is the space between PCs and the complex of SCs and ECs. BM. Basement membrane components; ECM, extracellular matrix. Senoo H, Yoshikawa K, Morii M, Miura M, Imai K, Mezaki Y (2010) Hepatic stellate cell (vitamin A-storing cell) and its relative--past, present, and future.Cell Biol Int (editor's special 70th birthday edition) 34, 1247-1272.

KCs are tissue macrophages and components of the diffuse mononuclear phagocyte system. They are usually situated on the endothelium with cellular processes extending between the underlying LSECs. The greater part of their irregular cell surface is exposed to the blood in the lumen of the sinusoid. Pit cells are natural killer cells. Dendritic cells locate in the portal triad in human liver (Prickett et al. 1988), and in periportal and central areas in rat liver (Steiniger et al. 1984) that capture and process antigens, migrate to lymphoid organs and secrete cytokines to initiate immune responses (Banchereau and Steinman 1998). The HSCs (Figs. 1 and 2) that lie in the space between LSECs and PCs are considered to be derived from mesenchymal origin. Both LSECs and HSCs are derived from mesenchymal tissue, namely, septum transversum. KCs are from monocyte-macrophage system.

Mesenchymal cells that store vitamin A in their cytoplasm have been found in extrahepatic organs (kidney, intestine, lung, pancreas, etc.) and characterized (Apte et al. 1998; Bachem et al. 1998; Matano et al. 1999. Nagy et al. 1997; Senoo et al. in press; reviewed by Wake, 1980a). The purpose of this monograph is to survey recent progress in studies of structure and function of the HSCs emphasizing the points mentioned above.

1.1. Discovery and Re-Discovery of Hepatic Stellate Cell (HSC)

The stellate cells ("Sternzellen") in the liver (hepatic stellate cells, HSCc) were discovered by Kupffer in 1876 (Kupffer 1876; reviewed by Wake 1980a) using the gold chloride method (Wake et al. 1986). A neuroanatomist, Kupffer tried to find nerve components in the liver of rat, mouse, rabbits, bovines, pigs, dogs, and humans using the gold chloride method at that time. Accidentally he found black-stained star-shaped cells in the liver and called the cells stellate cells ("Sternzellen"). The gold chloride reaction was specific; only HSCs were clearly stained black in the background of red-stained other liver cells such as liver PCs. Kupffer described correctly that HSCs located in the space between PCs and LSECs. Rothe, one of his students, applied the gold chloride method to livers of other mammals and found similar cells in these livers (Rothe 1882).

However, 22 years after the discovery, a misconception by himself (Kupffer 1898, 1899) generated new misconception and led to a great confusion in the liver histology (Wake 1974, 1978, 1982, 2009; reviewed by Wake 1980a). Kupffer "corrected" his description of 1876 on the stellate cells as a misconception in the 12th Congress of Anatomists held in Kiel in 1898 (Kupffer 1898, 1899). He compared the liver specimen stained by gold chloride method with the rabbit liver specimen that was injected India ink, and concluded that “Sternzelle” was a special endothelial cell that phagocytozed foreign materials. Although the research of phagocyic liver cells progressed even after Kupffer’s “correction”, the research contained errors; ”phagocytic liver cells” included both phagocytic KCs and HSCs. From Kupffer’s “correction” of 1898, the stellate cells of the liver (“Sternzellen”, HSCs) disappeared from the history of the research of the liver as mentioned above.

The true nature of these cells remained unknown for over several decades until it was re-discovered by Wake (Wake 1971). He used various morphological methods, namely, gold chloride method, silver impregnation, lipid staining, fluorescence microscopy, electron microscopy, and re-discovered the stellate cells (Wake 1971, 1980a, 1980b). He observed HSCs from various directions; he observed “old” phenomenon with “new” eyes and observed “new” phenomenon with “old” eyes. He has revealed that the HSCs are quite different from the phagocytic Kupffer cells located in the sinusoid formed by LSEC. HSCs locate in the space between the PCs and LSECs. HSCs are identical to the perisinusoidal cells such as fat-storing cells (Ito 1951) and interstitial cells (Suzuki 1958).

The history of the study of HSCs has been thoroughly described and discussed by Wake (review of Wake 1980a). The name of HSCs will be discussed in the section 1.2 in this article.

Wake divided the history of the study of HSCs into three periods. During the first period (1876-1897), HSCs were correctly recognized with regard to the cell shape, distribution, and localization, namely, in the perisinusoidal space. During the second period (1898-1970), due to Kuppfer’s “correction” in 1898, HSCs disappeared from the liver research. In Kupffer’s “correction”, he changed his earlier opinion and concluded that HSCs were the special endothelial cells of the sinusoids. During the third period (1970-present) HSCs have been recognized correctly. After the re-discovery of HSCs by Wake (Wake 1971), HSCs have reappeared and gained proper position in the liver research. During the misconception period, namely, second period, many researchers “found” HSCs and named the cells differently. Various names of HSCs became barriers for the researchers to enter the HSC study, and as will be discussed afterwards the standardization of the nomenclature was done in 1996 (Hepatology). Now many researchers use the common name of hepatic stellate cells (HSCs). The standardization promoted the entry of new researchers to this research fields and promoted communications among the researchers. After a long misconception period a “golden age” is now coming to the HSC research.

Until the Hepatology paper (1996), the name of "Ito cell" or fat storing cells (FSC, Fettspeicherung Zellen) was popular, because of the easiness of spelling, pronunciation, and nationalistic feeling. In 1951, Ito found the cell storing fat using lipid-staining method (Ito 1951). He named the cell fat-storing cell. The cell was also called Ito cell afterward. If he had examined thoroughly the literature of HSCs, he would have used the name of "Sternzellen" or the stellate cells instead of fat-storing cells. It is regret that he has not done so.

1.2. Nomenclature

HSCs those were originally designated as Sternzellen (Kupffer 1876) have been given various names as listed by Wake (reviewed by Wake 1980a). These names are stellate cells (Kupffer 1876; Wake, 1971), granular cells (Berkley 1893), pericytes (Zimmermann 1928), fat-storing cells (Ito 1951; Kobayashi and Takahashi 1971; Kobayashi et al. 1973), metalophil cells (Marshall 1956), interstitial cells (Suzuki 1958), lipophagic cells (Horiuchi 1960), perisinusoidal cells (Wood 1963), transmittal cells (Suzuki 1963), mesenchymal cells (Rhodin 1964), lipocytes (Brofenmajer et al. 1966), adventitious connective tissue cells (Schnack et al. 1967; Stockinger 1967), Disse-space cells (Takeuchi et al. 1967), sinusoidal mesenchymal cells (Rubin et al. 1970), Ito cells (Hruban et al. 1974), lipid-storing cells (Hruban et al. 1974; Yamamoto and Enzan 1975), lipocytes perisinusoideus (terminology in histology 1975), vitamin A-storing cells (Yamada 1982; Yamada and Hirosawa 1976; Matsumoto and Hirosawa 1983), extravascular cells (Purton 1976), and vitamin A-uptake cells (Kusumoto and Fujita 1977) (see references in the review of Wake 1980a).

The terminology of HSCs was discussed in Federation of American Society of Experimental Biology (FASEB), and HSC was judged as the most appropriate name, because this name had no personal names, indicating morphology and location of the cell (Norum 1984).

In 1996, 98 investigators in the field of liver non-parenchymal cell (NPC) biology and hepatic fibrosis sent a letter to the editor of Hepatology and proposed that the term "hepatic stellate cells" should be used in referring to the cell type formerly known as either the Ito cell, the lipocyte, the fat-storing cell, the perisinusoidal cell, the pericyte, or the parasinusoidal cell (Hepatic stellate cell nomenclature, 1996). The investigators hoped that the adoption of this proposal will eliminate a source of confusion in this rapidly growing field.

Their reasons for the choice of the term "hepatic stellate cells" included following:

1. It Is Historically Correct

Kupffer first used the term Sternzellen in his writings, although admittedly he misconstrued these cells as macrophages. The use of the term "hepatic" rather than "perisinusoidal" stellate cells distinguishes them from the stellate cells described in the nervous system, rheumatoid synovium, and elsewhere.

2. It Is Accurate

Unlike most of the other terms, particularly "fat-storing cell" or "lipocyte," the hepatic stellate cell engenders no confusion with adipocyte, as commonly occurs with the uninitiated or general audience. In view of the cells' shape and their luminescence, "stellate" is indeed an appropriate term.

3. The Term "Stellate Cell" Is Already Consistently Used in the Retinoid Field to Refer to These Cells

To this letter signed by 98 investigators, the editor commented as follows. The editor accepted the letter for publication in HEPATOLOGY because the journal believes the current widely varying nomenclature to be unnecessarily confusing and welcomes this concerned effort to achieve clarity. Future discussions among the growing numbers of workers in the field may achieve a broader consensus. Alternatively, consistent use of the term "hepatic stellate cell" by the large number of signatories to this letter, and by their colleagues and trainees, is perhaps the most effective way of moving the nomenclature toward an increasing consistent terminology.

After this correspondence of "Hepatic stellate cell nomenclature" appeared in Hepatology, using the term "hepatic stellate cell" has been increased. From this epoch-making standardization of the nomenclature, the number of studies of HSCs has increased.

1.3. Ontogeny and Phylogeny of HSC Ontogeny

In mammalian embryos, the liver arises as a ventral outgrowth—- -from the caudal or distal part of the foregut early in the fourth week (Du Bois 1968; Elias 1955; Fukuda-Taira 1981, Moore et al. 2008; Severn 1971, 1972; Varet and Grompe 2008; Zaret 2001). Fibroblast growth factors (FGFs) secreted by the developing heart, interact with the bipotential cells and induce formation of the hepatic diverticulum. The diverticulum extends into the septum transversum, a mass of splanchnic mesoderm between the developing heart and midgut. The septum transversum forms the ventral mesentery in this region. The hepatic diverticulum enlarges rapidly and divides into two parts as it grows between the layers of the ventral mesogastrium. The larger cranial part of the hepatic diverticulum is the primordium of the liver. The proliferating endodermal cells give rise to interlacing cords of PCs and to the epithelium-lining of the intrahepatic part of the biliary apparatus. The hepatic cords anastomose around endothelium-lined spaces, the primordial of the hepatic sinusoids. The fibrous and hematopoietic tissue and Kupffer cells of the liver are suggested to derive from mesenchyme in the septum transversum (Asahina et al. 2011; Yin et al. 2012)

Liver mesothelial cells give rise to mesenchymal cells which intermingle between the growing hepatoblast cords and become incorporated to the sinusoidal wall, contributing to both LSCE and HSC populations. HSCs which likely derive from pre-existing mesenchymal cells of the septum transversum are first detectable between 8 and 10 weeks of gestation; they slowly differentiate, as shown the progressive increase in the number of intracytoplasmic lipid droplets, a characteristic feature of fully mature HSCs (Collardeau-Frachon and Scoazec 2008). The developing liver is vascularized through a complex process of vasculogenesis that leads to the differentiation of the sinusoids. Both intrinsic or extrinsic mesothelium-derived cells have the developmental potential to contribute to the establishment of liver sinusoids (Pérez-Pomares et al. 2004). At day of 10 of gestation in mice and rats or at 5 weeks of gestation in humans, the hepatic cord grow into the mesenchymal tissue of the septum transversum, and the primitive sinusoid-like structure is simultaneously observed between the liver cell cords (Enzan et al. 1997).

In the margin of the growing liver primordium, mesenchymal cells in the septum transversum are trapped in the subendothelial space. These subendothelial cells are at the early stages of organogenesis and become progenitors of the HSCs.

Several reports have suggested that HSCs are derived from the neural crest (Yin et al. 2012) since HSCs express glial fibrillary acidic protein (GFAP; Buniatian et al. 1996; Gard et al. 1985; Neubauer et al. 1996; Niki et al. 1996) and nestin (Messing 1999; Niki et al. 1999), and that neural crest cells can differentiate into myofibroblasts expressing alpha smooth muscle actin (αSMA) which is a marker of the activated HSCs (Carlson 1999). HSCs are reactive to the Golgi staining which is usually used for neurofilament staining (Wake 1980a).

HSCs also display unique characteristics of gene expression similar to that of neural cell types; e.g., expression of neural cell adhesion molecule (N-CAM) (Knittel et al. 1996), synaptophysin (Cassiman et al. 1999), neurotrophins and neurotrophin receptors (Cassiman et al. 2001a; Trim et al. 2000), GFAP, or microtubule associated protein 2 (Sato et al. 2001). These findings also suggest the neural crest origin of HSCs. The activated HSC, a major extracellular matrix (ECM)-producing cell type in the liver fibrogenesis shows common phenotypic features to smooth muscle cells and myofibroblasts, both are originated from the neural crest and express vimentin, desmin, and αSMA.

However, yellow fluorescent protein (YFP) that is expressed in all neural crest cells and their derivatives, has not been detected in the developing liver or in HSCs from embryonic day 11.5 until adulthood of mice (Cassiman et al. 2006). This finding suggests that HSCs do not descend from the neural crest, and therefore may derive from the septum transversum mesenchyme (Kalinchenko et al. 2003; Varet and Grompe 2008), from endoderm or from the mesothelial liver capsule.

Recently, hematopoietic origin of HSCs has been proposed (Baba et al. 2004; Miyata et al. 2008; Suskind and Muench 2004). In mouse cirrhotic liver, the bone marrow contributes significantly to HSCs (68%) and myofibroblast (70%) populations (Russo et al. 2006). However, in response to the bile duct ligation-induced liver injury of mice, HSCs do not originate in the bone marrow, but collagen-producing fibrocytes are recruited from the bone marrow to damaged liver (Kisseleva et al. 2006). Contribution of bone marrow to HSC transdifferentiation might be different between the disease models. Additional works might be necessary for these studies.

A hypothesis that HSCs are a type of oval cell and capable of generating PCs to regenerate the injured liver was evaluated (Yang et al. 2008). The data suggest that HSCs are a type of oval cell that transitions through a mesenchymal phase before differentiating into PCs during liver regeneration. This report suggests that HSCs and PCs have the same progenitor, but more researches are needed to conclude this hypothesis is correct or not.

The phenotypic characteristics of HSCs in rat fetal livers, in which hepatic development and hematopoiesis occur in parallel, have been determined by using a strategy focused on vitamin A (Kubota et al. 2007). These results demonstrated that the vitamin A autofluorescence positive cells are fetal HSCs with extensive proliferative activity. Furthermore, the vitamin A autofluorescence positive cells strongly express hepatocyte growth factor, stromal-derived factor-1, and Hlx (homeobox transcription factor), indicating that they play important roles for hepatic development and hematopoiesis. Researches have been done studies as mentioned above, but the ontogeny of HSCs is still controversial (Geerts 2004).

Phylogeny

To demonstrate the origin of stellate cells (SCs) in phylogeny, SCs in non-mammalian and mammalian vertebrates have been investigated. We examined retinoid and retinoid-storing cells in arrowtooth halibut (*Atheresthes evermanni* Jordan Starks; Yoshikawa et al. 2006), lamprey (*Lampetra japonica*; Wake et al. 1987; Wake and Senoo 1986; Wold et al. 2004; Morii et al. 2010, 2011), ascidian (*Halocynthia roretzi*; Irie et al. 2004), and polar animals (Higashi and Senoo 2003; Senoo et al. 2012). In the arrowtooth halibut, the highest concentration of stored vitamin A is in retinoid-storing cells in the pyloric cecum, a teleost-specific organ protruding from the intestine adjacent to the pylorus. Considerable amounts of vitamin A were also stored in the cells in the lamina propria mucosae of the intestine and HSCs in the liver. In lamprey, retinoid is stored in retinoid-storing cells in the intestine, liver (HSCs), kidney, gill, and heart. In ascidian, retinal is the essential form of retinoid for storage, and no SCs are recognized (Irie et al. 2004). In arctic animals such as polar bears and arctic foxes a large amount of vitamin A is stored in the HSCs. However other organs store only a small amount of vitamin A (Higashi and Senoo 2003). Thus, the distribution of SCs with retinoid-storing capacity differs between non-mammalian vertebrates and mammals suggesting that the SCs appeared in lamprey, and vitamin A-storing site has shifted and concentrated from the whole body to the liver during vertebrate evolution.

Chapter 2

Morphology of HSCs

2.1. Light and Electron Microscopy of HSCs

2.1.1. Light Microscopical Observation of HSCs

Gold Chloride Method

After Kupffer (Kupffer 1876) and his pupil, Rothe (Rothe 1882) used the gold chloride method for the detection of HSCs, no one used this method for the research of HSCs until Wake used the method and re-discovered HSCs (Wake 1971, 1980a).

He improved the original method of Kupffer (Wake et al. 1986; Senoo and Wake 1988), because the original method of Kupffer was unstable (Wake et al. 1986). By this improvement, the gold chloride method has become stable and applicable to research of HSCs even in arctic animals in Greenland and Svalbard archipelago (Fig. 2; Higashi and Senoo 2003). By this method, HSCs are stained black in the red background of the other liver cells. The details of the gold chloride method and histochemistry of the gold chloride reaction were thoroughly described previously (Wake et al. 1986).

Silver Impregnation Method

Silver impregnation method also can demonstrate HSCs as described previously (Wake 1980a). In the silver-impregnated preparations, the stellate-shaped cytoplasmic processes of HSCs are obvious. Both in normal and hypervitaminosis A animals, a branching pattern and the fine structures of their dendritic processes are more clearly demonstrated with the silver impregnation method than the gold chloride method (Wake 1980a).

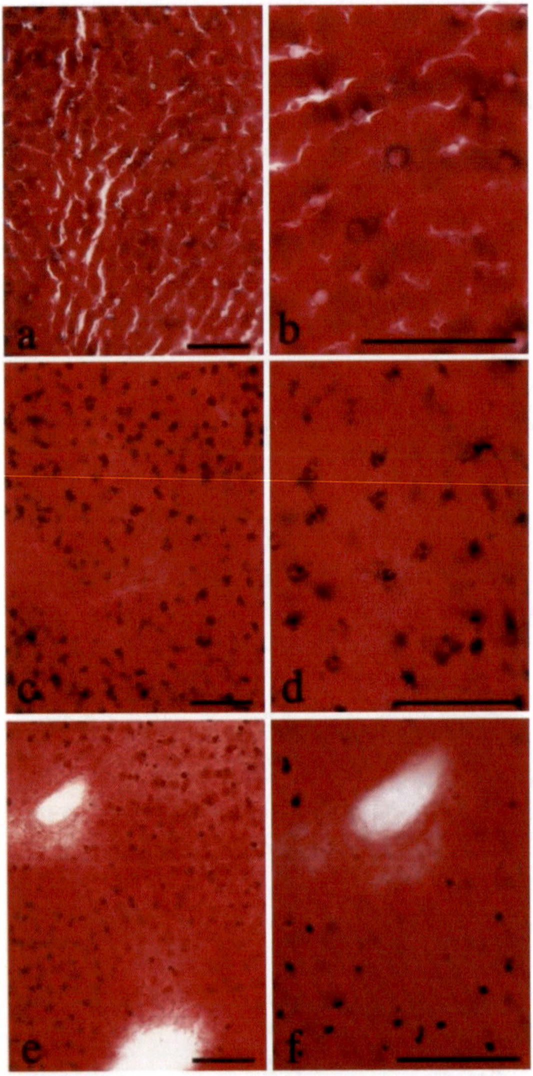

Figure 2. Gold chloride staining specifically demonstrating black-stained HSCs of polar bears (a and b), arctic foxes (c and d) and rats (e and f) Bars=100 μm. Reproduced, with permission, from Higashi N, Senoo H. Distribution of vitamin A-storing lipid droplets in hepatic stellate cells in liver lobules – a comparative study. Anat Rec 2003;271A:240-248, Wiley-Liss, Inc.

Lipid Staining and Hematoxylin and Eosin Staining

Lipid staining and hematoxylin & eosin staining are also able to demonstrate HSCs especially in hypervitaminosis A animals or arctic animals such as polar bears, arctic foxes, and bearded seals those store a large amount of vitamin A in the lipid droplet of the cytoplasm in HSCs (Higashi and Senoo 2003; Senoo et al. 2012).

Fluorescence Microscopy for Detection of Autofluorescence of Vitamin A

Fluorescence microscopy (Wake 1980a; Senoo and Wake 1988) is a useful tool for specific demonstration of autofluorescence of vitamin A emanating from the lipid droplets of HSCs (Fig.3: Higashi and Senoo 2003)

Autoradiography

Autoradiography using tritiated retinyl acetate demonstrates that the administered vitamin A is taken up by HSCs and localizes in the lipid droplets of the cytoplasm of HSCs (Hirosawa 1977; Hirosawa and Yamada, 1973; Hirosawa et al. 1988; Matsuura et al. 1993).

Immunofluorescence and Immunohistochemistry

Immunofluorescence and immunohistochemistry using specific markers of HSCs (such as desmin, α smooth muscle actin (αSMA), GFAP, αB crystallin) are useful methods for the demonstration of HSCs. The presence of desmin is used to identify HSCs in rat liver (Yokoi et al. 1984; Tsutsumi et al. 1987; Takase et al. 1988; Aimed et al. 1991) and to evaluate the purity of separated and cultured HSCs (Ballardini et al. 1994). HSCs express GFAP (Buniatian et al. 1996; Gard et al. 1985; Neubauer et al. 1996; Niki et al. 1996; Dack et al. 1997) and nestin (Messing 1999; Niki et al. 1999).

αSMA is known to be a marker of activated HSCs (Enzan et al. 1994b). Stromal cells around the hepatocellular cancer are frequently found and are strongly positive for αSMA (Enzan et al. 1994a). After necrosis of cancer tissue, they may become activated and actively participate in the fibrosis.

HSCs also express genes similar to that of neural cell types; e.g., neural cell adhesion molecule (N-CAM) (Knittel et al. 1996), synaptophysin (Cassiman et al. 1999), neurotrophins and neurotrophin receptors (Cassiman et al. 2001a; Trim et al. 2000), GFAP, or microtubule associated protein 2 (Sato et al. 2001). These molecules are also used as markers of HSCs.

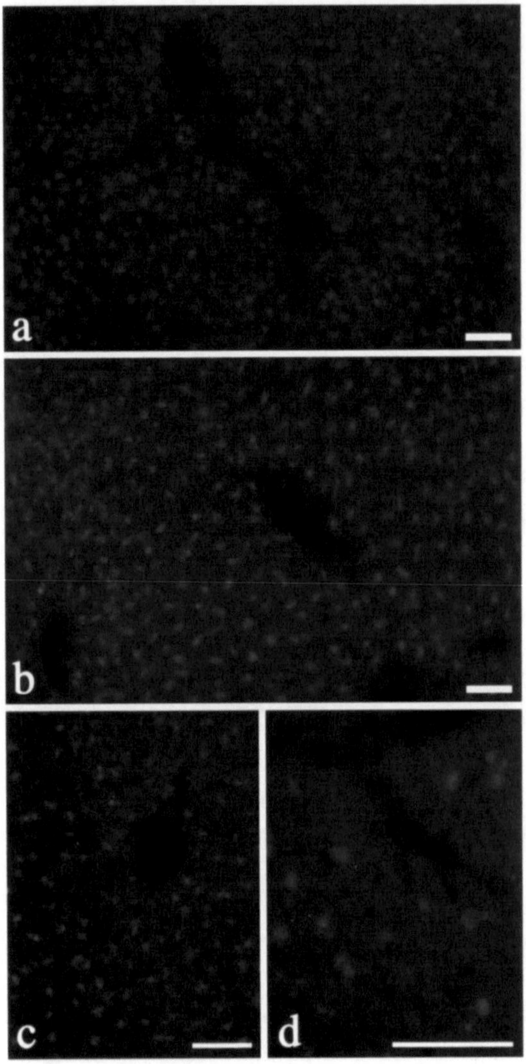

Figure 3. Fluorescence micrographs demonstrating vitamin A autofluorescence in HSCs of polar bears (a), arctic foxes (b) and rats (c and d) Bars=100 μm. Reproduced, with permission, from Higashi N, Senoo H. Distribution of vitamin A-storing lipid droplets in hepatic stellate cells in liver lobules – a comparative study. Anat Rec 2003;271A:240-248, Wiley-Liss, Inc.

An antibody specific to mouse and human lecithin:retinol acyltransferase (LRAT) was prepared based on the amino acid sequences. Antibodies to

LRAT were used for immunohistochemical studies to assess the distribution of LRAT-positive cells in the liver. LRAT-positive cells were found to be confined in the space of Disse, corresponding with the location of desmin-positive HSC in rodent and human livers. Furthermore, immune electron microscopic studies revealed that LRAT was mainly distributed in HSC within the rough-endoplasmic reticulum (RER) and multivesicular bodies (Nagatsuma et al. 2009). Thus, evidence has been accumulated that LRAT might serve as an excellent alternative marker for future structural and functional studies.

αB-crystallin, a small heat-shock protein and a chaperone (ABCRYS) is also expressed in HSCs. αB-crystallin is expressed in culture-activated but not quiescent rat HSCs (Lang et al. 2000). α B-crystallin is known to protect the cell against protein degradation in conditions of cellular stress and known to associate with various types of intermediate filaments. Expression of αB-crystallin is also induced in vivo activated HSCs from experimental cholestatic liver fibrosis. αB-crystallin represents an early marker for HSC activation (Cassiman et al. 2001b).

Laser-Induced Fluorescence Spectroscopy

Recently, the laser-induced fluorescence spectroscopy has been applied to investigate intestinal and liver tissue of normal and vitamin A-fed rats (Akhmeteli et al. 2008). A special procedure based on intensity spectral functions fitting was developed for the recognition of vitamin A in different tissues. However, the usefulness of this method is not yet fully confirmed.

2.1.2. Ultrastructure of HSCs (Fig. 4; See Summary of the Ultrastructure of HSCs by Wake1980b)

Vitamin A lipid droplets are conspicuous features of the cytoplasm of HSCs. Another conspicuous feature of HSCs is their well-developed rough endoplasmic reticulum (ER) with membrane-bound ribosomes. ER lumen or ER cisternal space is moderately expanded indicating active biosynthesis of secretory polypeptides or proteins. Development of smooth ER is poor.

A small amount of glycogen particles exists in the cytoplasm.

Several investigators have reported that HSCs display a conspicuous Golgi apparatus (Golgi complex), whereas a few investigators reported a small Golgi apparatus. Golgi apparatus may change its feature due to the functional status, namely, "quiescent" or "activated" status of HSCs.

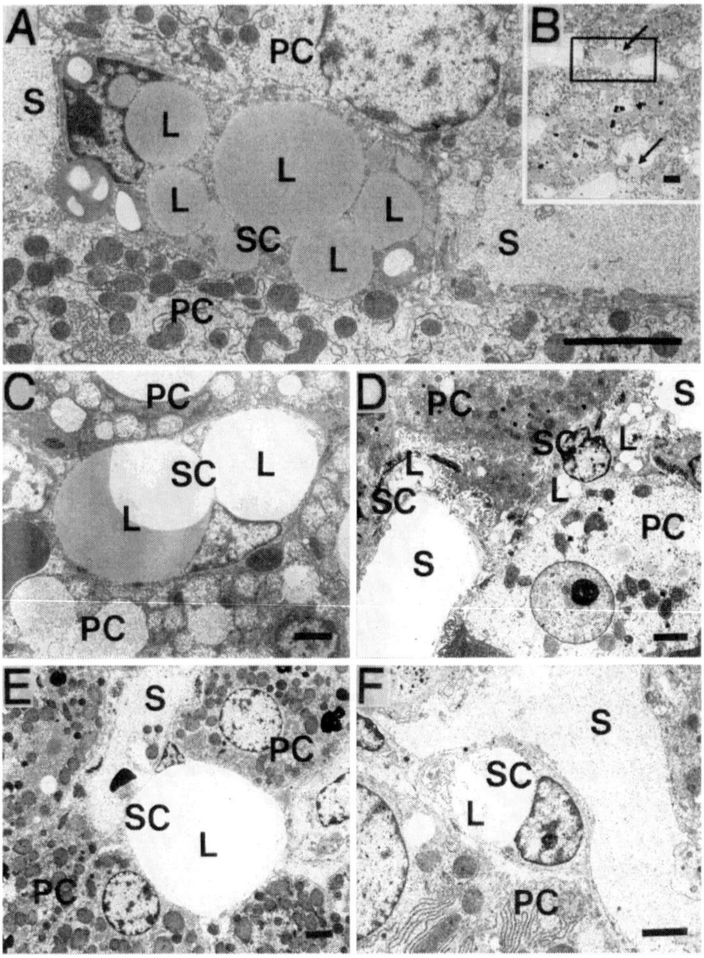

Figure 4. Transmission electron microscopy of the liver of arctic fox (A, B), polar bear (C), glaucous gull (D), bearded seal (E), and ringed seal (F). Panel A is a high magnification of a portion (rectangle) of B. Arrows in panel B indicate hepatic stellate cells. L: lipid droplet, PC: parenchymal cell (hepatocyte), S: sinusoid, SC: hepatic stellate cell. Scale bars for A, C, D, E and F: 2μm; for B: 5 μm. Senoo, H., Imai, K., Mezaki, Y., Miura, M., Morii, M., Fujiwara, M., Blomhoff, R (2012) Accumulation of vitamin A in the hepatic stellate cell of arctic top predators. Anat Rec. 295, 1660-1668, Wiley-Liss, Inc.

Lysosome exists in HSCs and HSCs have phagocyic activity (Mousavi et al. 2004). In extrahepatic SCs in the intestine of the lamprey have phagocytic activity during spawning migration stage (Higashi et al. 2005b). During this life stage of the lamprey, the intestine becomes atrophic, because the lamprey leaves the bigger fish that the lamprey sucked to take its blood, body fluid, and meat; necessity of the digestion and absorption decreased.

Activity of acid hydrolase has been demonstrated in the lysosome of the exrahepatic SCs in the intestine (Higashi et al. 2005b). Phagocytosis of collagen fibril was also demonstrated in the extrahepatic SCs in the intestine of the lamprey.

Early and late endosomes and multivesicular body (MVB) were demonstrated in HSCs; a function of other than action as phagolysosomes has been attributed to MVB (Wake 1974, 1980a). Retinol-binding protein (RBP) has been demonstrated in endosomes and MVB by immunoelectron microscopy (Senoo et al. 1990). MVB was proposed as an essential cell organelle for the development of the vitamin A-containing lipid droplets in HSCs (see Section 3.5).

Caveolae are small pits on the plasma membrane found in several, if not all, differentiated cells. They are involved in potocytosis, endocytosis, transcytosis, membrane trafficking, and signal transduction. Immunocytochemical analysis of caveolin in NPCs of the rat liver showed its presence in HSCs (Calvo et al. 2001).

Cytoskeleton

Actin filaments are distributed in the periphery of the cellular processes of HSCs (Sato et al. 1998). These filaments have been proposed to play pivotal roles during extension and retraction of the cellular processes (Sato and Senoo 1998; Imai and Senoo 1998, 2000). HSCs tend to project a cilium into the perisinusoidal space; the functional significance of the cilium is not yet clearly shown.

Microtubules have been shown to distribute in the core of the cellular processes of HSCs (Sato et al. 1998). These microtubules have been shown to play important roles in extension and retraction of the cellular processes of HSCs (Imai et al. 1997; Sato et al. 1998).

Intermediate Filaments

Desmin and GFAP are markers of HSCs, however the specific functions of these filaments are not yet thoroughly clarified.

Nucleus

The nucleus of HSCs is oval or elongated in EM. The nucleus is frequently indented by lipid droplets in the cytoplasm. One or more nucleoli can be seen in a HSC.

Thus, electron microscopy is one of useful techniques for demonstrating HSCs (Shin 1981).

2.1.3. Three-Dimensional Structure of HSCs

HSCs distribute regularly within hepatic lobules. The cell consists of a spindle-shaped or angular cell body and long and branching cytoplasmic processes which encompass the endothelial tubes of sinusoids (Wake 1995, 1998). Some processes penetrate the hepatic cell plates (structures formed by PCs. When PCs adhere each other, they become like a plate) to reach the neighboring sinusoids to taper off to several subendothelial processes. Accordingly, a single HSC wraps two or three, sometimes, four sinusoids with long processes. The total length of sinusoids surrounded by a single HSC is 60-140 μm in the rat liver.

The subendothelial processes of HSCs are flat and have three cell surfaces; inner, outer, and lateral. The inner one is smooth and adhere to the adluminal (basal) surface of the LSECs. Between the two cells, namely, HSCs and LSECs the basement membrane components such as type IV collagen, nidogen, and laminin are intercalated. The outer surface, facing the perisinusoidal space (space of Disse), is decorated with short microvillous protrusions. The lateral edges of the subendothelial processes are characteristically studded with numerous spike-like microprojections whose tips make contacts with the microvillous facets of the PCs (Fig. 1). HSCs adhere to LSECs through basement membrane components, and on the other hand, make spotty contacts with PCs.

Recently HSCs have been demonstrated at molecular and morphological levels to adhere each other by adherens junctions (Higashi et al. 2004).

2.1.4. Morphological Changes Caused by ECM Components in HSC Culture

Cultured HSCs exhibit mainly three types of morphology according to the substratum used for culture (Sato and Senoo 1998; Sato et al. 2003). The cells displayed a drastic change in cell shape accompanying the development of cytoplasmic processes by culturing in the presence of type I and type III collagen gel as a substratum (Fig. 5). On the other hand, HSCs have a flattened, fibroblast-like shape with well-developed stress fibers on the polystyrene surface, as well as on the lysine-or aminoalkylsilane-coated surface, and they show signs of neither cell spreading nor elongation of cell processes, and maintain a round shape in or on Engelbrech-Holm-Swarm murine tumor extracellular matrix containing the basement membrane components (Matrigel). Therefore, the ECM components can differentially regulate the morphology of HSCs, as well as at least a part of in vivo function (Senoo et al. 1996). Human fibroblasts also displayed a similar response to extracellular type I collagen to change their morphology to a rod shape with bipolar processes (Tomasek and Hay 1984) but the number of processes and the extent of secondary or tertiary branching in fibroblast culture was much less than those of HSC culture.

In HSC culture on a polystyrene surface, the time-lapse video recording demonstrated the cell surface ruffling activity of filopodia and lamellipodia, reflecting weak adhesion to the substratum (Fig. 6; Miura et al. 1997, 1999; http://www.med.akita-u.ac.jp/~kaibo2/default.html). All filopodia remained dynamic throughout the 3-hour video-recording, and repeatedly extended and retracted. On the other hand, HSCs were quiescent, but begin to elongate cytoplasmic processes within 1 hour after inoculating in or on type I collagen gel. The long processes appeared to contact with and extended along collagen fibril. After repeated extension and retraction of processes, HSCs display a number of processes with distal fine branching in 5-hour culture in type I collagen gel. After long term (over a week) culture in type I collagen gel, HSCs displayed three-dimensionally-developed processes with numerous secondary and tertiary fine branches. The cellular processes also extend in or on type III collagen gel but not on type IV collagen-coated surface or on Matrigel, indicating the different response of HSCs to collagen types or other extracellular matrix components. Such different response may be functionally important, since HSCs, as mentioned above, extend their processes in vivo along the perisinusoidal space of Disse containing mainly type I and type III collagen, whereas these cells display smooth cell surfaces in contact with the imperfect basal membrane components of LSECs (Wake 1980a). In vivo morphology of HSCs might be regulated by three-dimensional structure of ECM.

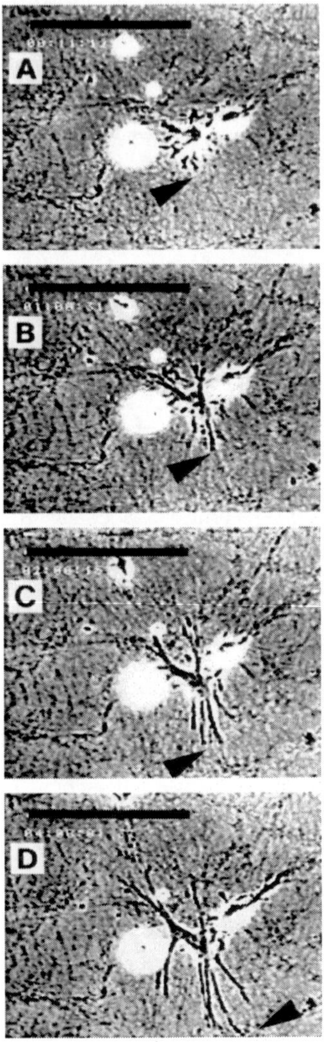

Figure 5. Extension of cellular processes in cultured rat HSCs on type I collagen gel. HSCs were cultured on type I collagen gel, and monitored by phase-contrast time-lapse video microscopy for up to 4 hours. Photographs were taken 71 minutes (A), 2 hours (B), 3 hours (C), and 4 hours (D) after inoculation. Scale, 200 μm. Miura M, Sato M, Toyoshima I, Senoo H (1997) Extension of long cellular processes of hepatic stellate cells cultured on extracellular type I collagen gel by microtubule assembly: observation utilizing time-lapse video-microscopy. Cell Struct Funct 22: 487-492.

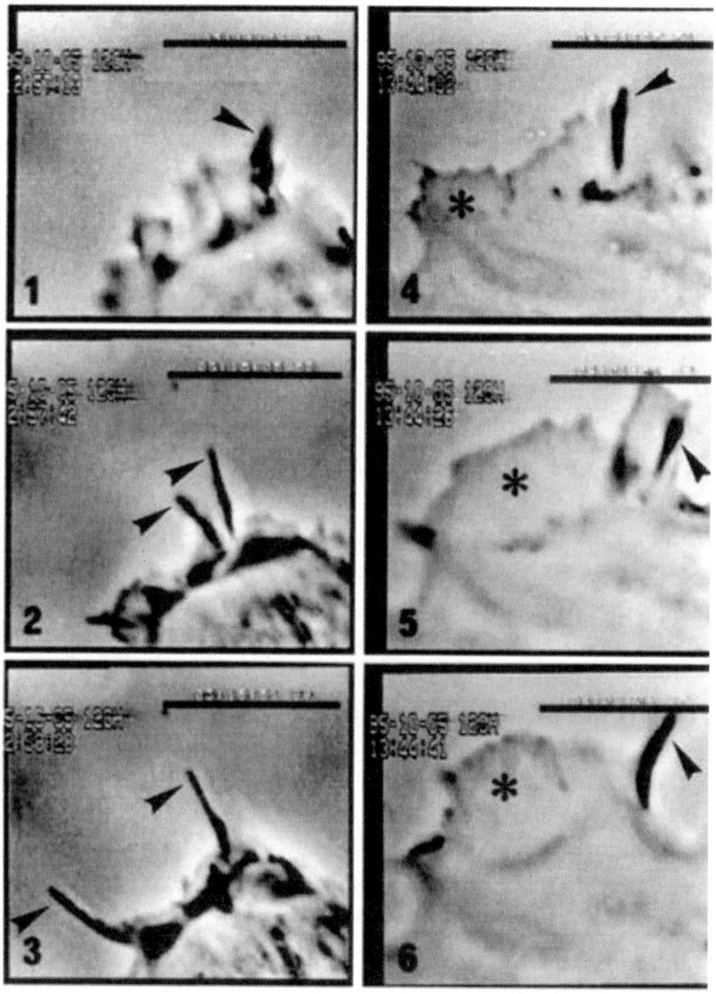

Figure 6. Motility of filopodia and lamellipodia in rat HSCs inoculated on polystyrene surface (http://www.med.akita-u.ac.jp/~kaibo2/default.html). The cells were monitored by phase-contrast video-enhanced microscopy. Photographs were taken at 29 seconds (Fig. 6-2) and 55 seconds (Fig 6-3) after taking a picture of Fig. 6-1, and at 24 seconds (Fig. 6-5) and 39 second (Fig 6-6) after taking a picture of Fig 6-4, respectively. Arrowheads indicate filopodia and asterisks indicate lamellipodia. Scale bars indicate 20 μm. Miura M, Sato M, Toyoshima I, Senoo H (1997) Extension of long cellular processes of hepatic stellate cells cultured on extracellular type I collagen gel by microtubule assembly: observation utilizing time-lapse video-microscopy. Cell Struct Funct 22: 487-492.

2.1.5. Molecular Mechanisms of Process Elongation

Cell surface integrin interactions with ECM are central to the migration, localization, and function of several types of cells within tissues (Jones et al. 1993; Hynes 1992; Kornberg et al. 1991; Rosales et al. 1995; Roskelley et al. 1995). Human HSCs have been reported to express integrin $\alpha1\beta1$, $\alpha2\beta1$, $\alpha(V)\beta1$ and $\alpha6\beta4$ (Carloni et al. 1996). The extension of the processes was inhibited by the addition of anti-integrin $\alpha2$ antibody or oligopeptide DGEA (Sato et al. 1998, 1999), which sequence in the type I or type IV collagen molecules has been reported to be responsible for cell surface integrin-binding (Staatz et al. 1991). Therefore the process elongation for HSCs appears to depend on integrin $\alpha2\beta1$-binding to extracellular collagen fibrils. Since no process elongation is seen in the culture on type I or type III collagen-coated surface (monometric collagen), a native fibrillar form of interstitial collagen is prerequisite for process elongation as reported for integrin-binding to a native form of collagen fibrils but not to monometric collagen in other cell type (Grab et al. 1996; Mercier et al. HSC 1996; Vogel et al. 1997).

Retraction of elongated processes is induced by the treatment with herbimycine A and staurosporin, a protein tyrosine kinase inhibitor and a general protein kinase inhibitor, respectively, or with wortmannin, a phosphatidyl inositol (PI) 3-kinase inhibitor (Miura et al. 1997, Sato et al. 1998; Kojima et al. 1998). When HSCs are inoculated in the presence of these inhibitors, the induction of process elongation is also inhibited, suggesting that both the induction and sustenance of processes depend on successive signaling events including protein and/or PI phosphorylation. Protein tyrosine phosphorylation was enhanced in HSCs cultured on type I collagen gel, when compared to the culture on the polystyrene surface (Kojima et al. 1998). In HSC culture, PI 3-kinase has been found to be involved in extracellular-signal regulated kinase (ERK) activation by platelet-derived growth factor (PDGF) (Marra et al. 1995). Interestingly, H-7 or hypericin, a specific inhibitor for protein kinase C, shows only a partial effect on the induction and sustenance of cytoplasmic processes in HSCs cultured on interstitial collagen gel, but H-7 or hypericin causes a significant morphological change in HSCs cultured on a polystyrene or molecular-coated surface accompanying the F-actin degradation. These results suggest a distinct pathway involving protein tyrosine kinase, PI kinase, and/or protein serine/threonine kinase is responsible for the cell spreading or the process elongation. It has been well documented that the reorganization of F-actin is triggered by integrin-binding to ECM components, followed by signal transduction mechanisms including protein phosophorylation (Yamada and Miyamoto 1995; Hynes 1992). In HSC culture, interstitial collagen signals triggered by cell surface integrin appear to finally result in the reorganization of microtubules, as well as F-actin assembly (Miura et al. 1997; Sato et al. 1998).

2.1.6. Cytoskeleton Organization in Cellular Processes of HSCs

The role of cytoskeleton organization in the sustenance of the process structure have been demonstrated by a video-recording of the HSC culture after the addition of cytoskeleton degrading drugs (Miura et al. 1997; http://www.med.akita-u.ac.jp/~kaibo2/default.html). Colchicine-treatment induces the retraction of the elongated processes. The effects are dose- and time-dependent, and almost all cells are changed to round shapes within a few hours in the presence of 1 μ M colchicine. The cold treatment at 4 °C, which is known to induce the degradation of a cold-labile form (dendritic type) of microtubules (Rosette and Karin 1995) also cause the retraction of elongated process within 3 hours. The elongated processes are also partly retract after the treatment with cytochalasin B (Sato et al. 1998). Although the effects of cytochalasin B appears to be weaker than that of colchicine, almost all cells are changed to a round shape after overnight treatment with cytochalasin B. Dual fluorescence staining of microtubule and F-actin in HSCs reveals that the core of processes consists of microtubules, while the periphery contain F-actin (Miura et al. 1997; Sato et al. 1998). Elongated front of the processes displays a similar filopodia and lamellipodia containing F-actin structure and microtubules to those of the growth cone of the extending neurites. These results, in addition to the effects of cytoskeleton degradation, suggest that the elongation of cellular processes results from F-actin and the microtubule assembly in the HSC culture.

2.1.7. Putative function of Cellular Processes of HSCs

Interstitial collagen gel induces the process elongation, mimicking the *in vivo* cell shape. It has been reported that interstitial type I collagen gel used as a substratum alters the HSC function to that of the quiescent, normal *in vivo* phenotype, such as the slight proliferation activity and the suppressed ECM production (Senoo et al. 1996). HSCs are unable to spread out or elongate their processes on or in Matrigel (Miura et al. 1997; Sato et al. 1998), but display rather normal *in vivo* functions (Friedman et al. 1989; Senoo and Hata 1994a, 1994b). Therefore, HSCs require the basement membrane components for a normal, inactivated phenotype, whereas they need interstitial collagen fibers for the process elongation, as mentioned above. Such an interpretation is consistent with the *in vivo* ECM status around HSCs in the liver tissue.

The primarily isolated and then repeatedly subcultured rat or human HSCs, as well as the established human cell line, LI90 (Murakami et al. 1995), retained at least some of the *in vivo* characteristic features by culturing in or on type I or type III collagen gel, such as the presence of long filamentous processes and the ability to store vitamin A in increased lipid droplets after the addition of retinyl acetate (Sato et al. 1998). HSCs cultured on interstitial collagen gel also expressed matrix metalloproteinase (MMP) 1 (Sato et al. 1998), which was demonstrable in cytoplasmic processes. HSCs are the primary ECM-producing cells in NPCs in liver fibrosis, and during liver injury HSCs undergo activation accompanying cell proliferation and enhanced fibrogenesis. Phenotypes including morphology of HSCs can be regulated by use of ECM components.

2.2. HSC Adhesion (Cell-ECM, Cell-Cell)

2.2.1. HSCs-ECM Adhesion

Extracellular matrix (ECM) is known to regulate a diversity of biological activities: cell proliferation, differentiation, migration, polarity, tumorigenesis and cancer metastasis (Alberts et al. 2008). The cells adhere to ECM by specialized cellular devices such as focal contacts, podosomes, point contacts, and hemidesmosomes (Senoo and Hata 1994b).

The ECM is composed of an insoluble complex of collagens, adhesive glycoproteins (e. g., fibronectin, laminin), proteoglycans (PGs) (e.g., heparan sulfate PGs, chondroitin sulfate PGs), glycosaminoglycans, and elastin. These ECM components construct an insoluble supramolecular complex (reviewed by Hata 1996). These molecules contain positional information and give it back as signals to the cells that produced them or to neighboring cells, as well as regulate their growth and metabolism (reviewed by Hata, 1996).

Integrins are the major family of cell surface receptors that mediate attachment to the ECM (Hynes 1992; Clark and Brugge 1995; Giancotti and Ruoslahti 1999). Formation of focal contacts is regulated by intracellular signals which promote integrin clustering and cytoskeletal associations. The relationship between the cells and ECM is one of the most important aspects with regard to the nature of the cells.

HSCs lie in the perisinusoidal space (space of Disse) (Wake 1980a, 1980b, 1995, 1997a, 1997b) and coexist with the three-dimensional ECM components within the space. The type of ECM components regulates behaviors of the HSCs (Senoo et al. 1991; Senoo and Hata 1994a, 1994b, 1995). The three-dimensional structure of substratum also reversibly regulates morphology, proliferation rate, and function of cultured HSCs (Senoo et al. 1996, 1997, 1998; Kojima et al. 1997; Imai et al. 1997). Adhesion between the HSCs and ECM is essential in the regulation of the cells by ECM.

The HSCs extend their thin membranous processes, dendritic processes, and fine fibrillar processes into the perisinusoidal space and coexist with the three-dimensional ECM components within the space (Wake, 1980a). The long three-dimensional processes of the HSCs and three-dimensional ECM form a complicated structure. Hence, it is difficult to analyze relationship between hepatic HSCs and ECM *in vivo* (Imai and Senoo 2000). As will be discussed later, we analyzed the relationship between HSC and ECM using cultured HSCs on or in various substrata.

2.2.2. ECM in the Perisinusoidal Space

The sinusoidal wall is consisted of three cell-layers; KCs and liver-associated lymphocytes layer, the LSEC-layer and the perisinusoidal HSC-layer (Wake 1995). Basement membrane-like structures interruptedly lie between the endothelial cell-layer and the HSC-layer (Wake 1997b). Small narrow strands of material resembling a basement membrane can be discerned underneath the endothelial lining or between the lining and the underlying subendothelial projections of the HSCs (Wake 1980a). The HSCs appear to adhere to the wall of sinusoids by the basement membrane. Collagen fibrils pass through the tunnels formed by the processes of the HSCs and the PCs (Wake 1995). Thus the HSCs adhere to the basement membrane-like matrix on one hand and the other hand contact with the collagen fibrils.

The normal perisinusoidal space contains type I, III, IV, V, and VI collagens, fibronectin, laminin, and proteoglycans (Martinez-Hernandez 1984; Geerts et al. 1986, 1990, 1994; Rojkind and Greenwel 1994; Martinez-Hernandez and Amenta 1993a, 1995). A matrix gradient in the space of Disse has been revealed by the detailed and extensive ultrastructural and immunochemical studies (Reid et al. 1992; Sigal et al. 1992). Fibronectin is present mainly in amorphous material in close contact with the microvilli of the PCs (Geerts et al. 1986; Martinez-Hernandez and Amenta, 1993b, 1995). Heparan sulfate proteoglycan is present in diffuse material associated with the surface of the PCs and LSECs (Geerts et al. 1986).

Immunofluorescence for type I collagen has been found to correspond with some of the coarse reticular fibers, while that for type III collagen has been found to correspond with most, but not all, reticular fibers of the liver in the snow monkey (Adachi et al. 1991). By immuno-electron microscopy, reaction products with anti-type III collagen antibody and anti-type V collagen antibody have been demonstrated on cross-striated collagen fibrils, about 45 nm in diameter, in the space of Disse in the liver of the monkey. Simultaneous localization of type I collagen and type III collagen in the same cross-striated collagen fibril has also been revealed in the space of Disse of normal rats (Geerts et al. 1986, 1990). In either case, each ECM component localizes three-dimensionally at a restricted region in the normal liver lobule.

Under pathological conditions such as liver fibrosis, activated HSCs lose their lipid droplets containing vitamin A, proliferate rapidly, and synthesize and secrete a large amount of ECM components such as type I, III, IV collagens, fibronectin, laminin, heparan sulfate, and dermatan sulfate (Clement et al. 1986; Gressner and Bachem 1990, 1995; Ramadori 1991; Geerts et al. 1994; Greenwel et al. 1994; Gressner et al. 1994; Martinez-Hernandez et al. 1995). The constitution of ECM components in the liver lobules and in the perisinusoidal space is altered according to pathological conditions (Gressner and Bachem 1995). As the liver becomes fibrotic, the total content of collagens and noncollagenous components increases 3-5-fold (Friedman, 2000). Therefore the three-dimensional ECM in the space of Disse is not static but dynamic.

ECM components interact with many types of cells and regulate cell shape, motility, growth, survival, differentiation and gene expression via integrin-mediated signaling processes. HSCs, which are located between PCs and LSECs, extend their long cellular processes around the sinusoid. HSCs alter their morphology with the elongation of long processes, as well as changes in collagen production and the proliferation rate, when cultured with type I collagen gel as a substratum (Senoo and Hata 1994a,1994b; Senoo et al. 1998). In cell culture, HSCs exhibit three different morphologies in response to the distinct substratum: (1) flattened shape with well-developed stress fibers on the polystyrene surface, on the aminoalkylsilane- or lysine-coated surface, and on the type I or type IV collagen-coated surface, (2) rod shape with well-developed cellular processes on or in type I or type III collagen gel, mimicking *in vivo* situation, (3) round shape with neither cell spreading nor process extension on or in Matrigel. The cellular processes are composed of microtubules as the core and F-actin at the periphery, and contain lipid droplets containing vitamin A and MMP1. The processes are induced by cell surface integrin-binding to interstitial collagen fibrils, followed by signaling processes including protein and/or phosphatidylinositol phosphorylation, and finally F-actin and microtubule organization.

Three-dimensional structure of substratum reversibly regulates morphology, proliferation rate and function of cultured HSCs (Senoo et al. 1996, 1997, 1998; Kojima et al. 1997; Imai et al. 1997). The molecular mechanisms in the regulation of HSCs by three-dimensional structure of the ECM imply that cell-surface integrin binds to the matrix components followed by signal transduction processes and cytoskeleton assembly (reviewed by Senoo et al. 1998).

2.2.3. Morphology of Adhesion between the HSCs and ECM

When the HSCs are isolated from the liver of rat and cultured in non-coated polystyrene culture dishes, the cells spread well and become flat (Imai and Senoo 1998). The size of cells is 50-100 μm (diameter). Only a few lipid droplets were retained within the cytoplasm. By scanning-electron microscopy (SEM), some lamellipodia are obvious in the peripheral portion of the cells.

When HSCs are inoculated on rigid type I collagen gel, the cells extend and become long polygonal. The cells sustain small lipid droplet within the cytoplasm and resemble the star-shaped HSCs as found *in vivo*. The cells cultured on type I collagen gel protrude their primary and secondary long cellular processes from the cell bodies onto the gel. These processes entangle and make contacts with fine type I collagen fibers of the gel.

When the HSCs are inoculated into type I collagen gel and cultured for 2 days, the cells are rod- or long spindle-like and 100-300 μm in length. By SEM examination at a lower magnification, the cell bodies and cellular processes of the HSCs cultured in the gel are seen to be entangled with three-dimensional collagen fibers of the gel. The collagen fibers attached to not only the lower side but also the upper side of both cell bodies and the cell processes. These data indicate that the HSCs cultured on or in type I collagen gel protrude long cellular processes from their cell bodies whereas the cells cultured in non-coated polystyrene culture dishes spread well and become flat.

The HSCs in the type I collagen gel are entangled three-dimensionally with the collagen fibers and make contacts with the fibers. These data strongly suggest that HSCs adhere directly to three-dimensional ECM.

Three-dimensional collagen fibers of type I collagen gel contact with cell bodies, cell processes, and a number of microprojections of the HSCs cultured in the collagen gel.

The morphology of the site of adhesion between networks of collagen fibers and the HSCs in type I collagen gel is revealed more precisely by transmission-electron microscopy (TEM). The collagen adhere directly to the surfaces of the cell bodies, of cellular processes, and of their thin microprojections. The area of these adhesion between the type I collagen fibrils and the HSCs formed a face but not a point at the electron microscopical level. The adhesive face measures 50-1,000 nm in length in thin TEM sections. Accumulations of actin-like thin filaments are observed beneath the surfaces of the cell bodies, although the cells do not show any cytoplasmic electron-dense plaques as seen in focal adhesion. There are some morphological differences in the adhesive structure between cells and collagen fibers (e.g., fibroblasts and HSCs). These differences may be due to species and cell type differences (Mercier et al. 1996; Tomasek et al. 1982).

2.2.4. Adhesion Molecules of HSCs for ECM

Integrins comprise a large family of transmembrane adhesion proteins composed of an α and a β subunit (Hynes 1992; Giancotti 2000). At least 24 integrin heterodimers, made from 9 types of βsubunits and 16 types of αsubunits, have been defined. Most integrins recognize several ECM proteins. Conversely, individual matrix proteins bind to several integrins: for example, at least eight integrins (α5β1, α4β 1 , α4β7, αvβ1, αvβ6, αvβ8, αvβ3, and αIIbβ3) bind to fibronectin and five integrins (α1β1, α2β 1 , α3β1, α6β1, and α6β4) bind laminin (Giancotti and Ruoslahti 1999; Giancotti 2000). HSCs express integrins α 1 β1, α2β 1 , αvβ1, α6β4, and α8β1 (Carloni et al. 1996; Levine et al. 2000). Integrin α2β 1 is defined as a specific receptor for type I collagen and type IV collagen (Takada et al. 1988) and it can also interact with laminin and fibronectin (Elices and Hemler 1989). The minimal active recognition sequence has been defined as a tetrapeptide of the sequence DGEA (Asp-Gly-Glu-Ala), corresponding to residues 435-438 of the type I collagen sequence (Staatz et al. 1991).

Localization of integrin α2 and β1 subunits in the human HSCs cultured in type I collagen gel has been examined by immuno-electron microscopy (Imai and Senoo 1998). Integrin α2 and β1 subunits were detected on the surfaces of the cell bodies, cellular processes, and microprojections. Thus the information of three-dimensional structures of ECM is transmitted to the HSCs by three-dimensional adhesive structures of the cells containing integrins.

2.2.5. Putative Role of Adhesion between HSCs and ECM

Synthetic oligopeptide DGEA from type I collagen molecule and anti-integrinα2 antibody inhibit the process elongation of HSCs cultured on type I collagen gel (Sato et al. 2003). These results suggest that the elongation of the cellular processes occurs via the integrin-binding to the sequence DGEA on extracellular type I collagen fibrils (Miura et al. 1997; Sato and Senoo 1998; Sato et al. 2003).

Ligand binding to the integrin family is currently thought to lead to integrin clustering and subsequent recruitment of actin filaments to the cytoplasmic domain of integrins. This recruitment is achieved via a complex of interacting cytoskeletal proteins, including talin, vinculin, α-actinin, and filamin (Critchley 2000).

Integrins transduce signals by associating with adapter proteins that connect the integrin to the cytoskeleton and cytoplasmic kinases. Integrin signaling and assembly of the cytoskeleton are intimately linked. As integrins bind to ECM, they become clustered in the plane of the cell membrane and associate with a cytoskeletal and signaling complex that promotes the assembly of actin filaments. The reorganization of actin filaments into larger stress fibers, in turn, causes more integrin clustering. Integrins activate various protein tyrosine kinases including focal adhesion kinase (FAK), Src-family kinases, and serine-threonine kinase. FAK also combines with, and may activate, phosphoinositide 3-OH kinase (PI 3-kinase). These interactions link FAK to signaling pathways that modify the cytoskeleton and activate mitogen-activated protein kinase (MAPK) cascades (Clark and Brugge 1995; Giancotti and Ruoslahti 1999).

Protein tyrosine phosphorylation is enhanced in HSCs cultured on type I collagen gel, while protein tyrosine kinase inhibitors or PI-3 kinase inhibitors retract the extended cellular processes and also inhibit the induction of cellular processes (Kojima et al. 1997; Miura et al. 1997; Sato and Senoo 1998). Therefore, the signal transduction mechanism including protein and phosphatidylinositol phosphorylation seems to be critical to induce and sustain the cellular process architecture.

Dual immunofluorescence staining of microtubule and F-actin in HSCs cultured on type I collagen gel has revealed that the core of elongated cellular processes of the cells consists of microtubules, while the periphery contains F-actin (Miura et al. 1997; Sato et al. 1998).

Well-developed cellular processes of cultured HSCs are retracted in the presence of colchicine. Cytochalasin B also destroy the cellular process architecture; the peripheral F-actin organization is necessary to sustain the microtubule core (Miura et al. 1997; Sato and Senoo 1998; Sato et al. 2003). These results indicate that the processes are induced by cell surface integrin-binding to interstitial collagen fibrils, followed by signaling processes including protein and/or phosphatidylinositol phosphorylation, and finally F-actin and microtubule organization.

In HSCs cultured in or on type I collagen gel, the time-lapse video-microscopy has demonstrated that the long processes appear to contact with and extend along collagen fibrils. The cellular processes also extended in or on type III collagen gel, but not in type IV collagen-coated dish or on Matrigel (Miura et al. 1997; http://www.med.akita-u.ac.jp/~kaibo2/default.html; Sato and Senoo 1998). Therefore, the morphological change in HSCs occurred by the recognition of fibrillar type I or type III collagen, but not type IV collagen and other Matrigel components.

The normal perisinusoidal space of Disse contains mainly type I and III collagen fibers (Clement et al. 1986) and each ECM component localizes three-dimensionally at a restricted region in the normal liver lobule (Reid et al. 1992; Sigal et al. 1992; Martinez-Hernandez and Amenta 1995). It is therefore concluded that HSCs in the space of Disse make multiple three-dimensional adhesive structures to three-dimensional ECM components and receive the information from ECM through the adhesive structures.

HSCs cultured on or in type I collagen gel are induced to elongate long cellular processes. The elongation of the processes occurs via integrin-binding to the sequence DGEA on type I collagen fibrils. The signal transduction mechanism including phosphorylation seems to be critical to induce and sustain the cellular process architecture. It is concluded that the multiple three-dimensional adhesive structures of HSCs to three-dimensional ECM participate in development and sustaining of three-dimensional processes of the cells within the perisinusoidal space as well as of the cells *in vitro*.

2.2.6. HSC-HSC Adhesion

Adherence Junctions

Intercellular junctions between mammalian HSCs have been investigated in cultured human and rat HSCs at the ultrastructural and molecular levels (Higashi et al. 2004). Intercellular junctions between cultured HSCs, which developed irrespective of the type of culture substratum, were detected by TEM. On the basis of their characteristic ultrastructure, these junctions were identified as adherence junctions. N-cadherin, α-catenin and β-catenin, and p120ctn were detected in HSCs as molecular components of the intercellular adhesive structure. HSCs may participate in the structural organization of the cells in liver lobules through the formation of intercellular adherence junctions.

Gap Junction

Cells of tissues are coupled by channel-forming junctions called gap junctions (Alberts et al. 2008). These take the form of plaques of clustered connexons (a gap-junction connexon is made up of six transmembrane connexin subunits) that usually allow molecules smaller than about 1000 daltons (such as inorganic ions, sugar, amino acids, nucleotides, vitamins, and the intracellular mediators cyclic AMP and inositol triphosphate) to pass directly from the inside of one cell to the inside of the next. The cell can regulate the permeability of these junctions. Cells connected by gap junctions share many of their inorganic ions and other small molecules and are therefore chemically and electrically coupled. Gap junctions are important in coordinating the activities of electrically active cells, and they have a coordinating role in other groups of cells as well.

HSC clones obtained from a CCl_4-cirrhotic rat expressed gap junction protein connexin 43 (Greenwel et al. 1993). The presence of functional intercellular channels between cultured HSCs was demonstrated by the accumulation of Lucifer Yellow in surrounding cells following ionophoretic injection of the dye into a single cell.

Protein expression of connexin 43 was upregulated in activated HSCs *in vivo* and *in vitro* and was mainly localized on the cell surface, where as connexin 26 was found intracellularly (Fischer et al. 2005). Increased connexin 43 expression and gap junctional communication between activated HSCs are suggestive of a syncytium-like organization of these cells in culture that may allow rapid signal propagation and coordination. The expression and function of adhesion apparatus and gap junction of HSCs have not been fully investigated.

Other Cell Adhesion Molecules of HSCs

HSCs express central nervous system typical adhesion molecules, namely, N-CAM (Knittel et al. 1996). N-CAM expression was increased during *in vitro* transformation of HSCs from resting to activated (myofibroblast-like) cells and by the fibrogenic mediator TGF-β1. Activated HSCs express intercellular adhesion molecule 1 (ICAM-1; Hellerbrand et al. 1996). ICAM-1 belongs to the immunoglobulin superfamily and is expressed on the cell surface. Functions of these molecules of HSCs are not yet fully clarified.

Chapter 3

Functions of HSCs

3.1. Isolation and Culture of HSCs

When morphologists re-discovered and identified PCs, and three NPCs (KCs, LSECs, and HSCs) in the liver lobule, researchers have started to isolate, purify, culture, and characterize functions of these cells.

Preliminary report for the isolation and purification appeared in 1982 (Knook et al. 1982). They made sinusoidal liver cell suspensions by the enzymatic preparation (Pronase and collagenase) and HSCs were purified by Metrizamide density centrifugation and centrifugal elutriation. Ultrastructure of the isolated HSCs was consistent with that of HSCs *in vivo*.

Culture of HSCs was reported separately (Senoo et al., 1984; de Leeuw et al. 1984). A cell fraction enriched with HSCs was prepared by collagenase perfusion of the liver and low speed centrifugation followed by Percoll density gradient centrifugation. Cells in the fraction were found to take up and store the largest amount of vitamin A per cell among the liver cells including PCs, when [^{3}H]retinol was injected through the portal vein of rats (Senoo et al. 1984). Analysis of collagen production by this fraction as well as another NPC fraction (rich in KCs and LSECs) in culture has shown that only the HSC-rich fraction produced collagen which was composed of type I (88.2 %), type III (10.4 %), and membraneous type (1.4 %). There was no indication of collagen production in other NPC fractions under the experimental conditions employed. Among NPCs, HSCs are primarily responsible for collagen production in the liver.

The typical morphological characteristics of HSCs *in vivo* were retained in the cells during primary culture (Senoo et al. 1984; de Leeuw et al. 1984). Vitamin A autofluorescence was associated with lipid droplets of the cells in culture. Vimentin, actin, and tubulin in the cells were demonstrated by indirect immunofluorescence. Collagen type I and IV and laminin were also demonstrated by indirect immunofluorescence.

By use of cell isolation method, newly administered [^{3}H]retinol was shown to be transferred from PCs to HSCs for storage (Blomhoff et al., 1982, 1984a).

By the collagenase perfusion from the portal vein and enzyme digestion method, different types of liver cells from rats fed a normal diet were isolated; and main retinoids, two intracellular retinoid-binding proteins, namely, cellular retinol-binding protein and cellular retinoic acid-binding protein (CRBP and CRABP) and the retinyl palmitate hydrolase and acyl CoA:retinol acyltarnsferase (ARAT) activities in each type of cell was quantified (Blomhoff et al. 1985a). The uptake of [^{3}H]retinol and retinol binding protein (RBP) was demonstrated in both PCs and HSCs using the technique of enzyme digestion method (Blomhoff et al. 1985b, 1988a).

The role of HSCs in retinoid metabolism was further analyzed by the cell isolation and purification method (Yamada et al. 1987; Hendriks et al. 1987). By these studies with isolated and purified cells up to 90% of the liver retinoids have been clearly demonstrated to present in HSCs in the form of retinyl esters, predominantly retinyl palmitate (Hendriks et al. 1987).

An overview of knowledge at that time about absorption, transport, storage, and metabolism of vitamin A was reported (Blomhoff et al. 1990). Cell isolation, purification, and culture of HSCs contributed to the progress of these studies (Blomhoff et al. 1988a, 1988b, 1988c, 1991, 1992a, 1992b).

HSCs were also isolated from normal rat liver by enzymatical digestion with Pronase and collagenase as described by Knook et al. (Knook et al., 1982) and discontinuous gradient of arabinogalactan (Stractan) (Friedman et al., 1985). HSCs in culture were demonstrated to secrete collagen type I, type III, type IV and laminin by immunofluorescence. Not only HSCs but also LSECs and PCs were shown to biosynthesize collagen.

Isolation and culture of liver NPCs (Hendriks et al. 1990) and HSCs (Blomhoff and Berg1990; Senoo and Hata 1993b) was reviewed.

From human liver, HSCs were isolated and cultured (Nakagawa et al. 1991; Friedman et al. 1992).

On the other hand, isolation, purification, and characterization of KCs and LSECs were developed by pioneer studies (Nilsson and Berg 1977; Knook et al. 1977; de Leeuw et al. 1982; Blomhoff et al. 1984b; Steffan et al. 1986; Brouwer et al. 1988a). These efforts also contributed to the establishment of HSCs isolation, purification, culture, and characterization of HSCs. Thus, contemporary research of HSCs at molecular cell biology levels has based on these pioneer studies mentioned above.

From the present to the future, new elaborated cell culture system for further investigation of functions of HSCs or development of an artificial liver will be developed such as three dimensional (3-D) culture or rotary culture.

3.2. Vitamin A Storage and Metabolism

Vitamin A (Fig. 7) is known to regulate diverse cellular activities such as cell proliferation, differentiation, morphogenesis, and tumorigenesis (Balmer and Blomhoff 2002; Blomhoff 1994; Blomhoff and Blomhoff 2006; Chawla et al. 2001). In physiological conditions, HSCs store 50-80 % of the total vitamin A in the whole body as retinyl palmitate in lipid droplets in the cytoplasm, and regulate both transport and storage of vitamin A (Blomhoff and Blomhoff 2006).

The liver has been demonstrated to be the main storage site of vitamin A in experimental animals (Moore 1931) and humans (Raica et al. 1972; Ralli et al. 1941; Underwood et al. 1970).

3.2.1. Morphology of Vitamin A storage in HSCs

It had been generally accepted that vitamin A was stored in KCs (reticulo-endothelial cells) belonging to the monocyte-macrophage lineage in the liver (Popper 1941; Popper et al. 1943) until Wake demonstrated that HSCs are the main storage site of vitamin A (Wake 1964). Wake injected excess vitamin A acetate to albino rats and rabbits, examined the liver by fluorescence microscopy, Suzuki's silver impregnation method (Suzuki 1958), Kupffer's gold chloride method, electron microscopy, and found that the liver of animals those were injected a large dose of vitamin A showed numerous scattered cells containing lipid droplets. Under a fluorescence microscope these droplets impart bright and quickly fading autofluorescence which is typical of vitamin A destroyed by ultraviolet light.

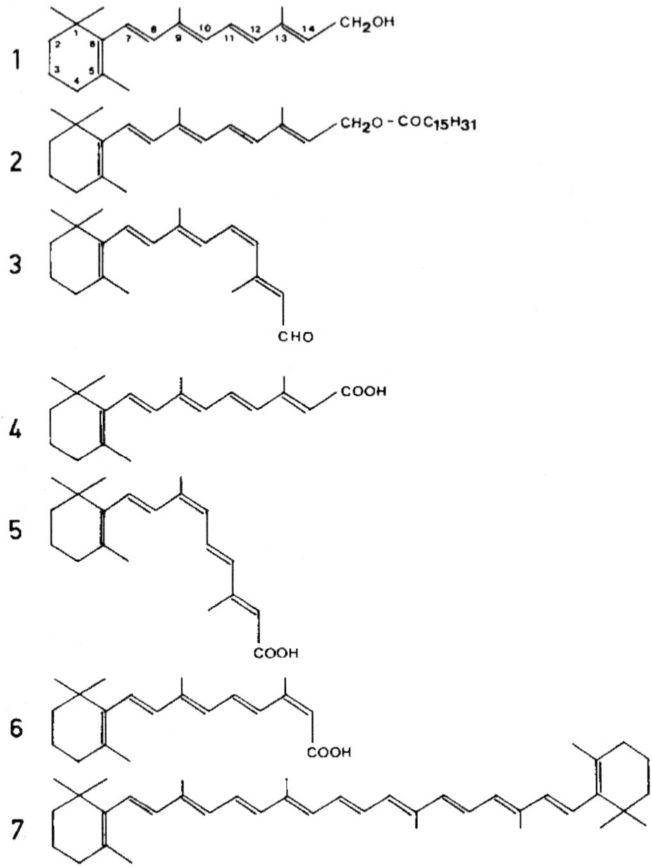

Figure 7. Structural formulas of some naturally occurring vitamin A and β-carotene. Vitamin A circulates in the plasma as retinol (1) that binds to a specific carrier protein, retinol-binding protein. Retinoid is stored as retinyl palmitate (2) in the HSCs. 11-*Cis*-retinal (3) exists in the retina with rhodopsin. All-*trans*-retinoic acid (4) binds to nuclear retinoic acid receptors (RARα, RARβ, RARγ), and 9-*cis*-retinoic acid (5) binds to nuclear retinoid X receptors (RXRα, RXRβ, RXRγ). These nuclear receptors regulate transcription of various genes. 13-*Cis*-retinoic acid (6) can bind to RARs. β-Carotene (7) forms two retinals and finally two retinols. Senoo H, Yoshikawa K, Morii M, Miura M, Imai K, Mezaki Y. Cell Biol Int (editor's special 70th birthday edition) 2010; 34, 1247-1272

Thus, he demonstrated that the cells which show vitamin A uptake and storage are interstitial cells, namely, HSCs of the liver. The "Sternzellen" (Kupffer 1876) in the liver are perisinusoidal HSCs located in the space between PCs and LSECs (Wake 1971). The cytoplasm of HSCs contains a number of lipid droplets which react intensely with gold chloride. These lipid droplets emit strong autofluorescence of vitamin A. Following the administration of excess vitamin A, the mass of these lipid droplets increase remarkably. These cells are quite different from the so-called KCs of the liver reticulo-endothelial system. In the gold chloride method, metallic gold deposition has been observed on the surface of the lipid droplets containing vitamin A in HSCs (Wake 1973). These lipid droplets develop in the multivesicular bodies (MVBs; Wake 1974). After losing the surrounding limiting membrane they are located in the cytoplasmic matrix and are stored for a long period (Wake 1975b, reviewed by Wake 1975a, 1975c). Two types of lipid droplets have been identified through histological analysis of HSCs: smaller droplets bounded by a unit membrane and larger membrane-free droplets (Wake 1971).

In mammals, 50-80% of the body's total vitamin A is normally present in the HSCs (Blomhoff and Blomhoff 2006). More than 95% of vitamin A in the HSC is present in the form of retinyl esters packed together in cytoplasmic lipid droplets. Retinyl esters account for 30-50% of the content of lipid droplets.

The normal reserve of retinyl esters in HSCs represents an adequate supply of vitamin A for most individuals for several weeks or months (Blomhoff et al. 1990b). This extensive storage of retinyl esters in HSCs, and the cells' ability to control mobilization of retinol, ensures a steady blood plasma retinol concentration of about 1-2 μ M in spite of normal fluctuation in daily intake of vitamin A. The mechanism responsible for retinol mobilization from HSCs has not been elucidated in detail. Results from knock-out mice indicate, however, that RBP is involved in this mechanism (Quadro et al. 1999).

Thus, HSCs have been explicitly demonstrated to be the main storage site of vitamin A (reviewed by Wake 1980).

3.2.2. Biochemical Analysis of Vitamin A Storage in HSCs

After establishment of the cell isolation and culture methods of HSCs, analysis of vitamin A uptake and storage has been started at the cell, cell organelle, and molecule levels.

To examine the distribution of vitamin A in the liver, radioactivity per cell was determined after cell fractionation (Senoo et al., 1984, 1991; Senoo and

Hata, 1993b). Specific activity of [^{3}H]retinol (per cell) was the highest in the HSC fraction, both 90 min and 6 days after the injection of [^{3}H]retinol into the portal vein. These results strongly support earlier morphological observations (Wake, 1971, 1980) that the HSC is the storage site of vitamin A in the liver, and are not inconsistent with reports on the retinol transfer from PCs to HSCs (Andersen et al. 1992; Blaner et al. 1987; Blomhoff et al. 1984a, 1984b; Gjøen et al. 1987; Malaba et al. 1995; Matsuura et al. 1989; Senoo et al. 1990, 1993).

Highly purified sinusoidal cells (HSCs, KCs and LSECs) and PCs were isolated to assess the cellular distribution of vitamin A in the liver of adult vitamin A-sufficient rats (Hendriks et al. 1985). HSCs have been shown to contain about 300-fold the amount of retinyl esters present in PCs on a mg cell protein basis. In HSCs, the same retinyl esters, namely, retinyl palmitate, retinyl stearate and retinyl oleate, were present as in the whole liver. It was also observed that, within 12 hours after intravenous injection of chylomicron [^{3}H]retinyl ester, most of the radioactivity had accumulated in the HSCs. Storage of retinol in PCs was proportional to the liver store of retinol, and less than 10% of retinol in the liver could be recovered in PCs. PCs play a minor role in liver storages of retinol, and HSCs store more than 90% of liver retinoid (Blomhoff et al. 1988a, 1988b, 1988c). Thus, HSCs have been demonstrated biochemically to be the main storage sites for vitamin A in the rat liver.

When chylomicron retinyl ester was injected intravenously into normal rats, the radioactivity was cleared from blood with t1/2 approximately equal to 10 min. Retinyl ester was taken up initially by the liver, which, after 30 minutes, contained 80-90% of the radioactivity injected. Initially, most of the radioactivity was in PCs, but after 30 minutes it disappeared from these cells and reappeared in NPCs. Newly administered retinol is initially taken up by the PCs, and subsequently (within 1–2 hours) transferred to NPCs (Blomhoff et al. 1982). When liver cells were prepared between 5 and 18 hours after intraduodenal administration of [^{3}H]retinol, the radioactive retinol was recovered mainly in the HSC. Other liver cells (i.e., PCs, LSECs, and KCs) contained only small amounts of [^{3}H]retinol. Newly administered [^{3}H]retinol, which is initially located in the PCs, is transferred to the HSCs and stored there (Blomhoff et al. 1988a). Chylomicron retinyl ester is not transported directly from PCs to HSCs without first undergoing hydrolysis to reinol (Blaner et al. 1987). Retinol delivered to HSCs from RBP is preferentially esterified, and that the retinol and RBP complex is handled differently to free retinol by the HSCs (Trøen et al. 1994).

Dietary retinoid intake but not triglyceride intake markedly influences the number and size of HSC lipid droplets (Moriwaki et al. 1988). The lipids present in rat HSC lipid droplets include retinyl ester, triglyceride, cholesteryl ester, cholesterol, phospholipids, and free fatty acids. Retinyl ester and triglyceride are present at similar concentrations, and together these two classes of lipid account for approximately three-quarters of the total lipid in HSC lipid droplets (Blaner et al. 2009).

It is suggested that CRBPs are important for intracellular metabolism of retinol. Retinol bound to CRBPs may be esterified with long chain fatty acids by the enzyme, LRAT or may be oxidized to retinoic acid metabolites are used in the mechanism of action of vitamin A. HSCs transfected with the vector for sense CRBP-I esterified more retinol than cells transfected with the expression vector for antisense CRBP-I, while retinol esterification in control cells was intermediate. CRBP-I influences retinol esterification in HSCs. Retinyl ester storage is altered in HSCs transfected with CRBP-I (Nilsson et al. 1997). Roles of retinioid-binding proteins in HSCs will be discussed in the chapter 3.

3.2.3. Regulation of Vitamin A Homeostasis by HSCs

The concentration of vitamin A in the bloodstream is regulated within the physiological range in the body. Cellular uptake mechanism of vitamin A is still controversial. By receptor-mediated endocytosis, the cells take up retinol from the blood, where it circulates as a complex of retinol and a specific binding protein called RBP (Fig.8; Blomhoff 1994). Once inside the cell, free retinol has several fates, one of which is reformation of the complex with RBP and returns to the bloodstream (Blomhoff et al. 1991, 1992a, 1992b; Senoo 2000).

Thus, the HSCs are important for the regulation of homeostasis of vitamin A. Immunoelectronmicroscopic studies suggest that RBP mediates the paracrine transfer of retinol from PCs to the HSCs and that HSCs bind and internalize RBP by receptor-mediated endocytosis (Malaba et al. 1995; Senoo et al. 1990 1993).

Recently, RBP receptor was cloned and characterized (Båvik et al., 1991, 1992, 1993; Smeland et al., 1995; Sundaram et al. 1998; Kawaguchi et al. 2007; Pasutto et al.2007). The HSCs may have pivotal roles in type 2 diabetes, because RBP was reported to contribute to insulin resistance in obesity and type 2 diabetes (Yang et al. 2005; Cho et al. 2006). This problem will be discussed in the section 3.3.

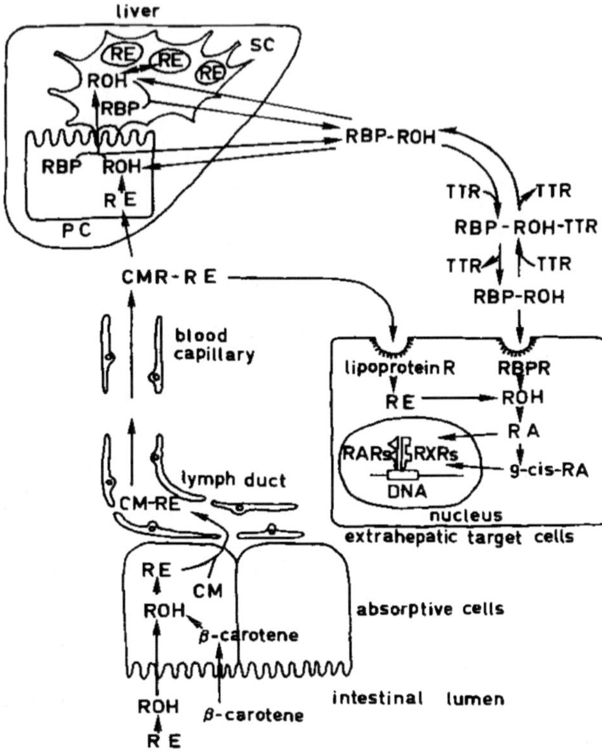

Figure 8. Major pathway for vitamin A transport in the body. Dietary retinyl esters (RE) are hydrolyzed to retinol (ROH) in the intestinal lumen before absorption by enterocytes, and carotenoids are absorbed and then partially converted to retinol in the enterocytes. In the enterocytes, retinol reacts with fatty acid to form esters before incorporation into chylomicrons (CM). Chylomicrons then reach the general circulation by way of the intestinal lymph, and chylomicron remnants (CMR) are formed in blood capillaries. Chylomicron remnants, which contain almost all the absorbed retinol, are mainly cleared by the liver parenchymal cells or hepatocytes (PC) and to some extent also by cells in other organs. In liver parenchymal cells, retinyl esters are rapidly hydrolyzed to retinol, which then binds to retinol-binding protein (RBP). A complex of retinol-RBP (RBP-ROH) is secreted and transported to hepatic stellate cells (SC). Hepatic stellate cells store vitamin A mainly as retinyl palmitate and secrete retinol-RBP directly into the blood. Most retinol-RBP in the bloodstream is reversibly complexed with transthyretin (TTR). The uncomplexed retinol-RBP is presumably taken up in a variety of cells by cell surface receptors specific for RBP. RA, retinoic acid; 9-*cis* RA, 9-*cis* retinoic acid; RARs, retinoic acid receptors; RXR, retinoid X receptors; lipoprotein R, lipoprotein receptor; RBPR, retinol-binding protein receptor. Senoo H, Yoshikawa K, Morii M, Miura M, Imai K, Mezaki Y. Cell Biol Int (editor's special 70th birthday edition) 2010; 34, 1247-1272.

3.2.4. Storage of β-carotene

HSCs are the site of the liver β-carotene storage and release, which can be used for retinoic acid production as well as for maintenance of the homeostasis of circulating carotenoids in periods of low dietary uptake. GRX is a permanent murine myofibroblastic cell line, derived from HSCs, which can be induced to display the vitamin A-storing phenotype by treatment with retinoids. β-Carotene induced a full cell conversion into the retinoid-storing phenotype. β-Carotene was directly converted to retinoic acid, which was found in total cell extracts and in the nuclear fraction, promoting the phenotype conversion but could not convert it to retinol nor produced retinyl esters (Martucci et al. 2004).

3.2.5. Release of Vitamin A

Mechanisms of release of vitamin A from HSCs to plasma is still controversial. Molecular mechanism for mobilization of retinol from HSCs has been studied (Andersen et al. 1992). HSCs isolated from liver contained RBP mRNA. By Western blot analysis, cultivated HSCs were found to secrete RBP into the medium. Cultivated HSCs loaded *in vitro* with [^{3}H]retinyl ester mobilized radioactive retinol as a complex with RBP. Furthermore, exogenous RBP added to the medium of cultured HSCs increased the secretion of retinol to the medium. These data suggest that HSCs *in vivo* mobilize retinol directly to the blood and that a transfer to PCs for secretion as holo-RBP is not required. The direct mobilization of retinol from HSCs as retinol-RBP to blood is indirectly supported by the demonstration of RBP mRNA production and RBP secretion by lung SCs. The data suggest that the same mechanism for retinol mobilization may exist in hepatic and extrahepatic SCs. Vitamin A-storing stellate cells in the liver, lungs, and probably also in other organs may synthesize their own RBP (or alternatively use exogenous RBP) and mobilize holo-RBP directly to the blood (Andersen et al. 1992).

The opposite data have been reported (Sauvant et al. 2001). Primary cultures of HSCs have been demonstrated to express immunoreactivity against RBP when cultured in a medium containing RBP but were unable to synthesize RBP transcripts and proteins. Pulse and chase-type experiments demonstrated that radioactive retinol was released in culture medium without any binding proteins. Inhibition of protein secretion by brefeldin A did not modify quantitatively retinol release. These data ruled out the direct involvement of RBP in retinol mobilization from HSCs. Moreover, HSCs co-cultured with primary isolated PCs displayed an increase of retinol transfer from HSCs to PCs when they established direct physical contacts as compared with co-cultures without contact. Based on this latter data, a mechanism of retinol mobilization from HSCs via the PCs using retinol transfer through cellular membranes is proposed (Sauvant et al. 2001). Activation of cultured HSCs by KCs-conditioned medium is accompanied by serum- and platelet-derived growth factor (PDGF)-dependent release of retinol; a similar mechanism may underlie retinoid loss by activated HSCs *in vivo* (Friedman et al. 1993).

3.2.6. Lecithin-Retinol Acyltransferase (LRAT)

Lecithin:retinol acyltransferase (LRAT), an enzyme responsible for all retinyl ester synthesis within the liver, is required for HSC lipid droplet formation, since LRAT-deficient mice completely lack HSC lipid droplets. When HSCs become activated in response to hepatic injury, the lipid droplets and their retinoid contents are rapidly lost. HSC lipid droplets are suggested to be specialized organelles for hepatic retinoid storage and that loss of HSC lipid droplets may contribute to the development of hepatic disease (Blaner et al. 2009).

Vitamin A is stored as retinyl esters in the lipid droplets in the cytoplasm of HSCs. Retinol esterification is performed by enzymes such as acyl-CoA:retinol acyltransferase (ARAT) (Ross 1982) and LRAT (Ong 1994). It is now well documented that LRAT is the physiologically important enzyme involved in the esterification of retinol in the liver. LRAT activity present in microsomes prepared from each of liver cell (PCs, HSCs, KCs, LSECs) fractions has been determined (Blaner et al. 1990). Among them, HSCs are found to contain the highest level of LRAT specific activity. The KS and LSEC microsome fractions are found to contain LRAT at low levels of the activity. HSCs are very enriched in LRAT but PCs also possess significant levels of LRAT activity.

Immunohistochemical studies to assess the distribution of LRAT-positive cells in the liver has been performed with the aid of fluorescence and immunogold electron microscopy (Nagatsuma et al. 2009). LRAT-positive cells have been found to be confined in the space of Disse corresponding with the location of desmin-positive HSC in rodent and human livers. LRAT in HSCs is mainly distributed within the rough ER and multivesicular bodies.

Hepatic LRAT activity is negligible during vitamin A deficiency, and all-*trans*-retinoic acid rapidly induces the activity of liver LRAT in retinoid-deficient rats. Retinol and all-*trans*-retinoic acid strongly induce LRAT activity. RARs are implicated in the induction of hepatic LRAT that is suggested to play a predominant role for RAR-α-active ligands (Shimada et al. 1997).

Retinol esterification activity of LI90 (Murakami et al. 1995), a human HSC-like cell line, is demonstrated to be similar to that of primary cultures of rat HSC and higher than that of a human hepatoma cell line (Matsuura et al. 1999). It is likely that LRAT contributes to retinol esterification in LI90. Both retinol and esterified retinol in LI90 cells increase in a manner dependent of retinol concentration in culture medium. The percentages of esterified and unesterified retinol in LI90 cells and of retinol in medium are linearly dependent on the logarithm of the initial concentration of retinol in the medium. Retinol esterification activity might contribute to retinol uptake by HSC and maintenance of non-toxic retinol levels in plasma.

Mouse Lrat gene expression has been disrupted by targeted recombination and a homozygous Lrat knock-out (Lrat-/-) mouse is generated (Batten et al. 2004). Despite the lack of expression of LRAT in multiple tissues, the Lrat-/- mouse develops normally. Lrat-/- mice have trace levels of all-*trans*-retinyl esters in the liver, lung, eye, and blood, whereas the circulating all-*trans*-retinol is reduced only slightly.

The level of cytosolic retinol-binding protein type III (CRBPIII) has been upregulated (3-4-fold) in adipose tissue of Lrat-/- mice (O'Byrne et al. 2005). Examination by electron microscopy reveals a striking total absence of large vitamin A lipid droplets that normally seen within the HSCs of mice. Lrat-/- mice absorb dietary retinol primarily as free retinol in chylomicrons; however, retinyl esters are also present within the chylomicron fraction obtained from Lrat-/- mice. The fatty acyl composition of these chylomicron retinyl esters suggests that they are synthesized via an acyl-CoA-dependent process suggesting the existence of a physiologically significant ARAT (O'Byrne et al. 2005).

Retinol esterification has been examined in the established GRX cell line, representative of HSCs, and in primary cultures of *ex vivo* purified murine HSCs. The metabolism of [^{3}H]retinol was compared in cells expressing the myofibroblast or the retinoid-storing phenotype under the physiological retinol concentrations. Retinyl esters were the major metabolites whose production was dependent upon both ARAT and LRAT. HSCs had a significantly higher esterification capacity than myofibroblasts. Both LRAT and ARAT activities were induced during the conversion of myofibroblasts to HSCs. LRAT induction was dependent upon retinoic acid, while that of ARAT was dependent upon the overall induction of the vitamin A storing phenotype. The fatty acid composition of retinyl-esters suggested a preferential inclusion of exogenous fatty acids into retinyl esters. Both LRAT and ARAT participate in retinol esterification in HSCs; LRAT's activity correlates with the vitamin A status, while ARAT depends upon the availability of fatty acyl-CoA and the overall lipid metabolism in HSCs (Fortuna et al. 2001).

3.2.7. Effects of Retinoid to HSC Function

Effects of vitamin A on HSC function both *in vivo* and *in vitro* are still controversial.

Okuno et al. (1990) reported that acyclic retinoid (polyprenoic acid) reduced the development of hepatic fibrosis induced by CCl_4 in rats. The rate of collagen synthesis in the liver was decreased which was consistent with histological findings.

In rats shows that vitamin A status, reflected by hepatic retinoid content (retinol and retinyl esters), modulates the development of hepatic fibrosis induced by CCl_4. In rats with low hepatic retinoid levels, CCl_4-induced liver fibrosis was more pronounced than in rats with sufficient hepatic retinoid levels. Vitamin A status of the liver plays an important role in hepatic fibrogenesis. Low hepatic vitamin A levels, which can be the result not only of low dietary intake but also of interference with vitamin A metabolism by agents such as ethanol and CCl_4, may be a risk factor for the development of liver fibrosis. Retinoids modulate collagen synthesis and deposition irrespective of the degree of hepatocellular necrosis induced by CCl_4. The reduction of retinoid levels in HSCs and fibroblast-like cells by an enhanced secretion of retinol from the liver into the circulation during CCl_4 treatment may stimulate the transformation of these cells to fibroblasts and, in this way, contribute to fibrogenesis of the liver (Seifert et al. 1994).

HSC collagen synthesis may be altered by underlying ECM and exogenous retinol (Davis et al. 1987). When grown on a type IV collagen matrix, the cells produced relatively equal amounts of types I and III collagen. The absolute amounts of type I collagen produced were greater when cells were grown on type IV versus type I matrix. When 10^{-5} M retinol was added to cell cultures, there was a uniform increase in type III collagen regardless of matrix type but a decrease in type I collagen when cells were grown on a type

IV matrix and a large increase in type I collagen when cells were grown on a type I collagen matrix. HSCs on a type I matrix contain more CRBP than do cells grown on a type IV matrix. Thus, HSC collagen synthesis may be altered by exogenous retinol (Davis et al. 1987).

Cultured HSCs were re-exposed to an increased concentration of retinol in vitro. Passaged HSCs (grown on a type I or type IV collagen matrix) which lack vitamin A droplets were exposed to media containing 10^{-5} M retinol. Cell proliferation was markedly inhibited for the 2 weeks of observation without apparent loss of cell viability. The effect was noted to be reversible and dose related with a submaximal effect at 10^{-6} M retinol. When cultured HSCs were grown on a type I collagen matrix and re-exposed to an increased concentration of vitamin A, the production of interstitial collagen was reduced. However, when the vitamin A-enriched HSCs were exposed to TGF, the production of interstitial collagen was increased, similar to cells that had not received vitamin A (Davis 1988). Thus, retinol can modulate HSC proliferation *in vitro* (Davis and Vucic 1988). However, the effects of retinoid to the HSC function are not yet thoroughly clarified.

The GRX cell line is derived from murine liver connective tissue cells. It has myofibroblastic characteristics and can be induced to display a phenotype analogous to HSCs. Retinol inducted vitamin A-storing phenotype to the GRX cells. Retinoid-induced changes in GRX cells provide a model for studying *in vitro* the interconversion of liver connective tissue cells between the myofibroblastic and retinoid-storing phenotypes. This interconversion is considered to be one of the major control points of normal homeostasis and of pathological modifications of liver connective tissue (Margis and Borojevic 1989).

Retinol (1 μM) and retinoic acid (1 μM) supplementation of primary rat HSC cultures inhibited the spontaneous increase in collagen synthesis associated with HSC activation. Cell proliferation was also inhibited by retinol. Extracellular retinoids suppress HSC-activated collagen synthesis and cell proliferation and support the interpretation that retinoids themselves are regulatory factors in maintenance of the HSC in its native, differentiated state (Sato et al. 1995).

Pure HSCs were isolated from rats with cholestatic liver fibrosis induced by bile duct ligation (BDL) and sham-operated animals (Sham). Diminished retinoic acid signaling in HSC from cholestatic liver fibrosis which appeared to have resulted from retinoic acid deficiency and suppressed expression of RAR-β and RXR-α. Furthermore, the reciprocal enhancement of AP-1 activity and coordinately increased expression of an AP-1 responsive gene, TGF-β1, suggest a permissive role of the diminished retinoic acid signaling in promoting AP-1 activity and TGF-β1 expression (Ohta et al. 1997).

In HSCs isolated from rat fibrotic livers, the amount of RXR-α mRNA is greatly reduced. However, the effectiveness of retinoids in the treatment of liver fibrosis is controversial. Increasing the expression levels of RXR-α in livers improves the response of liver fibrosis to retinoids treatment. Hepatic fibrosis of RXR-α-transfected group, tapered off remarkably (Chen et al. 2004).

Retinoic acid suppresses α2(I) collagen expression in HSCs through the binding of RARβ and RXRα to retinoic acid response elements (RAREs) in the α2(I) collagen promoter. This study determined the influence of coactivators and corepressors to RARβ and RXRα on the regulation of the α2(I) collagen promoter. In the presence of retinoic acid, the coactivators steroid receptor coactivator-1 (SRC-1) and growth hormone receptor interacting protein-1 (GRIP-1) augment, while the corepressor N-CoR abolishes the suppressive effects of RARβ and RXRα on α2(I) collagen promoter activity (Wang et al. 2004).

All-*trans* retinoic acid exerted a significant inhibitory effect on the synthesis of procollagens type I, III, and IV, fibronectin, and laminin of cultured HSCs, but did not influence HSC proliferation, whereas 9RA showed a clear but late effect on proliferation. 9-*cis* retinoic acid increased procollagen I mRNA 1.9-fold, but did not affect the expression of other matrix proteins. Results showed that ATRA and 9RA exert different often contrary effects on activated HSCs. These observations may explain prior divergent results obtained following retinoid administration to cultured HSCs or in animals subjected to fibrogenic stimuli (Hellemans et al. 1999).

However the opposite results have been reported as follows. Although there is strong implication that retinoids regulate HSC proliferation and collagen synthesis, results from *in vivo* studies on the relationship between vitamin A and liver fibrosis are conflicting.

In animals with high dietary hepatic retinoid levels, liver fibrosis was more pronounced and was associated with an increased CCl_4-toxicity resulting in high mortality (73%). It was further associated with decreased bile flow and increased PC damage. CCl_4 reduced hepatic retinoid levels in high vitamin A diet-fed animals, but restored hepatic retinoid levels in animals fed with a vitamin A-deficient diet implying major interference of vitamin A metabolism with hepatotoxic agents such as CCl_4. Low vitamin A feeding did not modulate liver fibrogenesis and caused no mortality. These results show that the vitamin A status of the liver plays an important role in liver fibrogenesis. While dietary vitamin A shortage does not promote liver fibrogenesis, high levels of vitamin A have the potential to increase systemic and hepatic toxicity of CCl_4. Thus, the narrow therapeutic window for nutritional vitamin A substitution must take into account that liver fibrotic patients may display enhanced susceptibility to the adverse effects of vitamin A (Vollmar et al. 2002a).

Recently, the role of retinoic acid receptors in activated HSCs has been shown (Mezaki et al. 2013a, in press).

3.2.8. Lipids and HSCs

Sphingolipids play a relevant role in cell-cell interaction, communication, and migration. Sphingolipid content in the murine HSC line GRX, has been studied. GRX expresses the myofibroblast phenotype, and can be induced *in vitro* to display the vitamin A-storing phenotype. Lipid modifications along this induction were investigated. Myofibroblast and HSCs can use distinct ceramide pools for sphingolipid synthesis. Differential ganglioside expression and presence of the long-chain saturated fatty acids suggested that they may participate in formation of distinct membrane microdomains or rafts with specific functions on the two phenotypes of GRX-cells (Andrade et al. 2003).

Adipogenic/lipogenic-related transcription factors and downstream-regulated genes were evaluated in a murine HSC cell line.

GRX-HSC cells are transitional myofibroblasts that differentiate into HSCs following retinol or indomethacin treatment.

PPAR-γ and Pex16 transcripts were increased either by retinol or indomethacin. Retinol induced a minor increase in C/enhancer binding protein α transcripts, while only indomethacin increased adipsin transcripts.

Myofibroblast to retinoid-storing phenotype switch follows partially different transcriptional pathways, according to the effector. Retinol induces lipid synthesis and storage without affecting characteristic adipocytic genes, while indomethacin treatment restores the lipocytic phenotype with increased adipsin expression (Guimarães et al. 2007)

PPAR in HSCs will be discussed in the Section 3.4 (nuclear receptor and HSCs)

3.2.9. CD36 on HSCs

CD36, identified as a platelet integral membrane glycoprotein (glycoproteinIV), was until recently best known as a receptor for thrombospondin-1 (TSP-1) (Febbraio et al. 2001). TSP-1 is found in ECMs and platelet α granules, and it participates in cell attachment, motility, and proliferation, as well as in modulation of protease activity, TGF-β activation, neurite outgrowth, and angiogenesis. CD36 has been implicated in multiple biological processes that define it as a multiligand scavenger receptor. These ligands appear remarkably diverse: In addition to TSP-1, they include long-chain fatty acids, modified LDL, retinal photoreceptor outer segments, Plasmodium falciparum malaria-parasitized erythrocytes, sickle erythrocytes, anionic phospholipids, apoptotic cells, and collagens I and IV. The biology of CD36 can be broadly divided in terms of functions that it mediates with or without TSP-1, but it is probable that it acts in concert with other proteins, such as fatty acid–binding proteins, caveola-associated proteins, integrins, cytoskeletal proteins, and signaling molecules, to effect its diverse functions.

CD36 belongs to the class B scavenger receptor family, which includes the receptor for selective cholesteryl ester uptake, scavenger receptor class B type I (SR-BI), and lysosomal integral membrane protein II (LIMP-II). The protein is heavily N-linked glycosylated, a modification that may provide proteins in this family some protection from degradation in proteinase-rich environments such as the lysosome and areas of inflammation or tissue damage (Febbraio et al. 2001).

Low concentrations of modified lipoproteins (oxLDL and MDA-LDL) represent fibrogenic mediators that bind to CD36 and stimulate matrix synthesis of HSC (Schneiderhan 2001). Cumulating evidence suggests that oxidative stress resulting in lipid peroxidation and protein modification is involved in the pathogenesis of chronic liver injury and fibrogenesis. The effects of oxidized low-density lipoproteins (oxLDL) on collagen and fibronectin synthesis of cultured human and rat HSCs have been investigated. As shown on protein and mRNA levels, oxLDL dose-dependently stimulated the synthesis of collagen types I and III and fibronectin of cultured HSC. LDL modified with malondialdehyde (MDA) stimulated ECM synthesis as well.

Preincubation of cultured human HSC with the monoclonal antibody, OKM5, known to block CD36-mediated oxLDL uptake, resulted in a reduction of the oxLDL-stimulated collagen type I synthesis by 56% (Schneiderhan 2001).

3.3. Retinoid-Binding Proteins and HSCs

3.3.1. Retinoids

Vitamin A (Fig. 7) and related molecules--the retinoids--play essential roles in vision, growth, reproduction, and cellular differentiation beginning in early development. Retinoic acid, a key regulatory retinoid formed intracellularly through the oxidation of retinol, functions as ligand for a family of nuclear retinoic acid receptors that regulate transcription from target genes. Nuclear retinoic acid receptors will be discussed in Section 3.4. Active vitamin A metabolites, known as retinoids, are essential for multiple physiological processes, ranging from vision to embryonic development. These small hydrophobic compounds associate *in vivo* with soluble proteins that are present in a variety of cells and in particular extracellular compartments, and which bind different types of retinoids with high selectivity and affinity (Noy 2000).

Dietary vitamin A gives rise to a variety of active metabolites, collectively known as retinoids. Chemically, retinoids are composed of three distinct structural domains: a β-ionone ring, an isoprenoid tail, and a polar end-group with an oxidation state that may vary: a hydroxyl group in retinols, an aldehyde in retinals, and a carboxylic moiety in retinoic acids. These small lipophilic compounds exhibit multiple and diverse biological activities. One retinoid, 11-*cis*-retinal, is critical for the visual function. Other vitamin A metabolites, i.e., all-*trans* and 9-*cis*-retinoic acids, are potent regulators of gene transcription, and play important roles in regulating cell proliferation and differentiation. Vitamin A-derived retro-retinoids were implicated in regulating immune function by controlling lymphocyte survival.

Traditionally, retinoid-binding proteins were viewed as transport proteins that act by solubilizing and protecting their labile ligands in aqueous spaces. It is becoming increasingly clear, that, in addition to this general role, retinoid-binding proteins have diverse and specific functions in regulating the disposition, metabolism and activities of retinoids.

The multiple biological actions of retinoids are mediated by two classes of proteins: retinoid receptors and retinoid-binding proteins. Retinoid receptors are ligand-inducible transcription factors that belong to the superfamily of nuclear hormone receptors, and which are activated by stereoisomers of retinoic acid. These proteins will be discussed in the section 3.4.

3.3.2. Retinoid-Binding Proteins

Metabolic events are critical to maintaining physiological concentrations of retinoic acid. In the cytoplasm, retinol, retinaldehyde, and retinoic acid are associated with retinoid-binding proteins, most of which are approximately 15-kDa proteins belonging to the fatty acid-binding protein/cellular retinol-binding protein family. The ligand binding properties and molecular features of these proteins have been well characterized. Recent experiments have highlighted the importance of the cellular retinoid-binding proteins in controlling the concentration of free retinoids and in directing protein-bound retinoids to key enzymes responsible for their metabolism. For example, CRBP has been implicated in retinol uptake, retinol esterification, mobilization of retinyl esters, and the initial oxidation of retinol to retinaldehyde. The ligands bound to other retinoid-binding proteins have also been shown to be available for enzymatic transformation. The new knowledge of the various ways these cytoplasmic proteins buffer the concentration of ligand, control their distribution, and determine their metabolism by specific enzymes is contributing to an improved understanding of the physiological control of retinoid action (Ross 1993).

Multiple types of retinoid-binding proteins that associate with different chemical and isomeric forms of retinoids have been identified both intracellular and extracellular compartments. Hence retinoids are found *in vivo* either associated with cellular membranes or bound to a specific retinoid-binding protein. The parent vitamin A molecule, all-*trans*-retinol, circulates in blood bound to serum retinol-binding protein (RBP, also called RBP4). Inside cells, all-*trans*-retinol and its oxidation product, all-*trans*-retinal, are associated with one of the two isoforms of cellular retinol-binding proteins (CRBP-I, CRBP-II, and CRBP-III, also called RBP1, RBP2, and RBP3, respectively). all-*trans*-Retinoic acid is found intracellularly bound to one of the two cellular retinoic acid-binding protein isoforms (CRABP-I and CRABP-II). The visual pigment 11-*cis*-retinal and its precursor, 11-*cis*-retinol, associate in several cell types in the eye with cellular retinal-binding protein (CRALBP; Saari et al. 1982). Another ocular protein that can bind retinoids, the interphotoreceptor retinoid-binding protein (IRBP), is present in the extracellular space separating pigment epithelium and photoreceptor cells. Intracellular lipid-binding protein (iLBP), and epididymal retinoic acid-binding protein (ERABP; Newcomer and Ong 1990; Ong et al. 2000) are also reported. Retinoid-binding proteins are believed to share a common role in that they act to solubilize and stabilize their hydrophobic and labile ligands in aqueous spaces. However, a growing body of information indicates that, in addition to this general role, specific retinoid-binding proteins have distinct functions in regulation of the transport, metabolism and action of the particular retinoids with which they associate.

3.3.3. Retinol-Binding Protein (RBP)

Retinol is secreted from its storage pools and circulates in blood bound to RBP (Kanai et al. 1968; Smith and Goodman 1979; Goodman 1984; Muto et al. 1982; Blaner 1989; Ross 1999). The main storage site for vitamin A and, correspondingly, the main site of synthesis of RBP, is the liver, although other tissues (including adipose tissue, kidney, lung, heart, skeletal muscle, spleen, eye, and testis) express this protein. Secretion of RBP from the liver is tightly regulated by the availability of retinol. In vitamin A deficiency, RBP secretion is inhibited and the protein accumulates in the endoplasmic reticulum of PCs. In the presence of retinol, RBP associates with retinol, moves to the Golgi apparatus and is secreted into blood in the form of the holoprotein. In blood, RBP is bound to transthyretin, which, in addition to associating with RBP, functions as a carrier protein for thyroid hormones. Binding of RBP to transthyretin serves to prevent the loss of the smaller protein from the circulation by filtration in the renal glomeruli. The ternary complex transthyretin+RBP+retinol thus serves to transport retinol in the circulation and to deliver it to target tissues.

The exact role that RBP plays in regulating vitamin A uptake by extrahepatic cells is controversial, and two alternative views have been presented. On the one hand it has been proposed that a receptor embedded in the plasma membranes of target cells mediates transfer of retinol from RBP, across the membrane and into cytosol, or perhaps directly to the protein that binds retinol in cells, CRBP. An alternative view regarding the mechanism by which retinol leaves RBP in the plasma and enters target cells stemmed from the consideration that, because of the hydrophobic nature of retinol, cellular membranes do not constitute a barrier to it.

In most cells the pools of retinol in blood and in cytosol will be near equilibrium, and retinol will be selectively taken up only by cells in which a retinol concentration gradient, directed inwards, can be created. Such a gradient will be generated in cells that actively utilize retinol, or in cells in which CRBP is up regulated, thereby decreasing the cytosolic concentration of free retinol.

Important insights into the biological role of RBP have been obtained recently by studies of mice and humans in which the RBP gene is disrupted. RBP-deficient mice display reduced blood retinol levels and impaired visual function during the first months of life. However, these mice are viable and fertile and, when maintained on a vitamin A-sufficient diet, they acquire normal vision by 5 months of age, even though their blood retinol level remains low. A striking phenotype of the RBP null mice is that they possess larger than normal hepatic vitamin A stores, but are nevertheless dependent on a continuous dietary intake of vitamin A (Quadro et al. 1999, 2003; Paik et al. 2004).

A recent study of two human siblings that harbor point mutations in their RBP gene and exhibit undetectable plasma RBP levels revealed that these sisters suffer from night blindness and mild retinal dystrophy but do not exhibit other clinical symptoms of vitamin A deficiency (Seeliger et al. 1999; Biesalski et al. 1999).

The observations obtained by examining RBP deficient mice and humans support the conclusions that RBP is critical for the mobilization of retinol from hepatic storage pools in times of insufficient dietary intake, but that the protein is not essential for the delivery of retinol to tissues. Supply of vitamin A to target tissues in the absence of RBP is likely to be accomplished via newly absorbed retinyl esters, or perhaps β-carotene present in circulating chylomicrons.

In patients with acute hepatitis, RBP concentrations correlated negatively with the levels of plasma bilirubin, glutamic-oxaloacetic transaminase, and alkaline phosphatase (Smith and Goodman 1971).

Piscine RBP is a prototype of the specific vitamin A-transporting protein in plasma of the vertebrates, being modified later in evolution, during phylogenetic development of the vertebrates, to acquire a binding site for prealbumin on the molecule (Shidoji and Muto 1977).

3.3.4. RBP 4

Recently, RBP has been named also retinol-binding protein-4 (RBP4), and studies using the name of RBP4 instead of RBP have been published. In obesity and type 2 diabetes, expression of the GLUT4 glucose transporter is decreased selectively in adipocytes. Adipose-specific Glut4 (also known as Slc2a4) knockout (adipose-Glut4-/-) mice show insulin resistance secondarily in muscle and liver. By using DNA arrays, that expression of RBP4 is elevated in adipose tissue of adipose-Glut4-/- mice (Yang et al. 2005). Serum RBP4 levels are elevated in insulin-resistant mice and humans with obesity and type 2 diabetes. RBP4 levels are normalized by rosiglitazone, an insulin-sensitizing drug.

Transgenic overexpression of human RBP4 or injection of recombinant RBP4 in normal mice causes insulin resistance. Conversely, genetic deletion of Rbp4 enhances insulin sensitivity. Fenretinide, a synthetic retinoid that increases urinary excretion of RBP4, normalizes serum RBP4 levels and improves insulin resistance and glucose intolerance in mice with obesity induced by a high-fat diet. Increasing serum RBP4 induces hepatic expression of the gluconeogenic enzyme phosphoenolpyruvate carboxykinase and impairs insulin signalling in muscle.

Thus, RBP4 is an adipocyte-derived 'signal' that may contribute to the pathogenesis of type 2 diabetes. Lowering RBP4 could be a new strategy for treating type 2 diabetes (Yang et al. 2005). Increased levels of RBP4 were also shown to cause insulin resistance in muscle and increased expression of the gluconeogenic enzyme phosphoenolpyruvate carboxykinase in the liver (Polonsky 2006).

Relation between plasma RBP4 concentrations and various metabolic parameters in humans has been examined (Cho et al. 2006). Plasma RBP4 concentrations were higher in the impaired glucose tolerance and type 2 diabetic groups than in the normal glucose tolerance group and to be related to various clinical parameters known to be associated with insulin resistance.

Elevated serum RBP4 was associated with components of the metabolic syndrome, including increased body-mass index, waist-to-hip ratio, serum triglyceride levels, and systolic blood pressure and decreased high-density lipoprotein cholesterol levels. Adipocyte GLUT4 protein and serum RBP4 levels were inversely correlated. RBP4 is an adipocyte-secreted molecule that is elevated in the serum before the development of frank diabetes and appears to identify insulin resistance and associated cardiovascular risk factors in subjects with varied clinical presentations. These findings provide a rationale for antidiabetic therapies aimed at lowering serum RBP4 levels (Graham et al. 2006).

Although the correlations of leptin, adiponectin, and high-sensitivity C-reactive protein concentrations with BMI in children (ages 9–15 years) are similar to those of adults, the correlations of RBP4 and lipocalin-2 with BMI in children are the inverse of those observed in adults. Thus, although systemic inflammation and mild insulin resistance are present in childhood obesity, RBP4 and lipocalin-2 concentrations are not increased in children as they are in obese adults with long-standing severe insulin resistance and type 2 diabetes (Kanaka-Gantenbein et al. 2008).

Subclinical hypothyroidism has also been associated with cardiovascular disease. Plasma RBP4 levels were associated with subclinical hypothyroidism independent of obesity in elderly subjects with normal glucose tolerance, indicating that RBP4 level could be used as an index of risk cardiovascular disease in subclinical hypothyroidism (Choi et al. 2008).

However, in patients with chronic liver disease, serum RBP4 was significantly reduced compared with healthy control subjects and closely correlated with the stage of liver cirrhosis (Yagmur et al. 2007). Chronic liver disease patients without cirrhosis showed normal RBP4 concentrations, which correlated with serum glucose and insulin secretion and inversely correlated with insulin sensitivity. In an animal model of experimental cirrhosis, hepatic RBP4 gene expression decreased in cirrhotic liver. RBP4 appears, unlike in obesity or type 2 diabetes, not to be a relevant systemic factor in the pathogenesis of insulin resistance in liver cirrhosis. Liver function has a tremendous impact on RBP4 levels, and future studies will need to take liver function into account when examining serum RBP4 levels (Yagmur et al. 2007). Mean values of serum RBP4 were similar in nonalcoholic fatty liver disease (NAFLD) and chronic hepatitis C (CHC), and both were significantly higher than in controls. RBP4 was higher in CHC patients with steatosis than in NAFLD. By linear regression, RBP4 was independently linked to steatosis only in CHC, and to elevated body mass index and low grading in NAFLD. By linear regression, steatosis was independently linked to homeostasis model assessment score and high RBP4 in CHC. By logistic regression, RBP4 was the only variable independently associated with moderate-severe steatosis in CHC (Petta et al. 2008; Blüher et al. 2008). RBP4 might contribute to the pathogenesis of NAFLD (Wu et al. 2008). Circulating RBP4 is not associated with the amount of fat in the classical depots or in the ectopic depots in muscle. However, it correlates positively with liver fat. Furthermore, metabolic parameters support the close relationship between circulating RBP4 with liver fat and, presumably, hepatic insulin resistance (Stefan et al. 2007).

3.3.5. Membrane receptor for RBP

STRA6

STRA6 (stimulated by retinoic acid 6) has been newly reported as the membrane receptor for RBP (Blaner 2007). The hypothesis that the cellular uptake of retinol involves the specific interaction of a plasma membrane receptor with RBP at the extracellular surface followed by ligand transfer to cytoplasmic CRBP has been investigated (Sundaram et al. 1998).

Optimal retinol uptake is achieved with holo-RBP, the membrane receptor, and apo-CRBP have been demonstrated. The RBP receptor, through specific interactions with the binding proteins, participates (either directly or via associated proteins) in the mechanism which mediates the transfer of retinol from extracellular RBP to intracellular CRBP (Sundaram et al. 1998).

Receptors for RBP have been reported previously (Båvik et al. 1991, 1992, 1993; Smeland et al. 1995), and a new receptor, STRA6, has been reported (Kawaguchi et al. 2007; Pasutto et al. 2007). In bovine retinal pigment epithelium cells, STRA6, a multitransmembrane domain protein, as a specific membrane receptor for RBP has been identified. STRA6 binds to RBP with high affinity and has robust vitamin A uptake activity from the vitamin A–RBP complex. It is widely expressed in embryonic development and in adult organ systems. The RBP receptor represents a major physiological mediator of cellular vitamin A uptake (Kawaguchi et al. 2007).

STRA6 mutations thus define a pleiotropic malformation syndrome representing the first human phenotype associated with mutations in a gene from the "STRA" group (Pasutto et al. 2007). Two unrelated consanguineous families with malformation syndromes sharing anophthalmia and distinct eyebrows as common signs, but differing for alveolar capillary dysplasia or complex congenital heart defect in one and diaphragmatic hernia in the other family have been reported.

RBP Knockout Animals

How retinol is taken up by cells has been an area of active research since the first report of a cell-surface receptor for retinol-binding protein (RBP) in the mid-1970s. Two recent reports, by Kawaguchi et al. (2007) and Pasutto et al. (2007), provide compelling data regarding the molecular identity and properties of a RBP receptor and open new research avenues for a better understanding of retinoid biology (Blaner 2007).

3.3.6. CRBPs

CRBP-I and CRBP-II (also called RBP1 and RBP2, respectively) are the first intracellular retinoid-binding proteins to be discovered (Ross 1993). The primary sequences of rat CRBP-I and CRBP-II show 56% identity, and each of these proteins is highly conserved among species, exhibiting 91-96% sequence identity among human, rat, mouse, pig, and chick. Both proteins interact with both all-*trans* retinol and all-*trans* retinal. It has been reported that the binding affinity of CRBP-I towards retinol is about 100-fold higher as compared with that of CRBP-II, that the two proteins display a similar binding affinity towards retinal, and that CRBP-II associates with retinol and retinal with similar affinities.

The two isoforms of CRBP display a strikingly different tissue distribution. CRBP-I is expressed in multiple tissues, both in the fetus and in the adult. In the adult, it is particularly abundant in the liver, kidney, lung, and reproductive organs, and is also expressed in the choroid plexus in the brain and in pigment epithelium cells in the eye. In contrast, in the adult, CRBP-II is restricted to the small intestine, where it is located in mature enterocytes on the villi of the mucosal epithelium. CRBP-II in the fetus is mainly localized in the intestine, but is also transiently expressed in the liver where, in the rat, it appears several days before birth and disappears shortly after birth.

Multiple enzymic activities that can catalyze metabolic conversions of free retinol and retinal have been reported. However, only specific enzymes recognize CRBP-bound retinoids, suggesting that CRBPs limit access of retinoids to some enzymes, while allowing metabolism by others to proceed. Such a role is deemed especially important in view of the need for tight regulation of cellular levels of the active vitamin A metabolite, retinoic acid.

Thus, CRBP-I seems to channel retinoids through the reactions of retinoic acid synthesis via a series of protein-protein interactions. CRABP-I facilitates retinoic acid metabolism by sequestering it and by acting as a low Km substrate, thereby also modulating the steady-state concentrations of retinoic acid (Napoli 1993). In the mammalian intestine, CRBP I and CRBP II levels are determinants of intracellular retinol accumulation and esterification (Levin 1993).

Recently phylogeny of CRBP has been reported (Mezaki et al. 2012a). Lampreys are ancestral representatives of vertebrates known as jawless fish. The Japanese lamprey, *Lethenteron japonicum*, is a parasitic member of the lampreys known to store large amounts of vitamin A within its body. How this storage is achieved, however, is wholly unknown. Within the body, the absorption, transfer and metabolism of vitamin A are regulated by a family of proteins called retinoid-binding proteins. Here we have cloned a cDNA for CRBP from the Japanese lamprey, and phylogenetic analysis suggests that lamprey CRBP is an ancestor of both CRBP I and II. The lamprey CRBP protein was expressed in bacteria and purified. Binding of the lamprey CRBP to retinol (Kd of 13.2 nM) was identified by fluorimetric titration. However, results obtained with the protein fluorescence quenching technique indicated that lamprey CRBP does not bind to retinal. Northern blot analysis showed that lamprey CRBP mRNA was ubiquitously expressed, although expression was most abundant in the intestine. Together, these results suggest that lamprey CRBP has an important role in absorbing vitamin A from the blood of host animals.

CRBP-I

Regulation of Vitamin A Storage

The processes by which vitamin A is taken up into the liver, the subsequent metabolism and disposition of retinol in this tissue, and the enzymic steps that have been proposed to be under regulation of CRBP-I. In vitamin A sufficiency, retinol accumulates in the liver, where it is stored in the form of retinyl esters. Two distinct enzymic activities that can catalyse the esterification of retinol with long-chain fatty acids to form retinyl esters have been identified: acyl-CoA: retinol acyltransferase (ARAT; EC 2.3.1.76), which is dependent upon the presence of CoA, and lecithin : retinol acyltransferase (LRAT; EC 2.3.1.135), for which the esterification reaction is coupled to hydrolysis of phospholipids. It has been demonstrated that, while both enzymes can metabolize free retinol, esterification of CRBP bound retinol is CoA-independent, implying that CRBP-bound retinol is metabolized by LRAT, but not by ARAT.

LRAT can recognize retinol when bound to CRBP-I, suggesting that the substrate is `channelled' between the binding protein and the enzyme via direct protein-protein interactions. While holo-CRBP-I presents its ligand directly to LRAT, apo-CRBP-I strongly inhibits this reaction. An additional enzymic activity that was reported to be affected by apo-CRBP-I is retinyl ester hydrolase.

In vitamin A sufficiency, CRBP-I will be largely saturated with retinol and will direct this ligand to storage by delivering it to LRAT. On the other hand, under conditions of vitamin A deficiency, the level of retinol and, consequently, the level of saturation of CRBP-I will decrease, resulting in an elevation in the level of the apoprotein. In turn, apo-CRBP-I will both inhibit retinol esterification and stimulate liberation of retinol from stored retinyl esters, thereby allowing retinol to be released into the circulation.

The gene encoding CRBP-I has been inactivated (Ghyselinck et al. 1999).

CRBP-I and LRAT are highly expressed in HSCs. These proteins play key roles in the storage of retinyl esters because mice lacking CRBP-I or LRAT both have impaired storage of HSC retinyl esters (Ghyselinck et al. 1999; Batten et al. 2004). Mutant mice fed a vitamin A-enriched diet are healthy and fertile. They do not present any of the congenital abnormalities related to retinoic acid (RA) deficiency, indicating that CRBPI is not indispensable for RA synthesis. However, CRBP-I deficiency results in an 50% reduction of retinyl ester accumulation in HSCs. This reduction is due to a decreased synthesis and a 6-fold faster turnover, which are not related to changes in the levels of retinyl ester metabolizing enzymes, but probably reflect an impaired delivery of retinol to LRAT. CRBPI-null mice fed a vitamin A-deficient diet for 5 months fully exhaust their retinyl ester stores. Thus, CRBP-I is indispensable for efficient retinyl ester synthesis and storage, and its absence results in a waste of retinol that is asymptomatic in vitamin A-sufficient animals, but leads to a severe syndrome of vitamin A deficiency in animals fed a vitamin A-deficient diet (Ghyselinck et al. 1999).

Retinoic acid is produced from retinol by two enzymic steps. The first step, catalyzed by retinol dehydrogenase, results in the formation of retinal, which is then converted, via the action of retinal dehydrogenase, to retinoic acid. Free retinol can be oxidized by multiple forms of alcohol dehydrogenases with broad substrate specificities that are present in both cytosol and membrane fractions. However, only distinct enzymes can gain access to CRBP-I bound retinol, suggesting that the binding protein delivers its ligand to enzymes in a specific manner which is likely to involve direct protein-protein interactions. As CRBP-I binds not only retinol but also retinal, it was suggested that retinal that is produced following oxidation of retinol also associates with CRBP-I and that the protein-bound retinal serves as a substrate for the subsequent reaction by retinal dehydrogenase. It has been shown in regard to this that CRBP-I-bound retinal is not readily accessible to cytosolic retinal dehydrogenase activity, but is efficiently metabolized to retinoic acid by microsomal enzymes.

Overall, current information implicates CRBP-I in regulating vitamin A storage, as well as in determining the specificity of the two enzymic activities that produce retinoic acid. It is worth noting, however, that while the proposed function for CRBP-I in regulating vitamin A storage has been strongly supported by studies of CRBP-I-null mice, these animals do not display abnormalities related to retinoic acid deficiency, at least under conditions of maternal vitamin A sufficiency. Hence, under these conditions, CRBP-I does not appear to be essential for retinoic acid synthesis during development.

CRBP-II

The exclusive expression of CRBP-II in the absorptive cells of the small intestine, and the high concentration of the protein in this location, suggests that CRBP-II has a role in the initial processing of retinol from food. Vitamin A is present in foods either as β-carotene, derived from plant sources, or as retinyl esters, originating from animal sources. The first step in the metabolism of β-carotene is an oxidative cleavage, generating retinal, which is subsequently reduced to retinol. Retinyl esters are hydrolyzed to produce free retinol upon entry into the enterocytes. Retinol, derived either from β-carotene or from dietary retinyl esters, is then esterified and the resulting retinyl esters are packaged into chylomicrons and secreted into blood via the lymphatic system. CRBP-II was also reported to block the re-oxidation of retinol to retinal, most likely because protein-bound retinol is not available to enterocyte retinol dehydrogenases. CRBP-II also participates in regulation of the esterification of retinol in the enterocyte. Similar to hepatic ARAT, intestinal ARAT is incapable of processing CRBP-II-bound retinol. In contrast, LRAT catalyzes retinol esterification more efficiently when the substrate is presented to the enzyme bound to CRBP as compared with free retinol. Unlike apo-CRBP-I, apo-CRBP-II does not inhibit the activity of LRAT, and thus formation of retinyl esters in the intestine is expected to proceed in times of low intake of vitamin A.

CRBP III

A novel fatty acid-binding protein (FABP) family member, cellular retinol-binding protein type III (CRBP III), has been identified (Vogel et al. 2001). Heart and skeletal muscle take up postprandial retinol but express little or no CRBP-I or CRBP-II. The 134-amino acid protein is encoded by a cDNA that is expressed primarily in heart, muscle, and adipose tissue. It shares 57 and 56% sequence identity with CRBP-I and CRBP-II, respectively, but less than 40% with other members of the FABP family. Fluorescence titrations of purified recombinant protein with retinol isomers indicates binding to all-trans-, 13-*cis*-, and 9-*cis*-retinol, with respective Kd values of 109, 83, and 130 nM. Retinoic acids (all-*trans*-, 13-*cis*-, and 9-*cis*-), retinals (all-*trans*-, 13-*cis*-, and 9-*cis*-), fatty acids (laurate, myristate, palmitate, oleate, linoleate, arachidonate, and docosahexanoate), or fatty alcohols (palmityl, petrosenlinyl, and ricinolenyl) fail to bind.

CRBP-III belongs to the family of intracellular lipid-binding proteins, which includes the adipocyte-binding protein aP2. In the cytosol, CRBP-III binds retinol, the precursor of retinyl ester and the active metabolite retinoic acid. CRBP-III is a PPAR target gene and plays a role in lipid and whole body energy metabolism (Zizola et al. 2008).

3.3.7. CRABPs

Two binding proteins with a high affinity for all-*trans*-retinoic acid have been identified, CRABP-I and CRABP-II. The two isoforms are highly similar, displaying 74% sequence identity between human CRABP-I and -II, and are also extremely conserved between species. For example, rat, mouse and bovine CRABP-I are all identical, and they differ from the human protein by a single amino acid residue. In the adult, CRABP-I is expressed almost ubiquitously, while CRABP-II is only expressed in the skin, uterus and ovary, and the choroid plexus. Both CRABPs are widely expressed in the embryo, although they do not usually co-exist in the same cells. It was reported that mice in which the genes for either CRABP-I or CRABP-II have been disrupted appear to be essentially normal, except for some defects in limb development. However, the molecular mechanisms underlying these effects remain to be clarified. Similarly to other retinoid binding proteins, it has been proposed that CRABPs serve to solubilize and protect their ligand in the aqueous cytosol, and that they transport retinoic acid between different cellular compartments. It was thus suggested that CRABPs act to deliver their ligand to the nucleus, where it will bind and activate retinoid receptors.

CRABP-I

CRABP-I has been shown to modulate the activities of enzyme(s) that catalyze the metabolic transformation of retinoic acid. It was reported that, when bound to CRABP-I, retinoic acid serves as a substrate for enzymes in rat testes microsomes, giving rise to the polar metabolites 3,4-didehydro-, 4-hydroxy-, 4-oxo-, 16-hydroxy-4-oxo- and 18-hydroxy-retinoic acids. These metabolites are likely to be products of members of the CYP26 family, cytochromes P450 that specifically metabolize retinoic acid. The details of the mechanisms by which CRABP-I regulates the activities of retinoic acid-metabolizing enzyme(s), and the identity of the specific enzyme(s) affected by this binding protein, remain to be clarified. Nevertheless, these observations suggest that CRABP-I acts to dampen cellular responses to retinoic acid, and that this effect reflects the ability of the binding protein to enhance the activity of an enzyme(s) that catalyzes the degradation of the hormone.

CRABP-II

Both CRABP-I and -II are present in the nucleus, implying that both proteins may serve to deliver retinoic acid to the transcription factor that is activated by it, namely the retinoic acid receptor (RAR). However, it was recently shown that the mechanisms by which CRABP-I and -II deliver their ligand to RAR are fundamentally different. Transfer of retinoic acid from CRABP to RAR may occur either via the aqueous phase or by `channelling' between the two proteins, i.e., through direct protein-protein interactions and in a way that bypasses the bulk solution. Kinetic studies of the processes through which retinoic acid moves from CRABP-I or CRABP-II to RAR revealed that, while CRABP-I acts as a passive vehicle which binds and releases its ligand according to concentration gradients, CRABP-II delivers retinoic acid to the RAR in a direct collisional process. It was shown further that channelling of retinoic acid between CRABP-II and RAR results in a significant facilitation of the formation of holo-RAR. These observations suggest that, in cells, expression of CRABP-II (but not of CRABP-I) would enhance the transcriptional activity of RAR. This conclusion has been supported by the observation that overexpression of CRABP-II (but not CRABP-I) results in a marked stimulation of transcription of a reporter gene driven by a RAR response element.

3.3.8. HSCs and RBP

Regulation of Vitamin A Homeostasis by HSCs

Vitamin A (Fig. 7) is known to regulate diverse cellular activities such as cell proliferation, differentiation, morphogenesis, and tumorigenesis (Blomhoff 1994; Chawla et al. 2001). In physiological conditions, HSCs store 50-80 % of the total vitamin A in the whole body as retinyl palmitate in lipid droplets in the cytoplasm, and regulate both transport and storage of vitamin A.

The concentration of vitamin A in the bloodstream is regulated within the physiological range. By receptor-mediated endocytosis, the cells take up retinol from the blood, where it circulates as a complex of retinol and a specific binding protein called RBP (Blomhoff 1994) (Fig. 8). Once inside the cell, free retinol has several fates, one of which is reformation of the complex with RBP and returns to the bloodstream (Blomhoff et al. 1992a, 1992b; Senoo 2000). Thus, the HSCs are important for the regulation of homeostasis of vitamin A.

As mentioned in the section 3. 2. 2, when [^{3}H]retinol was injected via portal vein, the largest amount of the labeled retinol was taken up by the liver within 90 minutes after injection, although the labeled material was detected in all organs examined (Senoo et al. 1984). The radioactivity of the retinol in the liver did not change until 6 days after the injection. These results were consistent with the reports that main storage site of vitamin A in mammals is the liver (Wake 1971, 1980a).

To examine the distribution of vitamin A in the liver, radioactivity per cell was determined after cell fractionation (Senoo et al. 1984, 1991; Senoo and Hata 1993b). Specific activity of [^{3}H]retinol (per cell) was the highest in the HSC fraction, both 90 minutes and 6 days after injection. These results strongly support earlier morphological observations (Wake 1971, 1980a) that the HSC is the storage site of vitamin A in the liver, and are not inconsistent with reports on the retinol transfer from PCs to HSCs (Andersen et al. 1992; Blomhoff et al. 1990; Gjøen et al. 1987; Malaba et al. 1995; Senoo et al. 1990, 1993).

Immunoelectronmicroscopic studies suggest that RBP mediates the paracrine transfer of retinol from hepatic PCs to the HSCs and that HSCs bind and internalize RBP by receptor-mediated endocytosis (Malaba et al. 1995; Senoo et al. 1990, 1993).

A study was conducted to determine the levels and distributions of retinoids, RBP, retinyl palmitate hydrolase (RPH), CRBP, and CRABP in different types of isolated liver cells (Blaner et al. 1985). Highly purified fractions of PCs, HSCs, LSECs, and KCs were isolated in high yield from rat livers. When these data were expressed on the basis of per unit mass of cellular protein, the concentrations of RPH, CRBP, and CRABP in the HSCs, which contain 10-fold less protein than the large PCs, were seen to be greatly enriched over PCs. The PCs contained approximately 9% of the total retinoids, 98% of the total RBP, 90% of the total RPH activity, 91% of the total CRBP, and 71% of the total CRABP found in the liver. The HSCs accounted for approximately 88% of the total retinoids, 0.7% of the total RBP, 10% of the RPH activity, 8% of the total CRBP, and 21% of the CRABP in the liver. The LSEC and KC fractions contained very low levels of all of these parameters. Thus, the large and abundant PCs account for greater than 70% of the liver's RBP, RPH, CRBP, and CRABP; but the much smaller and less abundant HSCs contain the majority of hepatic retinoids and greatly enriched concentrations of RPH, CRBP, and CRABP (Blaner et al. 1985)

HSCs contained 28-34 nmol of retinoids/10^6 cells, and PCs contained 0.5-0.8 nmol of retinoids/10^6 cells, suggesting that as much as 80% or more of total liver retinoids might be stored in HSCs with the rest stored in PCs (Blomhoff et al. 1985a). Isolated LSECs and KCs contained very low levels of retinoids. More than 98% of the retinoids recovered in HSCs were retinyl esters. Isolated PC and HSC preparations both contained considerable RPH and ARAT activities. PCs accounted for about 75-80% of the total hepatic content of these two enzyme activities, with the rest located in HSCs. On a cell protein basis, the concentrations of both these activities were much greater in HSCs than in PCs. Large amounts of CRBPs were also found in PCs and HSCs. Although PCs accounted for more than 90% of hepatic CRBP, the concentration of the protein in HSCs (per unit protein) was 22 times greater than that in PCs. HSCs were also enriched in CRABP. Thus, both PCs and HSCs contain substantial amounts of retinoids and of the enzymes and intracellular binding proteins involved in retinol metabolism. HSCs are particularly enriched in these several components (Blomhoff et al. 1985). Other report also demonstrated similar cellular distribution of retinoid and retinoid-binding proteins in the liver (Hendriks et al. 1988).

^{125}I-Tyramine cellobiose-labeled rat RBP has been prepared and studied its tissue uptake 1, 5, and 24 hours after intravenous injection into rats (Gjøen et al. 1987). The liver was the organ containing most radioactivity at all time points studied. After 5 and 24 hours, 30 and 22% of the injected dose were recovered in the liver, respectively. After separating the liver into PCs and NPCs in the 5-hour group, they found that both cell fractions contained approximately the same amount of radioactivity (per gram of liver). Most of the RBP radioactivity in the NPC fraction was in the HSCs (Gjøen et al. 1987).

We investigated *in vivo* uptake of RBP in liver cells by immunocytochemistry at the electron microscopic level using ultrathin cryosections. Ten minutes after injection, RBP was localized to PCs and HSCs. In these cells, RBP was detected on the cell surface and in vesicles near the cell surface. RBP was observed mainly in association with the membrane in these vesicles. Two hours after injection, RBP was localized not only on the cell surface and in vesicles close to the cell surface, but also in larger vesicles located deeper in the cytoplasm of these cells. RBP in larger vesicles was observed at a distance from the vesicular membrane. Finally, we compared the distribution of endocytosed RBP in PCs with that of asialo-orosomucoid, a ligand known to be internalized by receptor-mediated endocytosis. Both ligands on the cell surface and in small vesicles located close to the cell surface and in larger vesicles located deeper in the cytoplasm. Asialo-orosomucoid and RBP were seldom observed in the same small vesicles, but the larger vesicles contained both ligands. These data suggest that RBP is internalized in PCs and HSCs of the liver by receptor-mediated endocytosis (Senoo et al. 1990).

Although the major tissue site of RBP synthesis in the body is the liver, other sites of synthesis have been reported. A model a mouse strain (hRBP–/–) that expresses human RBP (hRBP) cDNA under the control of the mouse muscle creatine kinase promoter in an rbp-null background (RBP–/–) have been made. By comparing hRBP–/–, RBP–/–, and wild-type mice, extrahepatically synthesized hRBP has been shown, unlike RBP expressed in the liver, to be unable to mobilize liver retinoid stores. Consistent with this conclusion, circulating hRBP is not taken up by PCs. RBP has been proposed to play an essential role in distributing hepatic retinoids between PCs and HSCs (Quadro et al. 2004).

RBP Knock out Animals

RBP is the sole specific transport protein for retinol (vitamin A) in the circulation, and its single known function is to deliver retinol to tissues. RBP knockout mice (RBP-/-) were generated by gene targeting (Quadro et al. 1999; Paik et al. 2004). These mice have several phenotypes. Although viable and fertile, they have reduced blood retinol levels and markedly impaired retinal function during the first months of life. The impairment is not due to developmental retinal defect. Given a vitamin A-sufficient diet, the RBP-/- mice acquire normal vision by 5 months of age even though blood retinol levels remain low. Deprived of dietary vitamin A, vision remains abnormal and blood retinol declines to undetectable levels. The RBP-/- mice can acquire hepatic retinol stores, but these cannot be mobilized. Thus, their vitamin A status is extremely tenuous and dependent on a regular vitamin A intake. Unlike wild-type mice, serum retinol levels in adult RBP-/- animals become undetectable after only a week on a vitamin A-deficient diet and their retinal function rapidly deteriorates. Thus RBP is needed for normal vision in young animals and for retinol mobilization in times of insufficient dietary intake, but is otherwise dispensable for the delivery of retinol to tissues (Quadro et al. 1999, 2003).

3.3.9. CRBPs, CRABPs, and HSCs

CRBPs and HSCs

CRBP was demonstrated in HSCs by immunostaining using specific antibody. Diffuse cytoplasmic staining for CRBP was seen in all the PCs.

Much more intense staining for CRBP was seen in the HSCs. The prominence of the CRBP-positive HSCs changed markedly with vitamin A status. Thus, these cells were most prominent, and appeared most numerous, in the liver from rats fed excess retinol (Kato et al. 1984). CRBP in the rat liver was examined by the peroxidase-antiperoxidase immunolocalization technique. Positive cytoplasmic staining was seen in the liver when antiserum prepared against purified CRBP was used but not when antiserum absorbed with purified CRBP was used (Porter et al. 1983).

CRBP was reported to be localized in the PCs and in the HSCs (Eriksson et al. 1984). The appearance of high amounts of this protein in cells involved in the dietary uptake, storage, mobilization, and resorption of vitamin A suggests that one function of the CRBP is to act as a vehicle in the intracellular transport of retinol through these organs (Eriksson et al. 1984).

The concentration of retinoids in the bloodstream is regulated within the physiological range. By receptor-mediated endocytosis, the cells take up retinol from the blood, where it circulates as a complex of retinol and a specific binding protein called RBP (Fig. 8). Once inside the cell, free retinol has several fates, one of which is reformation of the complex with RBP and returns to the bloodstream. Thus, the HSCs are important for the regulation of homeostasis of retinoids. These findings reveal a striking functional difference between CRABP-I and CRABP-II, and point at a novel mechanism by which the transcriptional activity of retinoic acid can be regulated by CRABP-II (Dong et al. 1999).

CRBP-1 is involved in vitamin A metabolism because it mediates both retinol esterification to retinyl esters and retinol oxidation to retinal and retinoic acid. CRBP-1 is highly expressed in the liver, particularly in HSCs. The liver expression of CRBP-1 during experimental fibrogenesis has been investigated. The regulation of CRBP-1 expression in cultured HSC and portal fibroblasts, two fibroblastic cell types involved in liver fibrogenesis has been also studied. Fibrosis was induced in rats by CCl_4 or bile duct ligation. In normal liver, contrary to HSC, portal fibroblasts did not express CRBP-1. After CCl_4 injury, CRBP-1 expression was maintained in myofibroblastic αSMA-positive HSC. After bile duct ligation, portal fibroblasts (which proliferated around ductular structures) acquired expression of both CRBP-1 and αSMA. During HSC activation in culture, CRBP-1 expression gradually increased until day 5 when αSMA expression was obvious. Cultured portal fibroblasts developed both CRBP-1 and αSMA expression. In both cell populations, TGF-1 treatment increased CRBP-1 expression (Uchio et al. 2002).

In normal liver, quiescent HSCs expressed CRBP-1, while portal fibroblasts did not (Lepreux et al. 2004). In fibrotic or cirrhotic liver, activated HSCs co-expressed CRBP-1 and αSMA; a variable proportion of portal and septal (myo)fibroblasts, more important in cirrhosis, neo-expressed both CRBP-1 and αSMA. Biliary epithelial cells both in normal and pathological situations expressed CRBP-1. Neither KCs, nor LSECs showed CRBP-1 expression. CRBP-1 is a good marker to identify HSC in normal human liver. Furthermore, in fibrotic or cirrhotic liver, the different patterns of expression for CRBP-1 and αSMA allow the distinction of different subsets of fibroblastic cells involved in fibrogenesis and septa formation.

3.4. Nuclear Receptors and HSC

As mentioned above, HSC store vitamin A as a form of retinyl ester within the lipid droplets of their cytoplasm. This characteristic feature of HSC led to the idea that HSC functions are regulated by two types of transcriptional factors, retinoic acid receptors (RARs) and peroxisome proliferator-activated receptors (PPARs), both belonging to the nuclear receptor superfamily, because RARs mediate most physiological functions of vitamin A and PPARγ is known to be a master gene for the adipose cell differentiation. We first describe in this section the structure and function of nuclear receptor superfamily and then summarize the relationship between nuclear receptor superfamily members and HSC (Table 1).

3.4.1. Structure and Function of Nuclear Receptors

The cDNA clonings of nuclear receptors were done in mid 80's. They include steroid hormone receptors such as glucocorticoid receptor (GR) (Weinberger et al. 1985a; Hollenberg et al. 1985; Weinberger et al. 1985b), estrogen receptor (ER) (Green et al. 1986; Greene et al. 1986), progesterone receptor (PR) (Conneely et al. 1986), mineralocorticoid receptor (MR) (Arriza et al. 1987), androgen receptor (AR) (Chang et al. 1988; Lubahn et al. 1988), and thyroid hormone receptor α (TRα) (Weinberger et al. 1986), RARα (Petkovich et al. 1987), vitamin D receptor (VDR) (McDonnell et al. 1987), and so on.

The nuclear receptor proteins are divided into six regions A to F, according to the homology of their amino acid sequences (Krust et al. 1986). The highly conserved C region is a domain responsible for DNA binding, and the second highly conserved region E is a ligand-binding domain. Autonomous transcriptional activation functions are located in two separated regions A/B and E. The transcriptional activation by region E is ligand-dependent while that by region A/B is ligand-independent. Region E is a hinge region connecting DNA-binding domain and ligand-binding domain, and in some nuclear receptors, also includes a nuclear localization signal (Picard and Yamamoto 1987; Hamy et al. 1991; Ylikomi et al. 1992).

3.4.2. PPARs

Quiescent HSC store not only vitamin A but also triglycerides. Upon activation, both vitamin A and trigycerides are depleted from HSC. Therefore, there is an analogy between quiescence-activation transition of HSC and adipogenic-fibroblastic transition of adipocytes. Adipocyte differentiation is largely regulated by PPARγ. Three groups reported independently almost at the same time that PPARγ ligands could inhibit HSC activation (Galli et al. 2000; Marra et al. 2000; Miyahara et al. 2000).

PPARγ protein is present in quiescent HSC and it decreases drastically during HSC activation (Galli et al. 2000; Everett et al. 2000). Two PPARγ ligands, 15-deoxy-$\Delta^{12,14}$ prostaglandin J_2 (15dPGJ_2) and ciglitizone, suppress PDGF-induced HSC proliferation and αSMA expression in transdifferentiating HSC, and forced expression of PPARγ protein also down regulates PDGF-induced HSC proliferation (Galli et al. 2000). PDGF signal seems to be transduced to MAPK, which then phosphorylates ser^{112} of PPARγ and interferes PPARγ ligand-binding function, thus inducing HSC proliferation (Galli et al. 2000). Another PPARγ ligands, rosiglitazone and pioglitazone, inhibit TGF-β-induced collagen synthesis as well (Galli et al. 2002).

Another group reported that 15dPGJ_2 and troglitazone inhibited HSC proliferation induced by PDGF (Marra et al. 2000). These ligands also inhibited cytokine-induced secretion of monocyte chemotactic protein 1 (MCP-1), presumably suppressing hepatic inflammation. Decrease in protein levels of PPARγ during HSC activation was also reported.

Third group reported that HSC express PPARγ1 isotype, and PPARγ1 expression was reduced in HSC from fibrotic liver induced by bile duct ligation, or in culture-activated HSC (Miyahara et al. 2000). Two PPARγ agonist, $15dPGJ_2$ and BRL49653 inhibited DNA and collagen synthesis. Suppression of collagen synthesis by PPARγ was mediated by inhibition of NF-I binding to αI(I) procollagen promoter (Yavrom et al. 2005). $15dPGJ_2$ also suppressed αSMA and MCP-1 expressions. TNFα inhibited PPARγ function by MAPK-mediated phosphorylation of ser^{112} of PPARγ, and by suppression of PPARγ-DNA binding (Sung et al. 2004). Adenovirus-mediated overexpression of PPARγ (Hazra et al. 2004), sterol regulatory element-binding protein 1c, or treatment with the adipocyte differentiation mixture (isobutylmethylxanthine, dexamethasone, and insulin) (She et al. 2005), all induced a phenotypic switch from activated HSC to quiescent HSC (Tsukamoto 2005).

The inhibitory function of PPARγ ligands on HSC activation and liver fibrosis was confirmed by several other groups (Kon et al. 2002; Guo et al. 2005). It is also suggested that inhibitory effect of PPARγ on liver fibrosis is mediated by the suppression of TGF-β signaling (Zhao et al. 2006). Curcumin, an antioxidant included in curry, inhibits HSC growth and induces apoptosis by enhancing PPARγ activity (Xu et al. 2003; Zheng and Chen 2004). Curcumin-mediated activation of PPARγ down-regulates TGF-β, PDGF, and EGF signaling (Zheng and Chen 2006; Lin and Chen 2008).

On the other hand, limited effects of pioglitazone, a PPARγ ligand, on liver fibrosis are reported (Leclercq et al. 2006; Marra 2006). The anti-fibrotic effect of pioglitazone was observed only if the pioglitazone was introduced early in the course of disease progression (Leclercq et al. 2006). Furthermore, pioglitazone was not effective to bile duct ligation-induced liver fibrosis, though it is effective to CCl_4-induced or a choline deficient diet-induced liver fibrosis. Moreover, in mice, PPARγ agonists (pioglitazone and $15dPGJ_2$) prevent neither HSC activation nor hepatic fibrosis (Da Silva Morais et al. 2007).

The presence of PPARα mRNA in HSC (Miyahara et al. 2000) and suppressive effect of a PPARα agonist Wy-14,643 on liver fibrosis (Ip et al. 2004) were reported. Messenger RNA and protein of PPARβ/δ is detected in HSC, and L165041, a PPARβ/δ-specific agonist, promoted HSC proliferation and enhanced liver fibrosis induced by CCl_4 (Hellemans et al. 2003a). L165041 also regulates vitamin A metabolism-related gene expression toward the enhancement of vitamin A storage (Hellemans et al. 2003b).

3.4.3. RARs

HSCs store vitamin A-containing lipid droplets within the cytoplasm. The vitamin A (retinol) is hydrolyzed to retinal by retinol dehydrogenases and further hydrolyzed to all-*trans*-retinoic acid, an active form of retinoids, by retinal dehydrogenases (Napoli 1999). The retinoic acid binds to the RARα, β, and γ within the nucleus to enhance their transcriptional activity.

The presence of mRNA for RARα, β, and γ in HSC was reported (Weiner et al. 1992; Ohata et al. 1997; Hellemans et al. 2004). Protein presence was also evidenced by electrophoretic mobility shift assay (EMSA) (Ohata et al. 1997; Hellemans et al. 2004). RARβ mRNA is decreased in HSC isolated from fibrotic livers induced by bile duct ligation (Ohata et al. 1997), and decrease in RARα, β, and γ mRNA levels in culture-activated HSC was also reported (Hellemans et al. 2004). Both pro-fibrotic (Leo and Lieber 1983; Okuno et al. 1997; Okuno et al. 1999) and anti-fibrotic (Senoo and Wake 1985; Wang et al. 2007) functions of retinoids were reported, although it is not certain whether these effects were primarily mediated by RARs, because retinoids exert their physiological effects not only by transcriptional regulation but also by anti-oxidative mechanisms (Shiota et al. 2006). HSC growth was inhibited by retinoids (Pinzani et al. 1992). RARs in HSC are reported to down regulate α2(I) collagen expression (Wang et al. 2002; Wang et al. 2004), and to up regulate expressions of several genes such as the NK cell activating ligand, retinoic acid-induced early gene-1 (Radaeva et al. 2007), and the plasminogen activator (Okuno et al. 1997), which leads to the cleavage and activation of latent TGF-β (Okuno et al. 2002).

Recently, we have reported that RARs expression is suppressed in quiescent HSC at the post-transcriptional level, and only activated HSC are responsive to retinoids (Mezaki et al. 2007, 2009). Retinoids have many biological functions including cell growth and differentiation. The HSC must store large amount of biologically active retinoids safely. Nevertheless, the HSC have to release stored retinoids upon some situations such as decrease in serum vitamin A levels or liver fibrosis. We speculate that this quick response of the HSC is realized by their storage of mRNA for RARα, skipping the step of transcription of RARα gene. The upstream open reading frame at the 5' untranslated region of RARα gene, which is predicted to inhibit translation from the major ORF coding RARα (Kozak 1991), may contribute this type of translational regulation.

3.4.4. ER and PR

The inhibitory effect of estrogen on activation of rat HSC is reported (Shimizu et al. 1999; Shimizu 2003). This effect is mediated by ERβ subtype, because ERα is negative in both quiescent and activated rat HSCs (Zhou et al. 2001). Estrogen inhibits HSC activation by antagonizing oxidative stress-induced down regulation of antiapoptotic proteins, Bcl-2 and Bcl-X_L (Zhou et al. 2001), and also by suppressing oxidative stress-induced MAPK pathways (Itagaki et al. 2005). On the other hand, progesterone stimulates HSC activation by enhancing MAPK pathways, leading to the activation of AP-1 transcription factor (Itagaki et al. 2005), the factor which is responsible for αI(I) collagen gene expression in rat HSC (Chen and Davis 2000).

3.4.5. GR and MR

The presence of GR in HSC is demonstreted (Raddatz et al. 1996). In HSC, dexamethasone up-regulates alpha-2-macroglobulin, a plasma protein which inactivate many kinds of proteinase such as thrombin and plasmin, and down regulates apolipoprotein E, a chylomicron constituent (Ramadori et al. 1991). In contrast, MR mRNA is absent in rat HSC (Rombouts et al. 2001). However, quiescent HSC can respond to aldosterone and up regulate collagen type I expression (Rombouts et al. 2001). Moreover, an MR antagonist, spironolactone, reduces HSC activation during pig serum-induced hepatic fibrosis (Fujisawa et al. 2006). Corticosteroids (glucocorticoid and mineralocorticoid) induce TGF-β receptor type III expression, thus enhancing TGF-β signaling, leading to fibrosis (Wickert et al. 2004).

3.4.6. VDR

VDR content is very low in the liver compared to those in the small intestine and colon (Sandgren et al. 1991). However, HSC as well as other non-parenchymal cells such as LSECs and KCs harbor considerable amounts of VDR mRNA and protein (Gascon-Barre et al. 2003). In HSC, administration of $1,25(OH)_2D_3$, an active form of vitamin D, enhanced the expression of a VDR target gene, CYP24 (Gascon-Barre et al. 2003).

3.4.7. FXR

Bile acids work not only as a detergent which facilitates dietary fat absorption, but also as ligands for farnesoid X receptor (FXR) (Chiang 2002). FXR up regulates bile salt export pump (BSEP) in bile canaliculi, and down regulates cholesterol 7α-hydroxylase (CYP7A1), the rate-limiting enzyme for bile acid synthesis, thus reducing a concentration of toxic bile acids within the liver (Chiang 2002). Besides this bile acid homeostatic function of FXR in hepatic parenchymal cells or hepatocytes (PCs), there exist FXR in HSC, playing an anti-fibrotic roles in porcine serum-administrated, bile duct-ligated, and CCl_4-induced hepatic fibrosis (Fiorucci et al. 2004b; Fiorucci et al. 2005a). FXR up regulates small heterodimer partner (SHP), a transrepressional nuclear receptor which lacks DNA-binding domain, and SHP binds to and tether an AP-1 component JunD, thus inhibiting αI(I) collagen production (Fiorucci et al. 2004b), as well as reducing tissue metalloproteinase inhibitor-1 (TIMP-1) expression (Fiorucci et al. 2005a). Moreover, bile acids ameliorate decrease in PPARγ expression during HSC activation, and FXR and PPARγ ligands cooperatively suppress αI(I) collagen production (Fiorucci et al. 2005b).

On the other hand, there is a report stating that bile acids do not change the expression of collagen type I mRNA in HSC (Svegliati-Baroni et al. 2005). Instead, bile acids induce proliferation of activated HSC via EGFR phosphorylation, thus enhancing fibrosis (Svegliati-Baroni et al. 2005).

3.4.8. PXR

Pregnane X receptor (PXR), or steroid X receptor (SXR) in human, has been categolized in an orphan nuclear receptor, and its ligands include pregnane steroids, bile acids, and drug ligands such as rifampicin (Wright 2006). Recently, vitamin K is also shown to be a PXR ligand (Tabb et al. 2003; Igarashi et al. 2007). In rodent, pregnenolone-16α-carbonitrile, a PXR activator, inhibits liver fibrogenesis in spite of the absence of PXR expression in HSC (Marek et al. 2005). However, a recent report tells that PXR is actually expressed in quiescent rodent HSC but it suddenly decrease upon activation (Wright 2006), indicating that the antifibrogenic effect of pregnenolone-16α-carbonitrile might be mediated by PXR. In human, PXR is expressed constitutively throughout HSC activation, and rifampicin, a species-specific PXR activator, inhibits HSC activation as well (Haughton et al. 2006).

3.4.9. AR

There is no information so far whether AR is present in HSC or not. However, HSC from rats injected with testosterone-BSA does not show immunocytochemical localization of BSA (Nishimura and Nakano 2000), suggesting that HSC is not the target cell type of AR.

Table 1. Presence of nuclear receptors in HSC and effects of nuclear receptor ligands on HSC activation. See text for references

Ligand	Receptor	Receptor Presence	Effect on HSC activation
		quiescent → activated	
Retinoic acid	RARα	(- → +)[a], +[b]	↓ or ↑
Retinoic acid	RARβ	(- → +)[a], (+ → -)[b]	↓ or ↑
Retinoic acid	RARγ	-[a], +[b]	↓ or ↑
Wy-14,643[e]	PPARα	(+ → -)[b]	↓
L165041[e]	PPARβ	+[a,b]	↑
$15dPGJ_2$	PPARγ	(+ → -)[a,b]	↓
Estrogen	ERα	-[a,b]	n/a[d]
Estrogen	ERβ	+[a,b,c]	↓
Progesterone	PR	+[a,b,c]	↑
Androgen	AR	?	?
Glucocorticoid	GR	+[a,b]	?
Mineralocorticoid	MR	-[b] or +[c]	↑[c]
Vitamin D	VDR	+[a,b]	?
Bile acid	FXR	+[a,b]	↓ or ↑
Pregnenolone	PXR (rodent)	(+ → -)	↓
Rifampicin[e]	PXR (human)	+[a,b]	↓

[a] proved by western blotting or immunocytochemistry or EMSA.
[b] proved by RT-PCR or Northern blotting.
[c] proved by use of receptor antagonist.
[d] not applicable.
[e] synthesized compounds.

3.5. Lipid Droplets and HSC

HSCs store vitamin A as retinyl esters (RE) in their cytoplasmic lipid droplets (LDs) (Wake 1971, 1980a; Kobayashi and Takahashi 1971;

Kobayashi et al. 1973; Yamada et al. 1987; Blomhoff and Wake 1991; Senoo 2004, 2007b; Senoo et al. 2007; Friedman 2008b). Maintaining the homeostasis of vitamin A is important, because retinoic acids, one of vitamin A derivatives, bind with retinoic acid receptors (RARα, β, γ and RXRα, β, γ), which are members of nuclear receptor superfamily, and regulate cell proliferation, differentiation and tissue formation of the whole body including HSCs themselves (Balmer and Blomhoff 2002; Bastien and Rochette-Egly 2004; Blomhoff and Blomhoff 2006; Mezaki et al. 2007).

Two types of vitamin A-containing LDs have been described in HSCs. Type I LDs are membrane-bound (surrounded with unit membrane, namely phospholipid bilayer), whereas type II LDs are not membrane-bound (not surrounded with unit membrane) (Wake 1974, 1975b, 1980a; Yamamoto and Ogawa 1983, 1984; Yamada et al. 1987; Geerts et al. 1990; Blomhoff and Wake 1991; Friedman 2008a). The relation between the two LDs has not yet been elucidated. What kinds of molecules are involved in the formation of them is poorly understood. According to Wake type I LDs are derived from multivesicular bodies (MVBs), which belong to endosome-lysosome system, and type II LDs are derived from type I LDs after losing their surrounding unit membrane (Wake 1974, 1975b, 1980a). Matsuura et al. reported that MVBs are important organelles for retinoid storage as LDs (Matsuura et al. 1993). On the other hand, Yamamoto and Ogawa reported that type I LDs are autophagolysosome of type II LDs (Yamamoto and Ogawa 1983, 1984).

It is helpful to refer to the recent studies of the general LDs, because there are great progresses in this decade on the structure and the molecules involved in the development of them. In general, LDs exist in any kind of cells. Although LDs have long been regarded simply as depots of excess lipids and static organelle, recent studies have revealed that the general LDs harbor a number of functional proteins including signaling proteins, chaperones, cytoskeletal proteins and others. Thus it has been proposed that the LDs are more active organelle to control cellular events than they had been originally thought (Fujimoto and Ohsaki 2006; Fujimoto et al. 2008). It has been revealed that the surface of the general LDs, which have been recognized as lacking the unit membrane structure with transmission electromicroscopy of conventional ultrathin sections, is indeed made of the phospholipid monolayer (Murphy and Vance 1999; Brown 2001; Tauchi-Sato et al. 2002; Fujimoto et al. 2008). Namely, they are composed of a hydrophobic core (e.g., neutral fat and cholesterol esters) and a surface of the phospholipid monolayer. It is speculated that the phospholipid monolayer provides unique platform different from the phospholipid bilayer. The general LDs are assumed to be derived from endoplasmic reticulum (ER), though the mechanism of development is controversial (Blanchette-Mackie et al. 1995; Murphy and Vance 1999; Brown 2001; Robenek et al. 2006; Wolins et al. 2006; Fujimoto et al. 2008). In view of the research about the general LDs, it could be interpreted that the surface of type II LDs, which have no unit membrane, is indeed the phospholipid monolayer just like that of the general LDs. On the other hand, the surface of type I LDs could be the phospholipid monolayer surrounded with the unit membrane. In fact type I LDs have electron-dense three lines of phospholipid head group on the surface (Wake 1974; Yamamoto and Ogawa 1984).

The general LDs in adipocytes and other types of cells harbor PAT proteins, which are named after perilipin, ADRP (adipocyte differentiation-related protein or adipophilin) and TIP47 (tail-interacting protein of 47 kDa) (Greenberg et al. 1991, 1993; Jiang and Serrero 1992; Blanchette-Mackie et al. 1995; Servetnick et al. 1995; Brasaemle et al. 1997; Heid et al. 1998; Lu et al. 2001; Wolins et al. 2001, 2006; Miura et al. 2002). They are the representative proteins and assumed to be involved in the LDs formation from ER. Perilipin is expressed exclusively in adipocytes and steroidogenic cells (Greenberg et al. 1993; Servetnick et al. 1995), whereas ADRP (Brasaemle et al. 1997; Heid et al. 1998) and TIP47 (Wolins et al. 2001; Miura et al. 2002) are expressed in many cell types. PAT proteins are expressed in HSCs in vivo (Straub et al. 2008) and ADRP overexpression induces LDs in cultured HSCs (Fukushima et al. 2005), suggesting that the type II LDs, which would have the phospholipid monolayer on the surface, develop from ER like the general LDs do. Other than HSCs, involvement of PAT proteins on the vitamin A-containing LDs or vitamin A metabolism has been reported. In the retinal pigment epithelium, all-trans-retinol generated by photobleaching induces rapid translocation of TIP47 to the vitamin A-containing LDs (Tsuiki et al. 2007), whereas ADRP localizes constitutively on them (Imanishi et al. 2004, Tsuiki et al. 2007). In keratinocytes, TIP47 might function as a modulator of differentiation because of the inhibitory effect of retinyl ester hydrolases and lipases (Gao and Simon 2006).

Two retinol esterification enzyme activities have been identified, lecithin:retinol acyltransferase (LRAT) and acyl CoA:retinol acyltransferase (ARAT) activity. LRAT utilizes preferentially ROH bound to cellular retinol-binding proteins (CRBP-I in the liver, CRBP-II in the small intestine) as substrate (Ong et al. 1988; MacDonald and Ong 1988), whereas ARAT uses free ROH as substrate (Randolph et al. 1991). The molecular cloning of LRAT revealed it as an integral membrane protein (Ruiz et al. 1999). Although the molecular identity of ARAT has not known, several studies have suggested that diacylglycerol acyltransferase 1 (DGAT1) account for the majority of the activity (Orland et al. 2005; Yen et al. 2005; Yamaguchi et al. 2008). LRAT localizes at MVBs and ER in HSCs (Nagatsuma et al. 2009), and DGAT1 is ER resident protein (Cases et al. 1998). There may be two sources of vitamin A-containing LDs in HSCs. One is that type I LDs develop from MVBs and the other is that type II LDs develop from ER. The selected development course could be correlated with the location where ROH is esterified. There is a possibility that the manners of development are likely correlated with the manners of ROH uptake. It is assumed that there are two ways of ROH uptake in HSCs, endocytosis of ROH-RBP complex (Senoo et al. 1990, 1993) and transport of ROH into cytosol through plasma membrane (Mastuura et al. 1989). ROH-RBP complex taken in by endocytosis is transported to MVBs via endosome (Senoo et al. 1990, 1993). As a result, type I LDs would develop from MVBs (Wake 1974, 1975, 1980). In contrast, ROH passing through plasma membrane would be transported to ER by binding with or without cellular retinol-binding protein I (CRBP-I). Consequently, type II LDs would develop from ER into cytosol like the general LDs develop.

It is well known phenomenon that the activation of HSCs often coincides with decrease of the vitamin A-containing LDs. Administration of RE to the experimental rats of cirrhotic liver suppresses the decrease of RE and hepatic fibrosis (Senoo and Wake 1985). Could the vitamin A-containing LDs control the cellular behavior of HSCs? As mentioned previously, recent studies have revealed that overexpression of PPARγ or administration of the agonists of it induces quiescent phenotype for the activated HSCs (Galli et al. 2000, 2002; Marra et al. 2000; Miyahara et al. 2000). Other than the mechanisms through the direct effect as a transcription factor, the LDs induced might have some functions to control the behavior of HSCs. If it is in the case, the types I and II LDs would have different functions. Containing large amount of retinyl ester in the LDs might have different function from the general LDs. Elucidating whether the vitamin A-containing LDs are involved in the cellular behavior of HSCs would be very important.

3.6. Signal Transduction of HSCs

HSCs are presently regarded as one of the key cell types involved in the progression of liver fibrosis and in the related pathophysiological and clinical complications. Following acute or chronic liver tissue damage, HSCs undergo a process of activation towards a phenotype characterized by increased proliferation, motility, contractility, and synthesis of ECM components as will be mentioned in section 8. Several factors have been shown to play key roles in the promotion of the full-blown picture of activated HSCs. These include extensive changes in the composition and organization of the ECM, the secretion of several growth factors, cytokines, chemokines, products of oxidative stress and other soluble factors. It is evident that each cellular response to extracellular stimuli must be framed in a scenario where different forces modulate one another and result in a prevalent biological effect (Pinzani et al. 1998).

Different groups of soluble factors may be classified according to their prevalent biological effect: (a) factors promoting HSC proliferation and/or migration (i.e., PDGF, basic FGF, insulin-like growth factor-1); (b) factors promoting fibrillar ECM accumulation, particularly TGF-β1; (c) factors with a prevalent contractile effect on HSCs, such as endothelin-1, thrombin, angiotensin-II, and vasopressin, although all these agents also may promote HSC proliferation; (d) proinflammatory cytokines and chemokines; and (e) cytokines with a prominent antiinflammatory/antifibrogenic activity, such as interleukin-10 and interferon-γ. Additional important issues are represented by the relationship between cytokine and integrin signaling, and by the effects of oxidative stress-related molecules on cytokine signaling (Pinzani and Marra 2001). HSCs *in vivo* and in culture extend many cellular processes. Wortmannin, as well as staurosporin and herbimycin A, inhibits the elongation process and induced the retraction of elongated processes. The wortmannin treatment also resulted in an alteration in focal adhesion distribution from the cell processes to cell bodies. Thus, the cellular processes of HSCs are induced through signaling events (Kojima et al. 1998).

3.6.1. Leptin and HSCs

Leptin is a peptide hormone that appears critical in regulating fat metabolism. Circulating leptin levels are reported higher in patients with alcoholic cirrhosis. Leptin expression was not found in freshly isolated quiescent HSCs. Treatment of activated HSCs with either 1 μM retionic acid or 10 μM retinol acetate resulted in the inhibition of leptin mRNA expression. The observation that activated HSCs in culture can express leptin has implications for understanding adipocyte biology in liver disease and treatment of malnutrition in cirrhotics (Potter et al. 1998).

Leptin behaves as a profibrogenic cytokine. In fact, increased fibrosis and greater expression of procollagen type I were observed when leptin was injected into rats receiving CCl_4 or thioacetamide to produce an acute or chronic liver damage, respectively. Remarkably, leptin injection also increased the expression of TGF-β and of αSMA. Ikejima et al. (2002) used Zucker (fa/fa) rats, which are resistant to the biologic actions of leptin as a consequence of a mutation in the functional leptin receptor Ob-Rb, and found a dramatic reduction of the fibrogenic response to thioacetamide intoxication. In fact, when compared with wild-type littermates, Zucker rats had lower levels of procollagen I and TGF-βI mRNA and a markedly reduced expression of αSMA, despite long-standing liver injury. In addition, they identified LSECs and KCs as the main cellular targets of the profibrogenic actions of leptin within the liver. Both these cell types expressed Ob-Rb and, when studied in culture, responded to recombinant leptin with increased expression of TGF-β. Exposure of LSECs to leptin was also associated with increased tyrosine phosphorylation and DNA-binding activity of the transcription factor Stat3, a signaling intermediate of Ob-Rb signaling. These data are of outstanding relevance because they identify a complex paracrine loop involving the actions of leptin, produced by HSC, on other NPCs resulting in TGF-β expression, which in turn stimulates fibrogenesis in HSC. This mechanism may be particularly relevant in those conditions characterized by perisinusoidal fibrosis, such as alcoholic liver disease (Marra 2002).

3.6.2. Prostanoid and HSCs

Prostanoids produced by NPCs modulate the function of PCs and NPCs during homeostasis and inflammation through eight classes of prostanoid receptors coupled to different G-proteins.

HSCs have the highest levels of mRNA for the prostacyclin receptor. The mRNAs for the Gq-linked prostaglandin E2 receptor subtype 1 and the Gi-linked prostaglandin E2 receptor subtype 3 are expressed in PCs and all NPCs at similar high levels, whereas the mRNA of the Gs-linked prostaglandin D2 receptor is expressed in all NPCs at very low levels. The thromboxane receptor and the prostacyclin receptor in LSECs and the prostacyclin receptor in HSCs may be involved in the regulation of sinusoidal blood flow and filtration (Fennekohl et al. 1999)

Recent studies suggest that prostaglandin E may have the ability to suppress cytokine responsiveness. Effects of prostaglandin E administration on several parameters of acute and chronic liver injury induced by bile duct ligation have been examined (Beno et al. 1993). Enisoprost, a prostaglandin E1 analog, was found to suppress early hepatic and HSC type I collagen gene expression without diminishing the induction of TGF-β. Overall liver inflammation and cell proliferation were not altered, suggesting that prostaglandin E acts distal to the initial injurious event(s) (Beno et al. 1993).

Pretreatment with prostaglandin E markedly suppressed the PDGF response in HSCs. The PDGF-induced cascade was studied with or without PGE to determine the level of regulation which induced the observed suppression. PGE caused no apparent diminution in the abundance of the surface PDGFβ receptor nor its subsequent activation and tyrosine phosphorylation following PDGF stimulation. The cytoplasmic 'secondary messengers' mitogen-activated protein kinase pp42–44 and raf kinase, appeared to be comparably induced and therefore unaffected by PGE. Raf perinuclear translocation was also intact and comparable degrees of nuclear egr, fos, and jun expression occurred. Since other studies have suggested that many of these features of the PDGF cascade may be causally and sequentially linked, the data collectively suggests that the dominant PGE mitogenic suppressive effect resides at a raf-MAP parallel pathway or at a nuclear level distal to the induction of these early growth response genes (Beno et al. 1994)

HSCs could be involved in the nervous signal chain; during sympathetic nerve action the neurotransmitter noradrenaline and the cotransmitter ATP cause increases in prostaglandin F2 and prostaglandin D2 release from HSCs within 30 to 60 seconds by way of 1 and p2 receptors, respectively (Athari et al. 1994).

In the perfused rat liver, the anaphylatoxin C5a has been shown to enhance glucose output. In isolated HSCs but not in LSECs, recombinant rat C5a induced a time- and dose-dependent release of thromboxane B2 and prostaglandins D2, E2, and F2a. The rate of prostanoid release was maximal within the first two minutes and then declined again. C5a-induced prostanoid release from HSCs was smaller than that from KCs and it differed in the prostanoid ratios. Hepatocellular glycogen is activated phosphorylase via prostanoid release in cocultures of PCs with HSCs but not with LSECs. Thus, the part of glucose output in the perfused rat liver, which was not abrogated by elimination of the KCs with gadolinium chloride, most likely was mediated by prostanoids released from HSCs (Schieferdecker et al. 1998).

3.6.3. Reactive Oxygen Species (ROS) and HSCs

Following liver injury, HSCs undergo changes toward a myofibroblast-like phenotype and secrete ECM components. In addition, activated HSCs are involved in ECM degradation by providing MMPs. During liver fibrogenesis, a number of MMPs, such as MMP-1, MMP-2, and MMP-13, are expressed in the liver by HSCs. Therefore, it has been suggested that the activation mechanism of HSCs and the secretion of MMPs may contribute to the process of liver fibrosis (Migita et al. 2005).

Evidence of oxidative stress has also been detected in clinical condition of liver fibrosis with different etiology. It has become obvious that an increase in the levels of ROS occurs in the process of liver fibrosis. ROS include superoxide, hydrogen peroxide, hydroxyl radicals, and a variety of reaction products. Several differentially localized and expressed enzymatic systems contribute to ROS formation in the liver, including endothelial NO synthetases, mitochondrial uncoupling, cytochrome P450 monoxygenases (CYP 2E1), and NADPH oxidase. In the normal liver, antioxidant systems such as superoxide dismutase and catalase efficiently remove excess ROS to maintain the normal cell homeostasis. In contrast, during chronic liver diseases, there is increased ROS production, as well as decreased activity of antioxidant systems, resulting in oxidative stress. ROS may represent direct or indirect pro-fibrogenic stimuli for HSCs.

Moreover, signs of oxidative stress and lipid peroxidation are concomitant or precede HSCs activation and collagen deposition. It was demonstrated that HSCs express non-phagocytic NADPH oxidase and inducible NO synthase (iNOS), which generate superoxide and NO, once exposed to effective stimuli. Furthermore, the simultaneous production of NO and superoxide by HSCs or KCs may lead to the generation of peroxynitrite.

To investigate whether HSCs alter their expression of MMPs after exposure to nitrogen oxide intermediate (NOI), a human HSCs, LI90 cells (Murakami et al. 1995), was stimulated with an NO donor, SNAP, or a peroxynitrite donor, SIN-1. Although SIN-1 did not enhance the secretions of MMP-1 and 13, SIN-1 induced the NF-κB activation, MT1-MMP expression, and the secretion of activated MMP-2 in LI90 cells. These results suggest that peroxynitrite may contribute to the remodeling of the ECM in liver by activating pro-MMP-2.

Phagocytosis of apoptotic bodies by HSCs induces procollagen 1 (I) and TGF-β expression *in vitro* have been investigated (Zhan et al. 2006). The downstream effects of phagocytosis was demonstrated by studying NADPH oxidase activation and its link to procollagen 1 (I) and TGF-β1 expression in an immortalized human HSC line and in several models of liver fibrosis. Phagocytosis of apoptotic bodies in LX-1 cells significantly increased superoxide production both in the extracellular and intracellular milieus. Increased intracellular ROS were detected in the cells with intracellular apoptotic bodies, and immunohistochemistry documented translocation of the NADPH oxidase p47phox subunit to the membrane. NADPH oxidase activation resulted in up regulation of procollagen 1 (I); in contrast, TGF-1 expression was independent of NADPH oxidase activation. This was also confirmed by using siRNA to inhibit TGF-1 production. Thus, a mechanistic link between phagocytosis of apoptotic bodies, production of oxidative radicals, and the activation of HSCs has been shown (Zhan et al. 2006).

NADPH oxidase is a multi-protein complex producing ROS both in phagocytic cells, being essential in host defense, and in non-phagocytic cells, regulating intracellular signalling. In the liver, NADPH oxidase plays a central role in fibrogenesis. A functionally active form of the NADPH oxidase is expressed not only in KCs but also in HSCs, suggesting a role of the non-phagocytic NADPH oxidase in HSC activation. Consistent with this concept, profibrogenic agonists such as angiotensin II and PDGF, or apoptotic bodies exert their activity through NADPH oxidase-activation in HSCs. Both pharmacological inhibition with DPI and genetic studies using p47phox knockout mice provided evidence for a central role of NADPH oxidase in the regulation of HSC-activity and liver fibrosis. In addition to the p47phox component, only Rac1 has been identified as a functional active component of the NADPH oxidase complex in HSCs (De Minicis and Brenner 2007). Among the mechanisms mainly involved in mediating the process of liver fibrosis, an important role is played by ROS. It has been proposed that ROS derived from damaged PCs through cytochrome P450 monoxygenases (CYP 2E1) can induce phenotypic activation, proliferation, and increased collagen synthesis in HSCs and thus contribute to liver fibrosis. In particular, ROS produced by CYP 2E1, expressed in PCs, are important in HSCs activation, as assessed by studies in which HSCs were cocultured with HepG2 cells over-expressing cytochrome P450 CYP 2E1. CYP 2E1 may produce diffusible mediators, most likely stable ROS such as H_2O_2 and lipid peroxidation metabolites, which up regulate important matrix-synthesizing genes and consequently play a role in liver injury. NADPH oxidase complex has been recently recognized as a critical mediator of liver fibrosis. Specifically, the phagocytic form of NADPH oxidase expressed in KCs has been proposed to indirectly activate HSCs contributing to liver fibrosis, while the non-phagocytic form of NADPH oxidase complex is directly expressed and functionally active in HSC.

3.6.4. NADPH Oxidase Activity in HSCs and Its Contribution to Fibrosis

Although the best defined activity of ROS is extracellular killing in response to exogenous insults, a more recent view proposes that NADPH oxidase exerts a second and important action in the liver by regulating cell biology. Thus, if high levels of ROS, from phagocytic cells such as KCs mainly protect the organism from external pathogens, a lower amount of ROS, mainly from non-phagocytic cells such as HSCs, actively participates in the regulation of intracellular signalling. This interpretation led researchers to investigate the role of ROS in liver diseases and evaluate the potential role of NADPH oxidase as a mediator of different profibrogenic agonists involved in liver fibrosis. Based on this hypothesis, HSCs were shown to express components of NADPH oxidase. Moreover, the functional activity of this complex in HSCs was also demonstrated. Ang II-induced HSC activation was mediated by NADPH oxidase function, introducing for the first time the new role of non-pahgocytic NADPH oxidase in HSCs. The importance of NADPH oxidase and the role of this molecule complex during liver injury were recently confirmed by microarray analysis in human liver tissues. The gene expression pattern of liver samples obtained from patients with alcoholic hepatitis was characterized by a significant up regulation of several components of the NADPH oxidase and related molecules. These findings clearly demonstrated that NADPH oxidase is involved in the process of liver fibrosis, as stated from *in vivo* study in rodents and in humans as well, and is also significantly associated to human liver diseases such as alcoholic hepatitis.

3.6.5. Chemokine and HSCs

Chemokine interactions with their receptors have been implicated in HSC activation. The hepatic expression of CXCR4 mRNA is increased in hepatitis C cirrhotic livers and plasma levels of its endogenous ligand, stromal cell-derived factor-1 (SDF-1), correlate with increased fibrosis in these patients. Immortalized as well as primary human HSCs express CXCR4, and cell surface receptor expression increases with progressive culture-induced activation (Hong et al. 2009). CXCR4 receptor activation by SDF-1 is profibrogenic through its effects on HSC activation, fibrogenesis, and proliferation. Extracellular signal-regulated kinase 1/2 and phosphoinositide 3-kinase pathways mediate SDF-1-induced effects on HSC expression of collagen I and proliferation. The availability of small molecule inhibitors of CXCR4 make this receptor an appealing target for antifibrotic approaches.

3.7. Production and Degradation of ECM by HSCs, Regulation of HSCs by ECM, and "Activation" of HSCs

3.7.1. Production and Degradation of ECM Components by HSCs

In pathological conditions such as liver cirrhosis, HSCs lose vitamin A, proliferate vigorously, and synthesize and secrete a large amount of ECM components such as collagen, proteoglycan, glycosaminoglycan, and glycoprotein. The structure of the cells also changes from star-shaped HSCs to that of fibroblast-like cells or myofibroblasts (Majno 1979) with well-developed rough-surfaced endoplasmic reticulum and Golgi apparatus (Senoo and Wake 1985; Blomhoff and Wake 1991; Senoo et al. 1997; Sato et al. 2003).

In order to elucidate cell type(s) responsible for collagen metabolism among NPCs in the liver, collagen production by HSCs, KCs, and LSECs was analyzed (Senoo et al. 1984). HSCs were found to produce collagen on day 8 in primary culture, although collagen production was not induced at an earlier stage of culture (day 2). Capability of collagen production by cells was retained in the secondary culture, suggesting that the HSC is a candidate cell responsible for collagen production. KCs and LSECs produced little collagen either on day 2 or day 8 in primary culture under the conditions employed.

Types of collagen produced by HSCs in secondary culture were analyzed by fluorography after SDS-polyacrylamide slab gel electrophoresis under non-reducing and reducing conditions (Fig. 9; Senoo et al. 1984). Type I collagen is the major component synthesized (Fig. 9, lane a). Minor components include type III collagen which remained at the γ-region under non-reducing condition (Fig. 9, lane a), but migrated to the α1-region after reduction (Fig. 9, lane b), and type IV collagen which remained slightly below the origin under non-reducing condition (Fig. 9, lane a), but migrated to α–region slightly lower than the β-region after reduction (Fig. 9, lane b). All these bands were susceptible to purified bacterial collagenase (Fig. 9, lanes c and d). Quantitation of these collagen bands by densitometry indicated that the percentage of type I, type III, and typeIV collagens was 88.2 %, 10.4 %, and 1.4 %, which is consistent with an observation on collagen types in human liver cirrhosis. The dysregulation of collagen gene expression in HSCs is a central pathogenetic step during the development of hepatic fibrosis (Davis et al. 1996). The causes of the dysregulation have been studied by proteome analysis and several candidates such as cytoglobin/STAP or galectin-1 and –3 were reported (Kawada et al. 2001; Maeda et al. 2003).

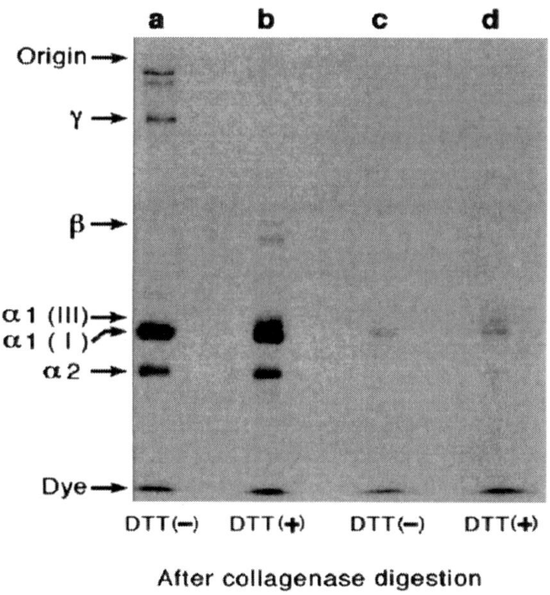

Figure 9. Fluorescence autoradiograms of [^{3}H]proline-labeled proteins. HSCs at confluency in the secondary passage were cultured in a medium containing [^{3}H]proline for 18 hours. Collagenous proteins were partially purified from the cell layer and medium with pepsin digestion after precipitation with ammonium sulfate. SDS-Polyacrylamide slab gel electrophoresis was performed before (a, b) or after (c, d) the treatment with purified bacterial collagenase, and processed for fluorescence autoradiography. b and d: electrophoresed after reduction with dithiothreitol. Arrows indicate the migration positions of carrier rat collagen chains. Senoo H Structure and function of hepatic stellate cells. Med Electron Microsc 2004; 37:3-15.

HSCs have the capacity to produce interstitial collagen types I and Ill as well as other matrix proteins and are involved in hepatic fibrogenesis. TGF responsiveness was evaluated during *in vitro* cell culture, since increasing evidence suggests that this ubiquitous polypeptide can stimulate the production of collagenous proteins in a variety of cell types. TGF induced marked inhibition of HSC proliferation for cells grown on either a type I or a type IV collagen matrix. In marked contrast, the collagen synthetic response was considerably different for cells grown on a type I versus a type IV collagen matrix. When cells were grown on a type I collagen matrix, TGF caused a significant increase in the accumulation of collagen type I and III. When HSCs were grown on a type IV collagen matrix, there was no stimulation of collagen production (Davis 1988; Davis et al. 1987; Davis and Vucic 1988).

Cultured HSCs contain large amounts of type I procollagen mRNA and lesser amounts of types III and IV, whereas freshly isolated cells contained more type IV procollagen mRNA than types I and III. TGF–β1-treated cells had an approximately threefold increase in their type I procollagen mRNA levels, whereas no increase in this mRNA level is found in TNF-α-treated cells. TGF-β1 treatment induces a twofold increase in TGF-β1 mRNA content in cultured cells (Weiner et al. 1990).

Expression of α2(I)collagen in HSCs is regulated by retinoic acid and retinoid X receptors (Wang et al. 2004b).

HSCs are the primary site of matrix glycoconjugate production (Bachem et al. 1989). The synthesis of total sulfated glycosaminoglycans (GAG) is stimulated by TGF α and β in primary cultures of rat HSCs. The combination of both TGFs results in an additively stimulated synthesis of total sulfated GAG, chondroitin sulfate and hyaluronate, respectively. HSCs can also produce proteoglycans (Gressner et al. 1994).

De Minicis et al. (2007) compare gene expression (Weiner et al. 1990) profiles between *in vivo*- and *in vitro*-activated HSCs. For *in vivo* HSC activation, mice underwent bile duct ligation for 2 weeks or received 4 intraperitoneal injections of CCl_4. Before RNA isolation, HSCs were cultured for 20 hours (quiescent HSCs or *in vivo*-activated HSCs) or for 5 days (culture-activated HSCs). The authors observed that bile duct liagation- and CCl_4-activated HSCs displayed an almost identical pattern of up and down regulated genes, whereas gene expression in culture-activated HSCs overlapped only partially with bile duct ligation- and CCl_4-activated HSCs. As noted by the authors, the finding that *in vivo* activation of HSCs regulates a different set of genes than culture activation is not entirely surprising, because others, using similar techniques, although with some methodologic differences, have shown that the current model of HSCs activated in culture does not reproduce exactly the activated HSC phenotype found in cirrhotic human livers (Minicis et al. 2007; Desmoulière 2007).

Relevance of TGFβ1 in Fibrosis

Cytokines of the TGF family influence a wide spectrum of cellular processes including differentiation, proliferation, apoptosis, and migration. In most cells TGF-β1 has anti-proliferative activity and is the most potent single profibrogenic factor known. TGF-β1 participates in initiation and maintenance of fibrogenesis in many organs including the liver. Accordingly, tissue and serum levels of active TGF-β1 are elevated in fibrosis, and overexpression of TGF-β1 in transgenic mice and application of exogenous TGF-β1 can induce organ fibrosis. Furthermore, experimental fibrosis can be inhibited by anti-TGF-β1 treatments, e.g., with neutralizing antibodies or soluble TGFβ receptors. The observed TGF-β1 expression of activated HSC/myofibroblast, the potency of TGF-β1 to up regulate ECM expression, and the expression of TGFβ receptors on HSC has led to a widely accepted model in which persistent auto-/paracrine stimulation of activated HSC/myofibroblast by TGF-β1 is the key fibrogenic response in liver fibrosis. Other cellular sources for TGF-β1 in liver are PCs, LSECs, platelets, and infiltrating mononuclear cells. Since specific inhibition of TGF-β1 seems to be a promising target for an anti-fibrotic therapy, the underlying molecular mechanisms of the profibrogenic effects of TGF-β1 are the focus of intense investigations.

TGF-β1-Induced Signal Transduction

TGF-β1 is synthesized as a precursor (latent TGF-β1) that has to undergo specific proteolysis, e.g., by plasmin, and dissociation from the latency-associated peptide moiety for activation. Our understanding of TGF-β-dependent signal transduction has been revolutionized in the past few years. Binding of active TGF-β1 to the cellular, constitutively phosphorylated TGF-β type II receptor (TGF-βRII) induces formation of heterotetrameric complexes with type I receptors (TGF-βRI). Upon phosphorylation of serine and threonine residues in TGF-βRI by ligand-activated TGF-βRII the thereby activated serine/threonine kinase domain of TGF-βRI phosphorylates the TGF-β-specific signal transducers Smad2 and Smad3. Whereas Smad2 requires presentation to TGF-βRI by the adapter protein Smad anchor for receptor activation (SARA), Smad3 works SARA-independent. Phosphorylated Smad2 and Smad3 dissociate from the (receptor) complex and form heterodimeric complexes with Smad4 or heterotrimeric complexes with Smad3 and Smad4. These complexes translocate into the nucleus where they act as transcriptional modulators on TGF-β responsive gene promoters, e.g., those for plasminogen activator inhibitor 1 (PAI-1), the K2 chain of collagen I, and Smad7. Smad2 seems to be the main signaling molecule for TGF-β1-induced ECM up regulation, since fibroblasts from Smad3 knockout mice still increase their ECM molecule production upon TGF-β1 treatment.

Expression of TGF-βRIII on the cell surface seems to be down regulated during transdifferentiation of HSC to myofibroblast (Bauer and Schuppan 2001). A Smad2 gene inactivation is embryonically lethal. The third TGF-β receptor (TGFβRIII or betaglycan) is a proteoglycan that binds TGF-β1 with high affinity, serving as a non-signaling co-receptor for TGF-βRI and TGF-βRII.

HSCs may enhance the deposition of ECM proteins by inhibiting their degradation (Schwögler et al. 1992). HSCs produce 2-macroglobulin, an important serine protease inhibitor (serpin), and C1-esterase inhibitor, another important serpin. C1-esterase inhibitor gene expression and synthesis are detectable in freshly isolated HSCs and increased distinctly during the time in culture. By inhibition of the N-glycosylation using tunicamycin, rat C1-esterase inhibitor is identified as a glycoprotein. C1-esterase inhibitor synthesis was increased by interferon-γ. Specific messenger RNA levels were also raised distinctly by this cytokine. In contrast, interferon-γ and dexamethasone did not alter C1-esterase inhibitor gene expression. Because C1-esterase inhibitor synthesis is increased by advancing culture time and by the inflammatory mediator interferon-γ.

Undulin and fibronectin are large ECM glycoproteins possibly involved in cell-matrix interactions. Since undulin is involved in the supramolecular organization of fibrillar collagens and in their enzymatic degradation, its acetaldehyde-induced inhibition may contribute to ECM rearrangement in the early stages of alcoholic liver fibrosis (Casini et al. 1994).

Thus, HSCs have been shown to be able to produce ECM components.

Degradation of ECM by HSCs

Matrix metalloproteinases (MMPs) and tissue inhibitor of metalloproteinases (TIMP) have been reported to be synthesized by HSCs and PCs (Montfort et al. 1990; Lindsay and Thorgeirsson 1995; Iredale et al. 1998;

Friedman 2000; Benyon and Arthur 2001; Pinzani and Marra 2001; Arthur 2002; Friedman and Arthur 2002; Poynard et al. 2002). Recent reports indicate that a differential expression of MMP activity, hence the remodeling of ECM components is dependent on the substratum used for the culture of HSCs (Li et al. 1999; Wang et al. 2003). Three-dimensional structure of ECM can regulate reversibly morphology, proliferation, and functions of HSCs (Senoo and Hata 1994a, 1994b; Senoo et al. 1996, 1998). HSCs can take up collagen fibrils by enodocytosis (Mousavi et al. 2005) and phagocytosis (Higashi et al. 2005a).

3.7.2. Reversible Regulation of Morphology, Proliferation, and Function of the HSCs by Three-Dimensional Structure of ECM

Tissues are not composed solely of cells. A substantial part of their volume is intercellular space that is largely filled by an intricate network of macromolecules constituting ECM. This matrix comprises a variety of polysaccharides and proteins that are secreted locally and assembled into an organized meshwork (Alberts et al. 2008). ECM was considered to serve mainly as a relatively inactive scaffolding to stabilize the physical structure of tissues until recently. But now it is clear that ECM plays a far more active complex role in regulating the behavior of the cells that contact; influencing their morphology, development, migration, proliferation, and functions (Hata and Senoo 1992; Senoo and Hata 1993b, 1994b; Senoo et al. 1996).

We reported that HSCs proliferated better and synthesized more collagen on type I collagen-coated culture dishes than on polystyrene dishes (Senoo and Hata 1994a). We also demonstrated that the HSCs formed a mesh-like structure, proliferated slowly, and synthesized a small amount of collagen on Matrigel (Senoo and Hata 1994a), a gel consisting largely of laminin, type IV collagen, heparan sulfate proteoglycan, and nidogen (Kleinman et al. 1986).

Other reports also indicate that ECM can regulate the functions of HSCs. The regulation of the retinol esterification activities, the central process in vitamin A storage, was evaluated in HSCs cultured on type I or type IV collagen-coated dishes in the presence of [^{3}H]retinol (Davis and Vucic 1989). Uptake of [^{3}H] retinol into the cells and esterification into retinyl palmitate was enhanced when the cells were cultured on type IV collagen-coated dishes. The Matrigel was reported to be able to maintain the differentiated phenotype such as storage of lipids in cultured HSCs (Friedman et al. 1989b). Types of collagen synthesized by HSCs were also modulated by ECM (Davis et al. 1987; Friedman et al. 1989a). The cells synthesized mainly type IV collagen on type I collagen-coated culture dishes, and synthesized equal amounts of type I and type IV collagen on type IV collagen-coated dishes. The total amount of collagen synthesized by HSCs was more on type I collagen than on type IV collagen. Thus, these studies support the idea that ECM regulates phenotypes of the HSCs such as collagen metabolism and storage of vitamin A in lipid droplets in the cytoplasm. Responses of the HSCs to cytokines are also modulated by ECM (Davis 1988). When TGF-β was applied to HSCs cultured on type I or type IV collagen-coated culture dishes, collagen synthesis of the cells inoculated on type I collagen-coated dishes was stimulated. On the other hand, there was no response to TGF-β in terms of collagen synthesis by the HSCs inoculated on type IV collagen. Thus, reactions of the HSCs to cytokines are modulated by ECM.

Our studies and other works clearly show that ECM can regulate morphology, proliferation, and functions of HSCs.

We reported recently that morphology, proliferation, and collagen synthesis of the HSCs were reversibly regulated by three-dimensional structure of ECM (Imai and Senoo 1998, 2000; Imai et al. 2000b; Kojima et al. 1998, 1999). The cellular processes of the HSCs were demonstrated to be extended and retracted according to the ECM, and speculated to have important functions in transport and storage of vitamin A and transport of metalloproteinases (Sato et al. 1997, 1998, 1999, 2001b, 2003, 2004). These data also indicate that the HSCs are not static, but dynamic in the changeable three-dimensional structure of ECM in the space between PCs and LSECs.

The dynamic movement of cultured HSCs was analyzed with a video-enhanced optical microscopy (Miura et al. 1997; http://www.med.akita-u.ac.jp/~kaibo2/default.html). When cultured on polystyrene surface, the HSCs spread well, flattened with extensive stress fibers. The cell surface ruffling activity of filopodia and lamellipodia was prominent (Fig. 6), reflecting weak adhesion to the substratum. All filopodia remained dynamic throughout the 4-hour recording, and extended and retracted repeatedly. Within 1 hour after inoculating in or on type I collagen gel, the HSCs began to extend cellular processes, and the cellular processes appeared to adhere to and extend along type I collagen fibers. After repeated extension and retraction of cellular processes, HSCs displayed a number of long cellular processes with distal fine branches by 4-hour culture on type I collagen gel. The cellular processes also extended in or on type III collagen gel, but not in type IV collagen-coated dishes or on Matrigel comprising from the basement membrane components.

The role of microtubule organization in maintenance of the cellular process structure was demonstrated by video-recording of the HSC culture after addition of colchicine (http://www.med.akita-u.ac.jp/~kaibo2 /default.html). In the presence of 1 μM colchicine, once extended cellular processes after overnight culture on type I collagen gel were time-dependently retracted. The effects of colchicine were also dose-dependent at a concentration of 0.1 to 1.0 μM, and almost all cells changed to round shapes within a few hours in the presence of 1 μM colchicine. Virtually no effects were seen after treatment with 1 μM γ-lumicolchicine as a control. The cold-treatment at 4 °C, which is known to induce the degradation of cold-labile form of microtubules, also induced the retraction of elongated cellular processes within 3 hours. The once extended cellular processes were also partly retracted 1 hour after treatment with 4 μg/ml cytochalasin B, as seen after treatment with 0.5 μM colchicine. The effects of cytochalasin B at the concentration of 4 μg/ml appeared to be weaker than that of 1 μM colchicine and a part of cellular processes still remained. However, almost all cells were changed to round shapes after overnight treatment with cytochalasin B.

Fibroblasts were also reported to change the phenotype according to three-dimensional structure of collagen (Cukierman et al. 2001; Grinnell et al. 2003; Kojima et al. 1999), and the integrin α2β1 was demonstrated to recognize three-dimensional structure of triple helical collagen peptide (Emsley et al. 2000).

Stimulation of Proliferation of HSCs and Tissue Formation of the Liver by a Long-Acting Vitamin C Derivative

A long-acting vitamin C derivative, L-ascorbic acid 2-phosphate (Asc 2-P), was found to stimulate cell proliferation, collagen accumulation, and tissue formation (Hata and Senoo 1989; Kurata et al. 1993). On the basis of this discovery, Asc 2-P was added to the medium in which HSCs were cultured (Senoo and Hata 1994a). The cells in the medium supplemented with Asc 2-P stretched better than the cells in the control medium. Asc 2-P stimulated cell proliferation and collagen synthesis of the HSCs, and formation of the liver tissue-like structure in coculture of PCs and fibroblasts (Senoo et al. 1989).

3.7.3. "Activation" of HSCs

Although several cell types in the liver contribute to fibrosis, it is generally accepted that the activated HSC is the source of the excess ECM. In the normal liver, the HSC is in a quiescent state where it is the primary storage site for retinoids. Following liver injury, the HSC undergoes an activation process with changes in cell morphology and gene expression, including increased cell proliferation, expression of new receptors, and synthesis of ECM of which type I collagen predominates (Rippe and Brenner 2004). "Activation" of HSCs to a myofibroblastic phenotype is a key event in liver fibrosis (Friedman 2006). Identification of transcription factors such as Zf9 (Ratziu et al. 1998) with activities that are modulated during HSC activation will improve our understanding of the molecular events controlling HSC activation. Thus, HSC is now well established as the key cellular element involved in the development of hepatic fibrosis and because of this there is considerable interest in establishing the molecular events that trigger and perpetuate HSC activation. Molecular mechanisms of the HSC activation are investigated vigorously as follows.

PDGF, epidermal growth factor (EGF), TGF-α and TGF-β, and basic fibroblast growth factor (bFGF) induced a dose-dependent increase in DNA synthesis of rat HSCs. TGF-β did not affect DNA synthesis of HSC; however, TGF-β markedly potentiated the stimulatory effects of both EGF and PDGF. PDGF is a key mitogen for HSC and that the coordinate release of other growth factors together with PDGF by inflammatory cells represents a potent potential stimulus for HSC proliferation in conditions of chronic self-perpetuating liver inflammation (Pinzani et al. 1989). HSC activation at the level of gene transcription requires the coordinated activity of several key transcriptional regulators of the HSC genome (Mann and Smart 2002).

Candidates of triggering or perpetuating of HSC activation are as follows: phosphatidylinositol 3-kinase (PI 3-K) (Marra et al. 1995), TGF-β1 induced activation of Ras, Raf-1, MEK and MAPK p42 and p44 (Reinmann et al. 1997), ibuprofen (cyclooxygenase-2 inhibitor) (Mallat et al. 1998), activation of NF-κB (Elsharkawy et al. 1999), TNF-α (Hellerbrand et al. 1998; Varela-Rey et al. 2002), TIMP-1 (Bahr et al. 1999), MyoD protein (Vincent et al. 2001), discoidin domain tyrosine kinase receptor 2 (Olaso et al. 2001), Smad 7 (Tahashi et al. 2002), p38 MAPK (Varela-Rey et al. 2002), connective tissue growth factor (CTGF) (Paradis et al. 2002), and FGF9 (Antoine et al. 2007).

A direct interaction between HCV proteins and HSCs may contribute to HCV-induced liver fibrosis (Bataller et al. 2004).

Transcriptional regulation plays a key role in the HSC activation process. Transcription factor myocyte enhancer factor 2 (MEF2) is correlated with HSC activation. MEF2 regulates multiple aspects of HSC activation. MEF2 is a key nuclear mediator that may participate in the pathologic process of liver fibrogenesis *in vivo* (Wang et al. 2004a).

The Forkhead box gene, group O (FoxO) family of Forkhead transcription factors, plays a crucial role in the transdifferentiation and proliferation of HSCs in liver fibrosis. Hyperinsulinemia inactivates FoxO1 in HSCs, resulting in HSC activation and may result in the fibrosis in nonalcoholic fatty liver disease (Adachi et al. 2007).

PC apoptosis and HSC activation are both features of chronic liver diseases. In macrophages, engulfment of apoptotic bodies induces expression of TGF-β. Whether a similar response occurs in HSCs has been examined (Canbay et al. 2003). Fluorescently labeled PC apoptotic bodies were added to cultures of primary and immortalized human HSCs. HSCs, but not PCs, readily engulfed apoptotic bodies in a time-dependent manner as assessed by confocal microscopy. The activation of primary and immortalized human HSCs after incubation with apoptotic bodies, as well as their fibrogenic activity, was indicated by an increase in αSMA (primary cells), TGF-β1, and collagen α1(I) mRNA (primary and immortalized cells). The profibrogenic response was dependent upon apoptotic body engulfment, because nocodazole (a microtubule-inhibiting agent) blocked both the engulfment and the increase of TGF-1 and collagen 1(I) mRNA. As described in primary rodent HSCs, up regulation of collagen 1(I) mRNA was inhibited by a PI-3K inhibitor and a p38 mitogen-activated protein kinase inhibitor in LX-1 cells. These data support a model in which engulfment of PC apoptotic bodies by HSCs leads to a fibrogenic response by eliciting a kinase-signaling pathway (Canbay et al. 2003).

Signals for HSC proliferation are transduced through FAK, PI3K, and Akt. Finally, expression of type I collagen is regulated by the PI3K-Akt signaling pathway (Reif et al. 2003).

In hepatic fibrogenesis, HSCs transform into myofibroblasts, which express αSMA and produce increased amounts of collagen. Morphological and biochemical differences between a population of vitamin A-poor HSCs (VAP-HSCs) from normal rat liver and vitamin A-replete HSCs (VAR-HSCs) have been examined. Both cell types were αSMA-negative; however, in contrast to VAR-HSCs, freshly isolated VAP-HSCs do not contain desmin. Desmin expression is induced in VAP-HSCs on activation. With time in culture, both VAP- and VAR-HSCs express αSMA and produce collagen, indicative of transformation to myofibroblasts. After 7 days, VAR- and VAP-HSCs are indistinguishable in terms of desmin and collagen production. Both populations of cells can be activated to myofibroblasts, the phenotype associated with hepatic fibrogenesis (Ramm et al. 1995). Antagonistic relationship between capability of storage of vitamin A lipid droplets and ability of ECM production in HSCs has been reported (Senoo and Wake 1985; Imai et al. 2000a).

Recently, protease-activated receptor 2 has been reported to promote experimental hepatic fibrosis in mice and activate human HSCs (Knight et al. 2012).

HSCs are responsible for liver fibrosis and are therapeutic targets for treatment of liver cirrhosis. Among the many molecular markers that define "quiescent" or "activated" states of HSCs, the characteristics of type III intermediate filaments are of particular interest. Whereas vimentin and desmin are upregulated in "activated" HSCs, glial fibrillary acidic protein is down regulated in "activated" HSCs. The functional differences between vimentin and desmin are poorly understood. By time-course quantifications of several molecular markers for HSC activation, we observed that the expression of vimentin preceded that of desmin during the transdifferentiation of HSCs. The immunoreactivity of vimentin in transdifferentiated HSCs was more intense in perinuclear regions compared to the immunoreactivity of desmin (Mezaki et al. 2013b, in press). We propose that the delayed expression of desmin following the expression of vimentin and the peripheral localization of desmin compared to vimentin are both related to the more extended phenotype of transdifferentiating HSCs observed *in vitro*.

3.8. STAP/Ctyoglobin Expression in HSCs

Recently proteome analysis (Kristensen et al. 2000; Kawada et al. 2001; Maeda et al. 2003; Nakatani et al. 2004) and gene expression analysis (Jiang et al. 2006; Minicis et al. 2007) have been induced to the study investigating molecular mechanisms of HSC "activation".

Proteome analysis was performed on cellular and secreted proteins of quiescent and activated rat HSCs using 2-dimensional polyacrylamide gel electrophoresis, and 312 polypeptides/proteins were identified (Kawada et al. 2001). The HSCs were activated either *in vitro* by cultivating quiescent HSCs or *in vivo* by injecting CCl_4 to rats. A total of 43 proteins/polypeptides were identified, which altered their expression levels when cells were activated *in vivo* and/or *in vitro*. Twenty-seven of them showed similar changes *in vivo* and *in vitro*, including up regulated proteins such as calcyclin, calgizzarin, and galectin-1 (all of them are growth- and proliferation-associated proteins) as well as down regulated proteins such as liver carboxyesterase 10 and serine protease inhibitor 3. Sixteen of them showed different expression levels between *in vivo* and *in vitro* activated HSCs. Recombinant galectin-1 and galectin-3 stimulated the proliferation of cultured HSCs through the MEK12-ERK1/2 signaling pathway (Maeda et al. 2003).

Using 2-dimensional polyacrylamide gel electrophoresis, a novel protein named STAP (stellate cell activation-associated protein) was reported (Kawada et al. 2001). STAP is a cytoplasmic protein with molecular weight of 21,496 and shows about 40% amino acid sequence homology with myoglobin. STAP is demonstrated to be induced in *in vivo* and *in vitro* activated HSCs. STAP, also called cytoglobin was demonstrated in fibroblast-like cells in splanchnic organs, namely, vitamin A-storing cells, but neither in epithelial cells, endothelial cells, muscle cells, blood cells, macrophages, nor dermal fibroblasts (Nakatani et al. 2004). Roles of STAP in HSCs will be clarified more in the near future.

Using DNA microarray analysis, expression of 31,000 genes was compared among quiescent, activated rat HSCs, and culture-activated rat HSCs (Jiang et al. 2006). Nine hundred genes were up regulated more than 4.6-fold and 500 genes were down regulated more than 5.7-fold in activated HSCs. The up regulated genes included Wnt receptor frizzled 2, ligands Wnt4 and Wnt5, which were confirmed in fibrotic livers. An important role of Wnt signaling in development of liver fibrosis was suggested.

Gene expression was analyzed by DNA microarray and confirmed by polymerase chain reaction and Western blot analysis after HSCs were isolated from normal mice, CCl_4-treated mice, and mice that underwent bile duct ligation (Minicis et al. 2007). Two thousand seventy-three probes sets were differentially expressed in at least 1 of 3 models of HSC activation, icluding novel genes that encode proinflammatory and antiapoptotic mediators; transcription factors; cell surface receptors; and cytoskeleton components. CCl_4- and bile duct ligation-activated HSCs showed highly correlated gene expression patterns, whereas culture activation only partially reproduced the gene expression changes observed during CCl_4- and bile duct ligation-induced activation.

Proteome analysis and gene expression analysis of the activation of HSCs are expected to bring more fruitful results in the future.

3.9. Cell Movement

3.9.1. Cell Migration

HSCs can migrate, contract, and stream. In liver fibrosis, alterations within the space of Disse microenvironment occur and facilitate further progression of chronic liver disease. The normal basement membrane–like matrix presents within the space of Disse converts to a matrix rich in fibril-forming collagens during fibrosis. In Boyden chamber, stimulation of HSCs with PDGF-BB, TGF-β1, and/or EGF resulted in an increase in their migratory capacity and up-regulated MMP-2 activity (Yang et al. 2003). An integrin-dependent, MMP-2–mediated migration of HSCs has been demonstrated. Basement membrane matrix integrity, composition, and cell-matrix interactions play an important role in anchoring HSCs and preventing them from spreading within the space of Disse and potentially elsewhere in the liver (Yang et al. 2003).

Trichostatin A (TSA), a histone deacetylase inhibitor, has been shown to exhibit strong antifibrotic characteristics in HSCs, which are known to play a central role in chronic liver diseases. TSA retains a more quiescent phenotype in spite of culture conditions that favor transdifferentiation into activated HSC. TSA treatment abrogates migration of quiescent HSC. TSA prevents new actin filament formation by down-regulation of two nucleating proteins, actin related protein 2 and 3, and by up regulation of adducin like protein 70 and gelsolin, two capping proteins (Rombouts et al. 2002).

3.9.2. Contractility

In the sinusoid, LSECs and HSCs have been identified as the cellular elements most likely to be important in regulation of resistance, with most data pointing to HSCs. Importantly, these two cells are intimately associated with each other and have paracrine effects on one another. For example, nitric oxide (NO) released by LSECs appears to have relaxing effects on HSCs. HSCs possess extensive long, branching, intersinusoidal, and perisinusoidal cytoplasmic processes and have been shown to contract in situ in the normal sinusoid. HSC contractility has been studied extensively in isolated cell systems and a number of vasoactive substances have been reported to have effects on HSCs. Although controversy exists regarding the magnitude of HSC contraction in the normal liver, available data emphasize that HSCs in the injured liver exhibit increased contractility and moreover, the degree of contraction appears to be proportional to the degree of liver injury. The mechanism for enhanced HSC contractility is coupled to enhanced expression of αSMA and modified signaling pathways after their activation.

A prominent role for HSCs has been suggested in the regulation of intrahepatic resistance. Cellular components of the intrahepatic vasculature (i.e., LSECs, smooth muscle cells, and HSCs) play an important role in vascular responses, as do the specific vasoactive compounds that exert effects on them. A number of vasoactive mediators have received attention, including vasoconstrictors such as endothelin (ET) and angiotensin II, and relaxing agents such as NO and carbon dioxide. Not only are HSCs thought to be an important functional component of the intrahepatic microcirculatory unit, but a large body of literature has emphasized their role in hepatic fibrogenesis. In this regard, a number of vasoactive agents appear to have potent fibrogenic effects on HSCs (Rockey 2003).

The nuclear area of the HSC is frequently located in recesses between PCs while the thin, multiple cytoplasmic processes of these cells course though the perisinusoidal space and extensively embrace the abluminal surfaces of the endothelium surrounding the sinusoid like a cylindrical basket (Wake et al. 1995, 1997, 1998). This close relationship of the processes of the HSC to the sinusoid wall, the presence of large numbers of cytoplasmic microtubules and microfilaments, and the positive immunostaining of desmin in the rat and αSMA, and the close association of nerve fibers coupled with the demonstration of contractile activity in these cells both *in vivo* and *in vitro*, strongly suggests that HSCs play a role in the local regulation of blood flow through the hepatic sinusoids (Pinzani et al. 1992; Kawada et al. 1993a, 1993b; Zhang et al. 1994; Rockey 1995, 2003; Rockey and Weisiger 1996; McCuskey 2008).

HSCs are considered to participate in the regulation of sinusoidal flow. Using a flexible silicone rubber substrate, Kawada et al. (1992, 1993a) have demonstrated that HSCs are able to undergo reversible contraction in primary culture, and the contraction of these cells may be mediated by eicosanoids that can be produced within the liver. Endothelin-1 (ET-1) is a potent stimulus for contraction in the perfused rat liver. On the other hand, extracellular Ca^{2+} and protein kinase C are involved in the signal transduction of ET-1. ET-1 action does not seem to be mediated by endogenous eicosanoids (Tran-Thi et al. 1993). In the normal rat liver, however, quiescent HSC are not involved in the regulation of sinusoidal blood flow in response to ET-1 (Oikawa et al. 2002). HSCs possess ET receptors and contract in response to ETs.

ET-1 and sarafotoxin S6C (a pure ETB receptor agonist) elicited similar contractile responses. The ETB receptor is a prominent mediator of HSC contraction (Rockey 1995). Sarafotoxin S6C has minor effects on portal pressure when perfused into normal livers at concentrations known to elicit HSC contraction. In contrast, both ET-1 and angiotensin II cause a rapid and pronounced rise in portal pressure. The effects of sarafotoxin S6C on portal pressure are greater in cirrhotic than normal liver, whereas those of angiotensin II are unchanged after liver injury. ET-1 and sarafotoxin S6C induced contractility of HSCs increased in proportion to the degree of liver injury. Contractility was greatest for HSCs isolated from cirrhotic livers, a population of cells that displayed the most activated phenotype, as measured by immunoblot of αSMA. Autoradiography of cirrhotic livers after perfusion with ^{125}I-ET-1 revealed binding to cells in both sinusoidal spaces and collagenous fibrotic bands, consistent with known locations of HSCs. The mixed endothelin-A (ETA) and ETB receptor antagonist, bosentan, reduced portal pressure in portal hypertensive animals, consistent with its inhibitory effect on HSC contraction. HSC contractility increases with progressive liver injury and is proportional to the degree of HSC activation, becoming most prominent in the cirrhotic liver. ET-stimulated contraction of HSCs in cirrhotic liver may contribute to increased intrahepatic resistance and portal pressure (Rockey and Weisiger 1996)

HSCs have been reported to contain voltage-operated Ca^{2+} channels. Furthermore, TGF-1 activates or up regulates these Ca^{2+} channels (Oide and Thurman 1994).

The tissue repair response to hypoxic stimuli during wound healing includes enhanced production of angiogenic factors, such as VEGF. HSCs are oxygen-sensing cells, capable of producing VEGF. Hypoxia induces VEGF mRNA in HSCs is dose- and time-dependent (Ankoma-Sey et al. 2000). Hypoxia stimulates cell signaling in HSCs, culminating in the rapid induction of VEGF and Flt-1 mRNA expression and VEGF secretion. The hypoxic induction of VEGF is mimicked by NO and may be of mechanistic importance in the pathogenesis of hepatic wound healing and hepatocarcinogenesis (Ankoma-Sey et al. 2000).

In the situation of hypoxia, the expression of MMP-2 protein was enhanced, while TIMP-2 protein was decreased in HSC and the activity of

MMP-2 declined obviously. HSC is sensitive to the oxygen, hypoxia enhances the expression of MMP-2 and the effect is more marked at the early stage; hyperoxia mainly raises the activity of MMP-2 (Chen et al. 2001)

In diethylnitrosamine (DEN)-treated rats, although the progression of liver fibrosis is associated with PC hypoxia and angiogenesis, VEGF and VEGF receptors, Flt-1 expressions in the liver are increased and correlated with the density of microvessels. *In vitro*, hypoxia induces the expression of VEGF, Flt-1, and type I collagen in activated HSCs. In addition, hypoxia-induced type I collagen expression in HSCs may occur independently of TGF-1 overexpression. Hypoxia may directly contributes to the progression of liver fibrosis (Corpechot et al. 2002).

HSCs possess ET and adrenergic receptors and contract in response to the corresponding agonists. NO inhibits the contraction of HSCs. HSCs thus appear to be involved in the regulation of hepatic sinusoidal microcirculation by contraction and relaxation. In the cirrhotic liver, intralobular innervation is decreased, but ET, ET receptors, and NO are overexpressed in the HSCs. HSCs in cirrhotic liver may play an important role in the sinusoidal microcirculation through agents such as ET or NO rather than through intralobular innervation (Ueno et al. 2004).

Norepinephrine stimulates the secretion of inflammatory chemokines (RANTES and interleukin-8) in a dose-dependent manner. Prazosin blocks norepinephrine-induced chemokine secretion. Norepinephrine stimulated NF-κB activation. BAY 11-7082, a specific NF-κB inhibitor, blocked norepinephrine-induced chemokine secretion. Norepinephrine stimulates NF-κB and induces cell contraction and proinflammatory effects in human HSC. Catecholamines may participate in the pathogenesis of portal hypertension and liver fibrosis by targeting HSC (Sancho-Bru et al. 2006)

The contractile force generated by HSCs in response to ET-1 contributes to sinusoidal blood flow regulation and hepatic fibrosis. Changes in $[Ca^{2+}]_i$ are neither necessary nor sufficient for contractile force generation by rat HSCs (Melton et al. 2006).

3.9.3. Streaming

The liver is proposed as a stem cell and lineage system with many parallels to lineages in the bone marrow, gut, and epidermis, varying from them only in kinetics. All are organized with three compartments: (1) a slow cycling stem cell compartment with cells expressing a fetal phenotype and responding slowly to injury; (2) an amplification compartment with cells of intermediate phenotype rapidly proliferating in response to regenerative stimuli or acute injuries; and (3) a terminal differentiation compartment in which cells increasingly differentiate and gradually lose their ability to divide (Reid et al. 1992; Sigal et al. 1992).

A lineage model involving a maturation process beginning with stem cells and precursors in the periportal zone and ending with senescencing parenchyma near the central vein has been proposed (Arber et al. 1988, 1992; Zajicek et al. 1985, 1988). If this hypothesis is correct, HSCs also stream in the perisinusoidal space.

Chapter 4

Relation with other Cells in the Liver

The hepatic parenchyma consists of PCs (epithelial cells) and NPCs associated with the sinusoids: LSECs, KCs, pit cells, dendritic cells, and HSCs (Fig. 1; Wake 1971, 1980a; Senoo et al. 1997). LSECs (Wisse 1970, 1972; Wanless 1999; Braet et al. 2001) express lymphocyte co-stimulatory molecules (Kojima et al. 2001) and form the greater part of the extremely thin lining of the sinusoids, which are larger than ordinary capillaries and more irregular in shape.

KCs are tissue macrophages and components of the diffuse mononuclear phagocyte system. They are usually situated on the luminal side of endothelium with cellular processes extending between the underlying LSECs. The greater part of their irregular cell surface is exposed to circulating blood in sinusoid. Dendritic cells capture and process antigens, migrate to lymphoid organs and secrete cytokines to initiate immune responses (Steiniger et al. 1984).

The HSCs (Wake 1980a; Senoo et al. 1997; Blomhoff and Wake 1991; Sato et al. 2003; Li and Friedman 2001; Friedman 2008a, 2008b) that lie in the space between LSECs and PCs are considered to be derived from mesenchymal origin. The goal of this chapter is to review and discuss the interaction of HSCs with neighboring cells, namely, LSECs, PCs, KCs, and nervous system.

4.1. Relation with Liver Sinusoidal Endothelial Cells (LSECs)

The hepatic sinusoidal wall is covered by a layer of LSECs which separates the lumen from underlying space of Disse (Wisse 1970, 1972; Wanless 1999). The hepatic sinusoids are unique among microvascular beds in that the endothelial lining lacks an organized basement membrane and possesses fenestrae without diaphragms (Braet et al. 2001). Immunofluorescence and immunohistochemical studies reveal the presence of basement membrane components such as type IV collagen and laminin, while TEM reveals basal lamina as a non-continuous basement membrane, with disruptions occurring under both fenestrated and non-fenestrated regions of the cytoplasm. Fenestrae are grouped into clusters called sieve plates. Mean fenestration diameter in the rat is 150 to 175 nm, occupying 6-8 % of the endothelial surface area (Wanless 1999; Braet et al. 2001). The fenestrae can change in size and number in response to various stimuli; agents that disrupt actin filaments can almost double the number of fenestrae within minutes (Wanless 1999; Braet et al. 2001).

On the basis of morphological and physiological evidence, it was reported that the grouped fenestrae act as a dynamic filter. Fenestrae filter fluids, solutes, and particles that are exchanged between the sinusoidal lumen and the space of Disse, allowing only particles smaller than the fenestrae to reach the PCs or to leave the perisinusoidal space.

Another unique functional characteristic of LSECs is their high endocytic capacity (Wanless 1999; Braet et al. 2001). This function is reflected by the presence of numerous endocytic vesicles and by the effective uptake of a wide variety of substances from the blood by receptor-mediated endocytosis.

Interactions between HSCs and LSECs play an important role in liver homeostasis (Wake 1995, 1998). The close association between these two cell types is similar to that observed with pericytes and endothelial cells in other capillary beds. A very close juxtaposition of LSECs and HSCs indicates a supporting function of the latter (Wisse 1970, 1972). In the normal rat liver, HSCs and LSECs are separated by basement membrane components. It is now clear that ECM plays an active and complex role in regulating the behavior of the cells they contact; influencing morphology, development, migration, proliferation and other functions. In non-mammalian vertebrates, the sinusoidal wall is less well organized, and the HSCs are often found in close contact with thick bundles of collagen fibrils. A similar arrangement has been observed in fibrotic livers (Senoo and Wake 1985). It appears that HSCs and

LSECs have established closer interactions (hence cross talk) during the evolution of vertebrates (Wake 1995, 1998).

Conventionally the perisinusoidal space has been understood as the space between the sinusoids and the PCs, in which the HSCs are present. There is no virtual space between the LSECs and the HSCs; the latter encircle intimately the endothelial tubes in normal mammalian livers. Thus, LSECs and HSCs form an inseparable entity. According to a revised model, the perisinusoidal space is bordered by the LSEC-HSC sheath on one side and PCs on the other (Wake 1995, 1998). Within this limited space are contained nerve fibers and various ECM components such as collagens (type I, III, V, and VI), glycoproteins, and proteoglycans. Interactions of HSCs and LSECs have been reviewed recently by Senoo (Senoo 2007a).

4.2. Relation with Parenchymal Cells or Hepatocytes(PCs)

In coculture of HSCs and PCs, an abubdant ECM deposits over PCs and between PCs and HSCs (Loreal et al. 1993). This matrix contains laminin, fibronectin, and procollagens III and IV. Thus HSCs and PCs interaction induces and promotes deposition of ECM. In this coculture system, functional gap junctions between PCs and HSCs have been demonstrated (Rojkind et al. 1995). PCs in the coculture system are polarized and maintain a cuboidal shape, and have a tendency to form cords.

PCs express nerve growth factor during liver injury and may regulate number of activated HSCs via induction of apoptosis (Oakley etal. 2003). Reversely, HSCs can regulate proliferation of PCs (Uyama et al. 2002). HSCs can stimulate proliferation of PCs through hepatocyte growth factor (HGF), extracellular heparansulfate, and heparansulfate proteoglycan. The cellular contact between PCs and HSCs may disturb the DNA synthesis of PCs via gap junctions.

Both TGF-β added exogeneously to the culture medium, and TGF-β produced endogeneously from HSCs after stimulation by retinoic acid, can suppress the production and secretion of albumin from PCs (Koda et al. 1996). TGF-β generated from HSCs facilitates the development of liver cirrhosis not only by inducing the production of fibrotic components from HSCs, but also by impairing the function of surrounding PCs.

The Stellate Cell Unit, the Stellon

A single HSC sends branching cytoplasmic processes to two, three, and sometimes more neighboring sinusoids. Conversly, a single LSEC receives cytoplasmic processes from one to three HSCs. On the other hand, subendothelial processes of a single HSC appear to make contacts through their spines with 20-40 PCs. The LSEC-HSC-PC (cell to cell to cell) complex may create a cellular unit in the liver tissue (Wake 2006). He calls this unit "the stellate cell unit", or in brief "the stellon". The stellon is not an independent unit, but a loosely overlapping unit with neighboring units.

The intimate association between HSCs and the neighboring cell types through the stellon may facilitate intercellular transport and paracrine stimulation by soluble mediators. When HSCs contract or relax, LSECs are contracted or relaxed. This wavy motion of HSCs is conducted to increased number of LSECs and PCs in a spreading manner. The stellon may be a transducer coupled between the blood stream and the hepatic parenchyma which regulates various functions in the liver (Wake 2006).

4.3. Relation with Kupffer Cells (KCs)

Direct contact between HSCs and KCs is rare in normal anatomical situation. The interaction of HSCs with KCs is important in pathological conditions such as hepatic fibrosis and inflammation.

HSCs exposed to KC culture medium exhibit cellular and nuclear enlargement associated with up to a threefold increase in collagen and total protein synthesis (Friedman and Arthur 1989). On the other hand, conditioned medium of KCs from normal rat liver has been reported to produce in culture two factors that inhibit fibroblast proliferation, but the KC conditioned medium obtained 48 hours after CCl_4 administration to rats stimulates proliferation of cultured HSCs (Armendariz-Borunda 1989).

Lipopolysaccharide stimulation of HSC/KC coculture, but not HSC monoculture, induces HSC death (Fischer et al. 2002). KC-induced HSC killing requires HSC/KC contacts and is prevented by dexamethasone, prostaglandin E2, tumor necrosis factor-related apoptosis-inducing ligand (TRAIL) receptor 2 antagonists, and down regulation of receptor-interacting protein, but not by antioxidants, tumor necrosis factor receptor, or CD95 antagonists. Activated KC can effectively kill HSC by a caspase 9- and receptor-interacting protein dependent mechanism. Thus, the interaction of HSCs with KCs is complicated.

Recently divergent roles of KCs on HSCs have been reported (Duffield 2005). KC function in a reversible model of liver injury in which the injury and recovery phases are distinct. CCl_4-induced liver fibrosis reveals scar-associated macrophages that persisted throughout recovery. A transgenic mouse has been generated in which macrophages could be selectively depleted. Macrophage depletion when liver fibrosis was advanced resulted in reduced scarring and fewer myofibroblasts. Macrophage depletion during recovery led to a failure of matrix degradation. These data indicate that functionally distinct subpopulations of macrophages exist in the same organ and that macrophage play critical roles in both the injury and recovery phases of inflammatory scarring.

4.4. Relation with Other Cells

Nerves and HSCs

HSCs are well innervated. During sympathetic nerve action the neurotransmitter noradrenaline and the cotransmitter ATP cause increases in prostaglandin F2 and prostaglandin D2 release from HSCs within 30 to 60 seconds by way of 1 and p2 receptors, respectively (Athari et al. 1994). The released prostaglandins then activate glycogenolysis in the PCs proper. Sympathetic hepatic nerves reach the liver through nerve bundles that accompany the large vessels in the liver hilus. They follow the vascular ramification until the portal fields. From there they penetrate to different extents into the acinus, where they end with varicosities in the space of Disse close to PCs (Reilly et al. 1978) and HSCs (Bioulac-Sage et al. 1990; reviewed by Püschel 2004).

Emerging evidence suggests that the sympathetic nervous system may play a role in the development of cirrhosis (Oben et al. 2003). Using cultured HSCs, the sympathetic neurotransmitters, norepinephrine and neuropeptide Y, markedly stimulate the proliferation of activated, myofibroblastic, HSCs have been shown (Oben et al. 2003). Norepinephrine, but not neuropeptide Y, also induces collagen gene expression. Physiologically relevant concentrations of sympathetic neurotransmitters directly modulate the phenotype of HSCs. This suggests that targeted interruption of sympathetic nervous system signaling in HSCs may be useful in constraining the fibrogenic response to liver injury (Oben et al. 2003).

The liver is innervated by aminergic, cholinergic, peptidergic, and nitrergic nerves. While innervation of structures in the portal tract is relatively similar between species, the extent and distribution of intralobular innervation are highly variable as well as species-dependent and may be inversely related to the density of gap junctions between contiguous PCs. In most mammals, including humans, these intralobular nerves course from the portal space through the space of Disse in close relationship to HSCs and PCs as well as LSECs and KCs.

Unmyelinated nerve fibres are visible in the human hepatic lobule. They extend through the Disse space, surrounded by Schwann cell processes, often close to perisinusoidal cell processes. A few bare nerve endings or varicosities are found contiguous to either PCs or perisinusoidal cells. These nerve endings or varicosities contain large and small granular vesicles and small clear vesicles. This heterogeneity probably corresponds to the presence of various neurotransmitters (noradrenaline, acetylcholine, various neuropeptides etc.). The effect of nerves on perisinusoidal cells has not yet been elucidated. However, the location, shape, morphology and origin of perisinusoidal cells would suggest that they play a role in the hemodynamic regulation of sinusoidal blood flow. It has recently been shown how important NPC-PC communication is in the action of nerves on glucose release by PCs; the cell to cell communications may also apply to nerves and sinusoidal cells for the hemodynamic regulation of sinusoidal blood flow (Bioulac-Sage et al. 1990).

Chapter 5

Extrahepatic Stellate Cells

Previous studies using fluorescence microscopy, TEM, and electron microscopic autoradiography, showed that cells that stored vitamin A distributed in extrahepatic organs, namely, lung, digestive tract, spleen, adrenal gland, testis, uterus, lymph node, thymus, bone marrow, adventitia of the aorta, lamina propria of the trachea, oral mucosa, urinary bladder, and tonsil (Popper 1941, 1944; Tanaka 1955; Kusumoto and Fujita 1977, Yamamoto et al. 1978; reviewed by Wake, 1980a; Yorifuji et al. 1980; Yamada 1982; Nagy et al. 1997; Matano et al. 1999; Senoo et al. 2013). Morphology of these cells is similar to that of fibroblasts. These cells emanate autofluorescence of vitamin A and contain lipid droplets in the cytoplasm. These cells and HSCs might form the SC system that regulates homeostasis of vitamin A in the whole body. Extrahepatic SCs also can synthesize and secrete ECM components. Pancreatic SCs (Apte et al. 1998; Bachem et al. 1998), one sort of extrahepatic SCs, are now considered to be responsible for the induction of chronic pancreatitis and pancreatic fibrosis. These extrahepatic SCs are now to be targets of the treatment of inflammation and organ fibrosis. Extrahepatic SCs and retinoid-storing cells in the extrahepatic organs will be summarized and discussed in this chapter.

Although HSCs are particularly important for vitamin A storage in many animals, some other cells in organs such as lung, kidney, and intestine of higher vertebrates may accumulate retinyl esters in lipid droplets after ingestion of large amounts of vitamin A (Nagy et al. 1997; Blomhofff and Wake 1991). Such extra-hepatic storage of retinyl esters may even be an important local supply of vitamin A to organs with a huge demand, for example, retinyl ester storage in retinal pigment epithelial cells as a prerequisite for normal visual function.

5.1. Pancreas

In humans, as mentioned above, pancreatic SCs (PSCs), one sort of extrahepatic SCs, are now considered to be responsible for the induction of chronic pancreatitis and pancreatic fibrosis (Apte et al. 1998; Bachem et al. 1998).

In pancreas sections, stellate shaped cells (SCs) are observed; these are positive for desmin and GFAP and negative for αSMA. PSCs have a periacinar and interlobular distribution. They comprise 3.99 % of all pancreatic cells. The PSCs from rat pancreas grow rapidly in culture. PSCs cultured for 24 hours have an angular appearance, contain lipid droplets manifesting positive vitamin A autofluorescence, and stained positively for desmin, but negatively for αSMA. At 48 hours, PSCs are positive for αSMA (Apte et al. 1998). The early primary cultured PSCs contain retinol and retinyl esters. Addition of retinol to the passaged cells results in retinol uptake and esterification (Bachem et al. 1998). During primary culture, PSCs change from a quiescent vitamin A-storing phenotype to a highly synthetic myofibroblast-like cell expressing α-SMA and desmin and biosynthesize collagen type I and III, fibronectin, and laminin. PSCs are now to be targets of the treatment of inflammation and organ fibrosis (Pinzani 1999, 2006; Wells and Crawford 1998).

As mentioned above, PSCs produce collagen and other ECM proteins, and respond to the cytokines PDGF and TGF-β by increased proliferation and increased collagen synthesis (Apte et al. 1999; Haber et al. 1999). TGF-β1 and TNF-α accelerate the change in phenotype from vitamin A-storing to αSMA-positive myofibroblast-like cells (Schneider et al. 2001). PDGF represents the most effective mitogen, and bFGF, TGF-β1, and, to a lesser extent, TGF-α stimulate ECM synthesis of cultured PSCs. PSCs can sythesize and secrete MMPs (Phillips et al. 2003a). However, the role of these cells in ECM protein degradation has not been fully elucidated.

Retinol and its metabolites all-*trans* retinoic acid, and 9-*cis* retinoic acid induce quiescence in culture activated PSCs associated with a significant decrease in the activation of all three classes, namely, extracellular regulated kinases a and 2 (ERK1/2), N-terminal c-Jun kinase (JNK), and p38 kinase, of mitogen activated protein kinases (MAPKs) in PSCs (McCarroll et al. 2006). Ethanol induced PSC activation is prevented by retinol supplementation.

PPAR-γ ligands (15-deoxy-Δ12, 14-prostaglandin J2 (15d-PGJ2) or with troglitazone) inhibited PDGF-induced PSC proliferation (Masamune et al. 2002). This effect is associated with inhibition of cell cycle progression beyond the G1 phase. PPAR-γ ligands decrease αSMA expression and α1(I) procollagen and proryl 4-hydroxhylase(A) mRNA levels. 15d-PGJ2, but not troglitazone, inhibits the degradation of IκB-α and consequent NF-κB activation. Thus PPAR-γ ligands are suggested to be a potential application in the treatment of pancreatic fibrosis and inflammation.

Phagocytosis by PSCs has been reported (Shimizu et al. 2005). PSCs act as resident phagocytic cells, and CD36 promotes troglitazone-induced phagocytic activity via PPASR-γ transactivation. Enhancement of phagocytic activity may provide an important approach to the treatment of pancreatic diseases.

PSCs have the capacity of migration (Phillips et al. 2003b). Activation of PSCs appears to be a prerequisite for migration. PDGF stimulates PSC migration and this effect is predominantly chemotactic. The PI3-kinase pathway is induced in PSCs after exposure to PDGF and this induction is sustained for at least 24 hours. The PI3-kinase pathway plays a role in PDGF-induced PSC migration and is partially involved in mediating ERK1/2 activation (McCarroll et al. 2004). PSC migration is dependent, at least in part, on cell proliferation.

PSCs actively proliferate in pancreatic cancer xenograft tumors and significantly contribute to the local invasive potential of the tumors (Neesse et al. 2007). Presence of PSCs enhances the pro-invasive effects of serine protease inhibitor nexin 2 (SERPINE2) expression and SERPINE 2 influences tumor growth only in the presence of PSCs. Thus, SERPINE2 has been suggested to be an important modulator of tumor/host interactions in pancreatic cancer.

Experimental acute pancreatitis was induced in rats by supramaximal doses of cerulein (Menke et al. 1997). The biological activity of TGF-β1 was inhibited by injections of neutralizing TGF-β1 antibody. TGF-β1 expression in pancreatic cells was suppressed after induction of acute pancreatitis by the application of neutralizing TGF-β1 antibody. Immunochemical analysis showed a clear reduction of ECM formation during the regeneration of the pancreas in antibody-treated animals. The hydroxyproline content and the concentration of collagen types I and III, fibronectin on protein, and mRNA level were significantly reduced in the pancreas of treated animals. These results provide evidence that TGF–β1 is involved in the regulation of ECM remodeling in the rat pancreas during regeneration from acute pancreatitis (Menke et al. 1997).

Expression of dominant-negative Smad2/3 inhibited PSC activation and enhanced their proliferation. TGF-1 differentially regulates PSC activation, proliferation, and TGF-1 mRNA expression through Smad2-, Smad3-, and ERK-dependent pathways, respectively (Ohnishi et al. 2004). Activin A is an autocrine activator of PSCs.

Follistatin can inhibit PSC activation and collagen secretion by blocking autocrined activin A and decreasing TGF-β expression and secretion of PSCs (Ohnishi et al. 2003). PSCs express IL-1 mRNA and secrete IL-1 peptide. Inhibition of TGF-1 activity secreted from PSCs by TGF-1-neutralizing antibody attenuated IL-1 secretion from PSCs. An autocrine loop might exists between TGF-1 and IL-1 in activated PSCs through Smad3- and ERK-dependent pathways (Aoki et al. 2006). Cyclooxygenase-2 (COX-2) was expressed in culture-activated PSCs but not in freshly isolated quiescent PSCs. TGF-1, IL-1, and IL-6 enhanced COX-2 expression in activated PSCs, concomitantly increasing the expression of αSMA, a parameter of PSC activation. The COX-2 inhibitor blocked culture activation of freshly isolated quiescent PSCs, and also inhibited the enhancement of αSMA expression by TGF-1, IL-1, and IL-6 in activated PSCs. Namely, COX-2 is required for the initiation and promotion of PSC activation. IL-1 and IL-6 promote PSC activation by enhancing COX-2 expression indirectly through Smad2/3-dependent pathway by increasing TGF-1 secretion from PSCs (Aoki et al. 2007).

Pancreatic cancer is characterized by excessive desmoplastic reaction and by a hypoxic microenvironment within the solid tumor mass. Chronic pancreatitis is also characterized by fibrosis and hypoxia. Fibroblasts in the area of fibrosis in these pathological settings are now recognized as activated PSCs. Hypoxia induced migration, type I collagen expression, and VEGF production in PSCs. PSCs expressed several angiogenesis-regulating molecules including VEGF receptors, angiopoietin-1, and Tie-2. Namely, hypoxia induced profibrogenic and proangiogenic responses in PSCs. In addition to their established profibrogenic roles, PSCs might play proangiogenic roles during the development of pancreatic fibrosis, where they are subjected to hypoxia (Masamune et al. 2008).

5.2. Kidney

The expression of STAP/cytoglobin (see section 3.8) was recently confirmed in all splanchnic vitamin A-storing cells including HSCs in normal conditions. In the hepatic fibrous lesion, the expression of STAP/cytoglobin has been shown to be in activated HSCs and myofibroblasts, which have synthesized ECM. Furthermore, splanchnic vitamin A-storing cells have been reported to be distributed in the kidney. The contribution of vitamin A-storing cells to renal fibrosis by focusing on STAP/cytoglobin has been studied (Kida et al. 2007). Adult mice were subjected unilateral ureteral obstruction (UUO) and kidneys were harvested. Numbers of STAP/cytoglobin-immuno positive cells as well as STAP/cytoglobin mRNA increased. STAP/cytoglobin and fibulin-2, a specific marker for distinguishing myofibroblasts from activated HSCs, revealed that the number of finbulin+ STAP+ cells (myofibroblasts) and finbulin- STAP+ cells (splanchnic vitamin A-storing cells) significantly increased in kidneys after UUO suggesting that splanchnic vitamin A-storing cells contribute to renal fibrogenesis in the obstructed kidney.

5.3. Lung

Physiologically the most important components of the lung are the thin-walled, terminal saccular compartments, the pulmonary alveoli (Fawcett 1986). The interstitium of the alveolar septa is the tissue between the two layers of pulmonary epithelium lining adjacent alveoli. It includes a very close-meshed network of capillaries, pericytes, septal cells (also called interstitial fibroblasts, interstitial contractile cells, interstitial myofibroblasts, or lipid-containing interstitial cells), mast cells, monocytes, and occasional lymphocytes. The most numerous of the cellular elements of the interstitium are the septal cells. They are considered to be a form of fibroblast and to function in maintenance and repair of the connective tissue of the lung. Actin and myosin have been found in the septal cells and it is speculated that contraction of these cells may decrease alveolar size and decrease capillary perfusion under certain physiological conditions. There is also some experimental evidence that they participate in resynthesis of elastin after enzymatic induction of emphysema.

The septal cells found in the connective tissue space of the alveolar septa are closely applied to the capillary endothelium and to the alveolar epithelium with elongated cell processes, and contain lipid droplets that incorporate ^{3}H-labeled vitamin A (Yamada 1982). CRBP, CRABP, and several isoforms of nuclear retinoic acid receptors are expressed in these cells (Chytil 1992; Redlich et al. 1996; Ross 2004). The septal cells that store vitamin A-lipid droplets in the cytoplasm are the lung stellate cells (LSCs),

The effect of vitamin A on the occurrence of lipid droplets in alveolar LSCs has been studied by light and electron microscopy on the lungs of Syrian golden hamsters fed on diets with a low, normal, or high vitamin A content for a period of 17 weeks (Spit 1983). The feeding of the high vitamin A diet results in a considerable increase in size and number of lipid droplets in LSCs.

The LSCs have lipoprotein lipase activity in the range of 3T3-L1 adipoctes (0.56 vs. 1.72 units/mg DNA) (Maksvytis et al. 1984). The LSCs have the potential of incorporating serum lipoprotein-triglyceride. The LSCs are probably a source of endothelial lipoprotein lipase in the developing lung.

The isolated rat LSCs grown in vitro retain well the overall morphology characteristic of the vitamin A-storing cells found in lung tissues (Okabe et al. 1984). The isolated cells grow well in vitro. The progeny of the cells still contains vitamin A lipid droplets after several transfer generations. Characteristic networks of fibronectin are also demonstrated around the cells. These cells possess fibroblast-like characters storing vitamin A in small lipid droplets.

Ultrastructural features of postnatal alveolar septal formation in rats from birth to 28 days of age have been examined (Vaccaro and Brody 1978). During development of the lung, lipid droplet-containing cells are found. At birth, the rat lung consists of large saccules with thick walls and cellular interstitium. Interstitial cells have large oval nuclei with scant cytoplasm containing few organelles and scattered lipid droplets. These cells appear to be poorly differentiated mesenchymal cells not engaged in active protein synthesis or secretion. Between 5 and 15 days of age, saccule walls are thin and many new alveolar septa form. Two types of interstitial fibroblast-like cells are present: one which appears at the tips of newly formed septa has the characteristics of a myofibroblast and appears to be engaged in synthesis and secretion of elastin; the other fibroblast appears at the base of new septa, is filled with lipid and contains few other cytoplasmic organelles. After 15 days of age, alveolar walls become thinner, few new septa form and interstitial fibroblasts begin to resemble the dormant type of fibroblasts seen at birth. Thus, the process of postnatal alveolarization of lung parenchyma involves differentiation of the interstitial fibroblast and elastogenesis. The lipid droplet-containing cells must be septal cells containing vitamin A.

A septal cell appears in the walls of alveoli during the period of postnatal lung growth associated with the formation of gas exchange surfaces (Maksvytis et al. 1981). This cell has been isolated from the 10-day neonatal rat lung by digesting the lung with trypsin and collagenase and using a 6 per cent metrizamide discontinuous density gradient. $5.0 \pm 0.4 \times 10^6$ septal cell per g of lung wet weight were isolated at 10 days. At this age, triglycerides accounted for 65 per cent of the septal cell lipid with 62 per cent of the triglyceride fatty acids being unsaturated. Linoleic acid is a prominent triglyceride moiety. Density profiles of septal cells isolated from 4-, 7-, 12-, 16-, and 21-day neonatal rats, using metrizamide continuous density gradients, revealed a 2-fold increase in septal cell numbers between 4 and 7 days, after which septal cell numbers decreased linearly until few septal cells were observed at the age of weaning. Mean septal density decreased, but thereafter increased suggesting accumulation and dissipation of cytoplasmic lipid by septal cells during the period of lung growth in which alveoli form. The cultured septal cells synthesize and secrete all-*trans* retinoic acid: its secretion is halved by dexamethasone, an inhibitor of alveolar formation (Dirami et al. 2004). The septal cells are suggested to be a source of retinoids for alveolus formation.

Alveolar interstitial septal cells are immunohistochemically labeled by total actin antibody but not by αSMA antibody (Kapanci et al. 1992). They stain for vimentin and gelsolin and, in rat lungs, most of them for desmin. Cells, identified as pericytes on the basis of their location, are intensely labeled by αSMA antibodies, whereas alveolar septal cells are not. In the lung interstitium pericytes and alveolar septal cells have distinct cytoskeletal features, αSMA antibody staining being a simple method to distinguish between them. Furthermore, it appears that alveolar septal cells have a peculiar pattern of cytoskeletal protein composition which, in the rat, is similar to that previously described for HSCs.

The majority of fibroblasts in alveolar septa are characterized by the presence of cytoplasmic bundles of microfilaments that contain cytoplasmic actin isoforms; these cells have been named contractile interstitial cells or V-type myofibroblasts. In the rat, they express desmin as intermediate filament protein. Experimental pulmonary fibrosis was produced by a unique intratracheal instillation of bleomycin to rats. αSMA appeared in desmin-positive alveolar fibroblasts as early as 24 hours after intratracheal bleomycin instillation; the modulation of αSMA in these cells was preceded by a lymphomonocytic infiltration of alveolar septa. Twenty-four hours to 3 days after bleomycin administration, a proliferation of alveolar myofibroblasts occurred. Fibrosis with laying down of collagen fibers took place after the above mentioned cellular modifications. Thus, septal fibroblastic cells can modulate into typical αSMA-containing myofibroblasts during experimental bleomycin-induced pulmonary fibrosis (Vyalou et al. 1993).

Collagen synthesis of the cultured LSCs is attenuated by bone morphogenetic protein (BMP)-7 and inhibitors of differentiation (Id) 2 (Izumi et al. 2006). Collagen production of cultured human lung fibroblasts is also inhibited by PPARγ agonist (Burgess et al. 2005). The PPARγ agonist has potent antifbrotic effects in human lung fibroblasts and may have potential for fibrotic diseases in the lung and other organs.

Thus, the septal cells that store vitamin A-lipid droplets in the cytoplasm and synthesize and secrete ECM components are the LSCs, one sort of extrahepatic SCs. However, the details of morphology, function, roles in pathogenesis, ontogeny, and phylogeny are unknown and remain to be investigated.

5.4. Intestine

The main sources of vitamin A in the diets are carotenoids (provitamin A) from vegetables and retinyl esters from animal tissues (Blomhoff 1987; Blomhoff and Blomhoff 2006). Vitamin A is absorbed mainly from the intestine (Drummond and Bell 1935; Popper and Volk 1944). Cellular and molecular mechanisms of the absorption of vitamin A and provitamin A by absorptive cells has been extensively investigated (Goodman et al. 1966; Lawrence et al. 1966; Hollander and Muralidhara 1977; Ong 1994).

Recently new information in several aspects of the mechanisms of the intestinal absorption of dietary vitamin A and provitamin A (carotenoids) has been reported (During and Harrison 2007). The new information suggests that (1) retinol enters intestinal absorptive cells by diffusion, (2) retinol efflux is partly facilitated, probably by the basolateral transporter, ATP-binding cassette, subfamily A, member 1 (ABCA1), (3) newly synthesized retinyl esters, but not preformed esters, are incorporated into chylomicron and secreted from the absorptive epithelial cells, and (4) in contrast to retinol transport, carotenoids uptake is mediated by the apical transporter, scavenger receptor class B type 1 (SR-B1), and carotenoid efflux occurs exclusively via their secretion in chylomicron.

Vitamin A is absorbed by absorptive epithelial cells in the intestine and transported to the lymphatic system, and stored as retinyl palmitate in lipid droplets in the cytoplasm in the HSCs. However, the route of the vitamin A to the lymphatics within the villi is still problematic like that of fat (Popper and Volk 1944). When the absorption of vitamin A was observed in the rat by fluorescence microscopy, Popper and Volk found that the cells in the lamina propria mucosae of the intestine emitted autofluorescence of vitamin A, and suggested that vitamin A is carried by mesenchymal cells, leucocytes or histiocytes to the lymphatics. It was also suggested that in those cells vitamin A might be stored for a considerable time. We have speculated that αSMA and desmin positive fibroblastic cells exist in the lamina proproa mucosae of the intestine of rats (Matano et al. 1999). We investigated the morphology and roles of these cells (Senoo et al. 2013). Vitamin A (retinyl palmitate) was injected subcutaneously or administered to rats by tube feeding. After subcutaneous injection, vitamin A was taken up and stored in cells of the lamina propria mucosae of the rat intestine. After oral administration, vitamin A was absorbed by the intestinal absorptive epithelial cells and transferred to cells of the lamina propria mucosae which cells took up and stored the transferred vitamin A. The morphology of these cells was similar to that of HSCs. Thus, these cells in the intestine could take up vitamin A from the systemic circulation and as well as by intestinal absorption, and store the vitamin in the lipid droplets in their cytoplasm. These data suggest that these cells are extrahepatic SCs of the digestive tract and may play roles in both the absorption and homeostasis of vitamin A.

Previously, we reported that retinoid-storing cells exist not only in the liver (HSCs) but other organs in lower vertebrates such as lamprey (*Lampetra japonica*; Wold et al. 2004; Higashi et al. 2005b) and arrowtooth halibut (*Atheresthes evermanni*; Yoshikawa et al. 2006). We also reported that SCs in the liver and other organs stored vitamin A in normal as well as vitamin A-fed rats, and proposed that extrahepatic SCs were playing an important role in vitamin A storage in normal rats (Matano et al. 1999; Nagy et al. 1997). The lamina propria mucosae of the digestive tract contains these retinoid-storing cells (Hirosawa et al. 1988; Matano et al. 1999; Nagy et al. 1997). The intestine of the digestive tract is the main site of absorption of vitamin A, but the role of these retinoid-storing cells of the intestinal in absorption, transport, and storage of vitamin A is not yet fully analyzed. As mentioned above, vitamin A distribution and content in tissues of a primitive vertebrate, lamprey (*Lampetra japonica*) have been reported (Wold et al. 2004; Higashi et al. 2005). HSCs show an abundance of vitamin A stored in lipid droplets in their cytoplasm. Similar cells storing vitamin A are present in the intestine, kidney, gill, and heart in lampreys. The highest level of total vitamin A is found in the intestine. The second and third highest concentrations of vitamin A are found in the liver and the kidney, respectively. These retinoid-storing cells are not epithelial cells, but mesoderm-derived cells.

We have proposed as a hypothesis that these retinoid-storing cells belong to the SC system (family) that stores vitamin A and regulates homeostasis of vitamin A in the whole body in these animals.

As discussed in the section 1.3, we have demonstrated that retinal is the essential form of vitamin A for storage and transport in the adults of the ascidian *Halocynthia roretzi*, and that there was no SC system in the ascidian indicating that the SC system appeared firstly in the lamprey in the phylogeny (Irie et al. 2004).

Other morphological studies on the mesenchymal cells in lamina propria mucosae of the digestive tract were reported (Popper and Volk 1944; reviewed by Wake 1980a; Hirosawa et al. 1988) but the systematic study was not yet performed.

Connective tissue growth factor (CTGF) is a 38-kd protein involved in several human fibrotic disorders including atherosclerosis and skin and renal fibrosis. The role of small intestinal carcinoid tumor-derived fibrotic mediators, TGFβ1 and CTGF, have been investigated in the mediation of fibrosis via activation of an "intestinal" stellate cell (Kidd et al. 2007). Gastrointestinal carcinoid tumors were collected and analyzed for CTGF and TGF-β1. Message levels of both CTGF and TGF-β1 in small intestinal carcinoid tumors were significantly increased versus normal mucosa and gastric (non-fibrotic) carcinoids. Small intestinal carcinoid tumor fibrosis is a CTGF/TGFβ1-mediated stellate cell-driven fibrotic response. The delineation of the biology of fibrosis will facilitate diagnosis and enable development of agents to obviate its local and systemic complications.

Retinoid-storing cells in the intestine of lamprey digest ECM and involved in the atrophy of the intestine in the lamprey during the spawning migration stage (Higashi et al. 2005). Phagocytosis by extrahepatic SCs was also reported in the pancreas (Shimizu et al. 2005).

The SC lipid droplet area in hepatic and extrahepatic SCs in control rats and in rats fed excess vitamin A has been quantified using TEM (Nagy et al. 1997). The SCs were identified by the gold chloride staining technique, specific autofluorescence of retinyl ester, and by electron microscopy. The SC lipid droplet area was then quantitated by the use of morphometric quantitation. Lipid droplet-containing SCs were identified using TEM in liver, lung, kidney, and intestine, in normal as well as vitamin A-fed rats. The area of lipid droplets in liver, lung (Maksvytis et al. 1981), and intestine SCs of normal rats was 0.2, 0.3, and 0.04 mm^2 per cm^2 tissue, respectively. When the rats were administered excess vitamin A, the hepatic, lung, and intestinal SC lipid droplet area increased about 10-fold, 2-fold, and 40-fold, respectively. Thus extrahepatic SCs in lung and intestine of normal rats contain lipid droplets, and that these lipid droplets increase in area when high doses of vitamin A are fed to the animals. These data suggest that not only HSCs but also extrahepatic SCs play an important role in vitamin A storage in normal as well as vitamin A-fed animals (Nagy et al. 1997).

5.5. Vocal Fold SCs

The maculae flavae of the human vocal folds include dense ECM and compacted cells with a stellate morphology (Fuja et al. 2005). These vocal-fold stellate cells (VFSC), are thought to participate in the metabolism of ECM essential in maintaining vocal-fold viscoelasticity required for phonation. Isolated and cultured VFSCs maintain a distinct cellular and biochemical phenotype. Vocal-fold stellate cells undergo culture-induced transdifferentiation to a myofibroblast-like phenotype with an altered phenotype resembling, but not identical to, activated HSCs and PSCs. These cells are capable of responding to exogenous all-*trans* retinol in culture. Exposure to this synthetic co-factor causes deactivation characterized by decreased proliferation, loss of the activated stellate cell marker, αSMA, and restoration of intracellular lipid and vitamin A metabolite storage.

The regulation of ECM consistency is critical in maintaining vocal cord biomechanical viscoelasticity required for phonation. VFSC are thought to play a central role in laryngeal ECM metabolism, aging, scarring, and cancer.

VFSCs maintain an ECM expression pattern similar to laryngeal cancer and scars but distinct from tracheal fibroblasts. Exposure to retinol differentially affects the VFSC expression of ECM components and matrix-regulating enzymes (Fuja et al. 2006).

Chapter 6

Aging and HSCs

A regularly reported finding has been the presence of fat engorged HSCs in old age, including mice, rats, and baboons (Martin et al. 1992; Vollmar et al. 2002b; Cogger et al. 2003; Grizzi et al. 2003; Warren et al. 2005; Ito et al. 2007; Le Couteur et al. 2008). Livers of mice were examined at 0.8 (pre-pubertal), 3 (young adult), 14 (middle-aged), and 27 (senescent) months of age using electron microscopic method (Ito et al. 2007). HSCs at 27 months were shown to contain numerous lipid droplets. Same lipid-engorged HSCs were found extensively in the old mice (Warren et al. 2005). Liver tissue from 5 young baboons (5.4 ± 05 years) and 5 old baboons (21.8 ± 0.7 years) was compared by TEM, SEM, and immunohistochemistry (Cogger et al. 2003). Lipid-engorged HSCs were prominent in the old baboons.

It has also been reported that vitamin A autofluorescence is increased in old age (Vollmar et al. 2002b). They assessed by HPLC, retinol, retinyl oleaote, retinyl palmitate and retinyl starate content of livers in rats of different age (1, 3, 12, and 24 months), and found that the vitamin A content markedly increased during the lifespan of the animals. Vitamin A in the HSCs was demonstrated to increase with age.

Thus, the content of vitamin A in HSCs increases with age, but the molecular mechanisms and biological meanings of this increase are still unknown.

Chapter 7

Roles of HSCs during Liver Regeneration

It is well known that liver cells including PCs and HSCs show a remarkable growth capacity after partial hepatectomy (PHx). Following 70% PHx in rodents, liver mass is almost completely restored after 14 days. PC proliferation starts after ~24 hours, in the areas surrounding portal tracts and proceeds to the pericentral areas by 36-38 hours. As a result of the early PC proliferation, avascular clusters of PCs are observed from 3 days after PHx. NPCs enter DNA synthesis ~24 hours after PCs, with peak activity at 48 hours or later. Not only proliferation of PCs but also activation of sinusoidal liver cells including HSCs are involved in the regeneration process through cell-cell interaction and cytokine networks (Mabuchi et al. 2004; Balabaud 2004). We investigated PCs and HSCs interaction and the HSC activation at different time points after 70% PHx in the rat (Mabuchi et al. 2004). At 3 and 7 days after 70% PHx the hepatic microcirculation was studied using intravital fluorescence microscopy. HSCs and PCs were isolated and liver tissue was processed for histology and immunohistchemistry using anti-desmin antibody and αSMA (a marker of "activated" HSCs) antibody. In the isolated PCs and HSCs, double immunostaining was used to establish the presence of activated HSCs [desmin and bromodeoxyuridine (BrdU); desmin and αSMA].

PC clusters were often seen *in vivo* at 3 days after 70% PHx. The distance between HSCs fell from 61.7±2.1 μm in controls to 36.1±1.4 μm ($p<0.001$) while the HSCs:PCs ratio rose (0.71±0.01 to 1.08±0.03 ($p<0.001$)). In >80% of *in vivo* microscopic fields at 3 days after 70% PHx, clusters of HSCs were observed especially near PC clusters. At 1 and 3 days after PHx, >20% of cells in the PC-enriched fraction were HSCs which adhered to PCs. At 3 days after PHx, in addition to desmin staining, isolated HSCs were also positive for BrdU and αSMA, and formed clusters suggesting that these HSCs were activated. At 3 days after PHx, HSCs in the HSC fraction were only positive for desmin which indicated that adherence to PCs is required for HSC activation. Thus, these data suggest that HSCs are activated by adhering to PCs during the early phase of hepatic regeneration.

As mentioned earlier, under physiological conditions, HSCs within liver lobules store about 50-80% of the total body vitamin A in lipid droplets in their cytoplasm, and these cells show zonal heterogeneity in terms of vitamin A-storing capacity. We have examined the status of vitamin A storage in HSCs in the liver regeneration (Higashi et al. 2005a). Morphometry at the electron microscopic level, fluorescence microscopy for vitamin A autofluorescence, and immunofluorescence microscopy for desmin and αSMA were performed on sections of liver from rats at various times after the animal had been subjected to 70% PHx.

Under the electron microscope the mean area of vitamin A-storing lipid droplets per HSC gradually decreased toward 3 days after PHx, and then returned to normal within 14 days after it. However, the heterogeneity of vitamin A-storing lipid droplet area per HSC within the hepatic lobule (Higashi and Senoo 2003) disappeared after PHx and did not return to normal by 14 days thereafter, even though the liver volume had returned to normal.

These results suggest that HSCs alter their vitamin A-storing capacity during liver regeneration and that the recovery of vitamin A homeostasis requires a much longer time than that for liver volume.

Chapter 8

Hepatic Diseases and HSCs

8.1. Hepatic Fibrosis and Liver Cirrhosis

8.1.1. General Aspects of Fibrosis and Cirrhosis

The overall prevalence of cirrhosis in the United States is estimated at 360 per 100,000 population, or 900,000 total patients, the large majority of whom have chronic viral hepatitis or alcoholic liver disease (Friedman 2003). In Japan, 16,000 patients die per year due to hepatic diseases. Cirrhosis affects hundreds of millions of patients worldwide. In the US, it is the most common non-neoplastic cause of death among hepatobiliary and digestive diseases, accounting for approximately 30,000 deaths per year. In addition 10,000 deaths occur due to liver cancer, the majority of which arise in cirrhotic livers, with the mortality rate steadily rising (Friedman 2003).

The increasing knowledge on the mechanisms responsible for hepatic fibrogenesis together with the introduction of potentially more effective therapeutic strategies for chronic liver diseases have led to the compelling need of acquiring more adequate clinical approaches for the evaluation of the fibrogenic progression of chronic liver diseases.

While millions of patients worldwide are affected by chronic liver diseases potentially leading to cirrhosis, only a minority (25–30%) are likely to develop significant fibrosis and cirrhosis. This is particularly true for hepatitis C virus-related liver cirrhosis, whose prevalence is predicted to peak between the years 2010 and 2015. Regardless, both in the US and Europe, liver cirrhosis is the most common non-neoplastic cause of death among hepatobiliary and digestive diseases. In addition, this condition is largely associated with primary liver cancer, with a further increase in the relative mortality rate.

Liver fibrosis, a wound-healing response to a variety of chronic stimuli including alcohol, persistent viral and helminthic infections, and hereditary metal overload, is characterized by excessive deposition of ECM proteins, of which type I collagen predominates. This alters the structure of the liver leading to organ dysfunction.

Critically re-evaluation of classic standard approaches such as liver biopsy and the search for non-invasive methods for the longitudinal follow-up of the disease are needed. Overall, the situation appears rather confused, prone to significant speculation and the urgent need for clarification and consensus. A similar consideration can be made for the area of the so-called 'anti-fibrogenic' drugs, where in spite of a remarkable number of proposed agents, no drugs have been so far thoroughly tested and approved for use in humans. Progressive accumulation of fibrillar ECM in the liver is the consequence of reiterated liver tissue damage due to infective (mostly hepatitis B- and C-viruses), toxic/drug-induced, metabolic and autoimmune causes and the relative chronic activation of the wound healing reaction. Liver fibrosis results from a dynamic process in which the accumulation of fibrillar ECM is associated with ECM degradation and remodeling in a balanced process that can result in an advanced stage defined as 'cirrhosis' or reversed to restore normal hepatic structure and function. Cirrhosis is characterized by the formation of regenerative nodules of liver parenchyma that are separated by and encapsulated in fibrotic septa and is associated with major angio-architectural changes. In light of these important structural changes, cirrhotic liver tissue can be 'remodeled' in response to removal of the primary cause of damage.

The third American Associated for the Study of Liver Diseases (AASLD)-sponsored Single Topic Conference on Hepatic Fibrosis was held in June 2006. New themes emerged about molecular, clinical, and regulatory aspects of the field, and a consensus emerged that hepatic fibrosis has matured into an integrated discipline that promises to significantly improve the prognosis of patients with fibrosing liver disease (Friedman et al. 2007).

8.1.2. Hepatic Fibrosis and HSCs

The activated HSC is primarily responsible for excess collagen deposition during liver fibrosis. Two important aspects are involved in mediating the fibrogenic response: first the HSC becomes directly fibrogenic by synthesizing ECM proteins; second, the activated HSC proliferates, effectively amplifying the fibrogenic response. Although the precise mechanisms responsible for HSC activation remain elusive, substantial insight is being gained into the molecular mechanisms responsible for ECM production and cell proliferation in the HSC. The activated HSC becomes responsive to both proliferative (PDGF) and fibrogenic (TGF-β) cytokines. It is becoming clear that these cytokines activate both mitogen-activated protein kinase (MAPK) signaling, involving p38, and focal adhesion kinase–phosphatidylinositol 3-kinase–Akt–p70 S6 kinase (FAK-PI3K-Akt-p70S6K) signaling cascades. Together, these regulate the proliferative response, activating cell cycle progression as well as collagen gene expression. In addition, signaling by TGF-β, mediated by Smad proteins, and p38 MAPK influence collagen gene expression. Smad and p38 MAPK signaling have been found to independently and additively regulate α1(I) collagen gene expression by transcriptional activation while p38 MAPK, but not Smad signaling, increases α1(I) collagen mRNA stability, leading to increased synthesis and deposition of type I collagen. It is anticipated that by understanding the molecular mechanisms responsible for HSC proliferation and excess ECM production new therapeutic targets will be identified for the treatment of liver fibrosis (Friedman 1993, 2000; Bauer and Schuppan 2001: Parsons et al. 2007).

The molecular composition of the scar tissue in cirrhosis is similar regardless of etiology and consists of the ECM constituents, collagen types I and III (i.e., 'fibrillar' collagens), sulfated proteoglycans, and adhesive glycoproteins. These scar constituents accumulate from a net increase in their deposition in liver and not simply collapse of existing stroma. Although the cirrhotic bands surrounding nodules are the most easily seen form of scarring, it is actually the early deposition of matrix molecules in the subendothelial space of Disse – so-called 'capillarization' of the sinusoid – that more directly correlates with diminished liver function.

Chronic tissue damage often results in a deregulated wound healing, characterized by an imbalance between ECM synthesis (fibrogenesis) and degradation (fibrolysis), that leads to scar formation. Excessive scarring finally results in architectural distortion and failure of organs such as lungs, kidneys, and liver. HSCs have been identified as an important cellular source of ECM in liver fibrosis. Upon injury (e.g., by toxins or chronic hepatitis) the normally "quiescent" HSC become "activated" and start to proliferate. The "activated" HSC undergo a phenotypic transdifferentiation to contractile myofibroblasts that express αSMA and an excess of ECM molecules.

Activation of HSCs and other resident mesenchymal cells into myofibroblasts expressing αSMA and collagen I is a key event in liver fibrogenesis. Using transgenic animals, heterogeneity of gene expression in myofibroblastic cells during active fibrogenesis has been demonstrated (Magness et al. 2004). The different cell types were distinguished on the basis of their immunophenotypic pattern with a combination of marker antibodies and on the basis of ultrastructural characteristics. Combined staining for αSMA and desmin revealed HSCs as desmin+ αSMA- and myofibroblasts around the central veins of the normal rat liver as desmin+ αSMA+. During the initial phase of CCl_4-induced hepatic fibrosis (week 1 and 2), the number of desmin+ αSMA+ cells (myofibroblasts) increased in the degenerating area around the central veins and desmin+ αSMA+ cells appeared in the very thin fibrotic septa at week 2. These αSMA+ cells proliferated. In degenerating parenchymal areas, desmin+ αSMA- HSC were present. The HSC in the perisinusoidal space of areas which were not affected by CCl_4 intoxification, remained desmin+ αSMA-. HSCs exist in both the degenerating areas and the perisinusoidal space of unaffected areas. After one week of CCl_4-treatment, enhanced deposition of procollagen type III was observed around the central veins. Enhanced deposition of collagen type IV was seen subendothelially along the sinusoids, notably in degenerating parenchymal areas where the septa were later formed. HSCs appear to be the principal source of collagen type IV during fibrogenesis. These observations further support and specify the role of HSCs in early fibrogenesis. With the progression of the CCl_4-induced fibrosis, desmin+ αSMA+ myofibroblasts remained localized in the fibrotic septa, but now along their outer edge. The majority of the cells in the septa was formed by desmin- αSMA- cells indicating a prominent role of fibroblasts in the septal formation. Myofibroblasts and HSC appear to be the main cell types involved in the initial phase of liver fibrogenesis induced by CCl_4. Both myofibroblasts and HSCs divide and transform (Seifert et al. 1994)

Substantial improvements in the treatment of chronic liver disease have accelerated interest in uncovering the mechanisms underlying hepatic fibrosis and its resolution. Activation of resident HSCs into proliferative, contractile, and fibrogenic cells in liver injury remains a dominant theme driving the field.

HSCs and rat liver myofibroblasts display mostly overlapping properties with four striking differences. The complement-activating protease P100 and the protease inhibitor α2-macroglobulin are preferentially expressed by HSCs, whereas interleukin 6–coding mRNAs and the ECM protein fibulin 2 are almost exclusively detectable in rat liver myofibroblasts. Morphologically and functionally different fibroblastic populations, HSCs and rat liver myofibroblasts, can be derived from liver tissue. HSCs may not represent the single matrix-producing cell type of the fibroblast lineage in the liver (Knittel et al. 1999).

Liver myofibroblasts of the portal field and of the pericentral area may also become "activated" by increasing protein synthesis, DNA synthesis, and cell division. They express the fibulin-2 gene and produce large amount of IL-6. In contrast to "activated" HSC they do not undergo spontaneous apoptosis *in vitro* and do not express the CD95-ligand gene. So far no definite prove has been found for a "transdifferentiation" of HSC to myofibroblasts. The conviction that HSC and myofibroblasts represents two similar but not identical cell populations the latter being comparable to those of other organs (Ramadori and Saile 2002).

Progress in understanding the cellular and molecular basis of hepatic fibrosis continues to accelerate, leading to an understanding that is increasingly nuanced. A clear example is the paper of Magness et al. (2004), which explores the topic of HSC heterogeneity using an elegant genetic approach in mice to unearth subtle differences in cellular phenotype and plasticity (Friedman 2004).

8.1.3. Hepatic Fibrosis and Other Cells

Another relevant aspect of the fibrogenic evolution of chronic liver diseases is the topographic distribution of fibrosis and the pattern of fibrotic development. Indeed, although cirrhosis is the common result of progressive fibrogenesis, there are distinct patterns of fibrotic development. These different patterns of fibrogenic evolution are related to different factors and particularly: (1) the topographic localization of tissue damage; (2) the relative concentration of pro-fibrogenic factors; and (3) the prevalent pro-fibrogenic mechanism(s). In addition, these different patterns imply the participation of different cellular effectors of the fibrogenic process. Although most of the knowledge on the cellular mechanisms of fibrogenesis derives from studies performed on HSCs, it is now evident that distinct ECM-producing cells, each with a distinct localization and a characteristic immunohistochemical and/or electron microscopic phenotype, are likely to contribute to liver fibrosis. These include: fibroblasts and myofibroblasts of the portal tract, smooth muscle cells localized in vessel walls, and myofibroblasts localized around the centrolobular vein. It is likely that the relative participation of these different cell types is dependent on the development of distinct patterns of fibrosis. It is likely that all these different ECM-producing cell types undergo a process of activation in conditions of chronic liver damage or, anyhow, in conditions in which the physiological homeostasis of the tissue is chronically perturbed (Pinzani et al. 2005).

Not only HSCs but also other cells are able to produce ECM components for hepatic fibrosis and cirrhosis (Friedman 2008a). Several new areas of rapid progress in the past 5–10 years also have taken root, including: (1) identification of different fibrogenic populations apart from resident HSCs, for example, portal fibroblasts, fibrocytes, and bone-marrow–derived cells, as well as cells derived from epithelial mesenchymal transition; (2) emergence of HSCs as finely regulated determinants of hepatic inflammation and immunity; (3) elucidation of multiple pathways controlling gene expression during HSC activation including transcriptional, post-transcriptional, and epigenetic mechanisms; (4) recognition of disease-specific pathways of fibrogenesis; (5) re-emergence of hepatic macrophages as determinants of matrix degradation in fibrosis resolution and the importance of matrix cross-linking and scar maturation in determining reversibility; and (6) hints that HSCs may contribute to hepatic stem cell behavior, cancer, and regeneration. Clinical and translational implications of these advances have become clear, and have begun to impact significantly on the management and outlook of patients with chronic liver disease.

Fibrotic septae in cirrhotic livers are populated by (myo)fibroblastic cells that lie embedded in large amounts of ECM. Exception made for alcoholic and metabolic liver disease, which in addition are characterized by the deposition of large amounts of ECM between and around PCs or hepatocytes (pericellular fibrosis), one may state that the major matrix-producing cells in fibrosis or cirrhosis are the cells that populate the fibrotic septa. Liver ECM constituents can be synthesized by PCs, bile duct epithelial cells, and LSECs, but the largest contribution to ECM production and therefore fibrogenesis is made by fibroblastic cell populations in the liver. In the last three decades, several fibroblastic cell types have been described in the liver. Typical HSC, transitional cells (intermediate between HSC and myofibroblast), and myofibroblasts have been reported to be present in the perisinusoidal space of Disse. Portal tracts were described to harbour portal (myo)fibroblasts. In addition, periductal (myo)fibroblasts and vascular smooth muscle cells residing in the walls of portal vein branches and portal arteries were considered to constitute distinct subpopulations of mesenchymal cells in the portal tract and it was suggested that these subpopulations would be implicated in for instance 'biliary type fibrosis' in the bile duct-ligation model and the portal/periportal fibrosis characteristic of chronic schistosomiasis, respectively. Another subpopulation of liver fibroblastic cells are the myofibroblasts located around the centrolobular vein: the so-called second-layer cells. These second-layer cells were suggested to proliferate in the livers of alcohol-fed baboons, causing typical 'alcoholic type' pericentral fibrosis. And finally, (myo)fibroblasts residing in the liver capsule (Glisson's capsule) form a potential source of ECM in the liver (Cassiman and Roskams 2002).

Myofibroblasts are absent from normal liver. They are produced by the activation of precursor cells, such as HSCs and portal fibroblasts. The portal fibroblasts are embedded in the portal tract connective tissue around portal structures (vessels and biliary structures). Differences have been reported between these two fibrogenic cell populations, in the mechanisms leading to myofibroblastic differentiation, activation and "deactivation", but confirmation is required. Second-layer cells surrounding centrolobular veins, fibroblasts present in the Glisson capsule surrounding the liver, and vascular smooth muscle cells may also express a myofibroblastic phenotype and may be involved in fibrogenesis. It is now widely accepted that the various types of lesion (e.g., lesions caused by alcohol abuse and viral hepatitis) leading to liver fibrosis involve specific fibrogenic cell subpopulations. The biological and biochemical characterization of these cells is thus essential if we are to understand the mechanisms underlying the progressive development of excessive scarring in the liver. These cells also differ in proliferative and apoptotic capacity, at least *in vitro*. All this information is required for the development of treatments specifically and efficiently targeting the cells responsible for the development of fibrosis/cirrhosis (Guyot et al. 2006).

In advanced fibrosis and in cirrhosis, regardless of cause or species, three distinct mesenchymal (myo)fibroblast-like liver cell subpopulations can be discerned: portal/septal myofibroblasts, interface myofibroblasts, and perisinusoidally located HSCs (Cassiman et al. 2002).

Circulating fibrocytes may be one of the ECM-producing cells in the liver. Long-term culture of adherent, human, and murine leukocyte subpopulations was combined with a variety of immunofluorescence and functional analyses to identify a blood-borne cell type with fibroblast-like properties. A population of circulating cells with fibroblast properties that specifically enter sites of tissue injury has been described (Bucala et al. 1994). This novel cell type, termed a "fibrocyte," was characterized by its distinctive phenotype (collagen+/vimentin+/CD34+), by its rapid entry from blood into subcutaneously implanted wound chambers, and by its presence in connective tissue scars. Thus, blood-borne fibrocytes contribute to scar formation and may play an important role both in normal wound repair and in pathological fibrotic responses. While initially described in the context of wound repair, fibrocytes have since been found to participate in granuloma formation, antigen presentation, and various fibrosing disorders (Quan et al. 2004). Fibrocytes produce matrix proteins such as vimentin, collagens I and III, and they participate in the remodeling response by secreting matrix metalloproteinases. Fibrocytes also are a rich source of inflammatory cytokines, growth factors, and chemokines that provide important intercellular signals within the context of the local tissue environment. Moreover, fibrocytes express the immunological markers typical of an antigen-presenting cell, and they are fully functional for the presentation of antigen to naïve T cells. Fibrocytes can further differentiate, and they may represent a systemic source of the contractile myofibroblast that appears in many fibrotic lesions (Quan et al. 2004).

Myofibroblasts are obviously also producing ECM components such as collagen and fibronectin, and it has become clearer that granulation tissue remodeling depends on the coordinate activities of intracellular and extracellular molecules. The interactions of these molecules are under the control of microenvironmental factors such as TGF-β or other cytokines and mechanical stress (Desmoulière et al. 2003).

The accumulation of ECM observed in fibrosis and cirrhosis is due to the activation of fibroblasts, which acquire a myofibroblastic phenotype. Myofibroblasts, which are absent from normal liver, are produced by the activation of precursor cells such as HSCs. It is generally accepted that activated HSCs are responsible for this ECM accumulation. Numerous observations suggest, however, that different liver fibroblast subpopulations are involved in deposition of the different ECM components or that there are different subpopulations of HSCs. Indeed, it has long been suggested that several subclasses of HSCs are present in the parenchyma.

The animal model of bile duct proliferation and fibrosis after common bile duct ligation has also attracted considerable attention because it simulates many histologic features of human chronic biliary fibrosis and cirrhosis. Few studies have examined the responses of different fibrogenic cells and the cellular origin of the ECM components in this model of fibrosis. It has been suggested that the fibrogenic cells involved are HSCs reaching the portal region by proliferation and migration. Portal fibroblasts are present in portal tracts, however, and they may also play a major role in liver fibrogenesis. TEM of normal rat and human liver has distinctly shown the presence of portal fibroblasts in the connective tissue around vessels and biliary structures, with a typical appearance of quiescent fibroblasts presenting few cytoplasmic processes, and constituting a major reservoir of fibrogenic cells. The involvement of portal fibroblasts around biliary structures in the portal fibrosis induced by bile duct ligation has now been clearly demonstrated, at least for the early stages. These portal fibroblasts acquire a myofibroblastic phenotype and are involved in the early deposition of ECM in the portal zones (Desmoulière 2007).

Activated HSCs, portal fibroblasts, and myofibroblasts of bone marrow origin have been identified as major collagen-producing cells in the injured liver. These cells are activated by fibrogenic cytokines such as TGF-β1, angiotensin II, and leptin (Bataller and Brenner 2005).

8.1.4. PCs and Hepatic Fibrosis

In 1976 PCs or hepatocytes were demonstrated to synthesize collagen for the first time (Sakakibara et al. 1976). Then Hata and his group analyzed collagen biosynthesis by PCs thoroughly (Hata et al. 1978, 1980, Hata and Nagai 1980; Hata and Ninomiya 1984). PCs and HSCs were demonstrated to be able to biosynthesize collagen type XVIII (Musso et al. 1998). The role of PCs in hepatic fibrosis is intriguing.

Epithelial-Mesenchymal Transition

Epithelial to mesenchymal transition (EMT) is a central mechanism for diversifying the cells found in complex tissues. This dynamic process helps organize the formation of the body plan, and while EMT is well studied in the context of embryonic development, it also plays a role in the genesis of fibroblasts during organ fibrosis in adult tissues (Kalluri and Neilson 2003).

The role of adult PCs as contributors to the accumulation of fibroblasts in the fibrotic liver is yet undetermined. Zeiberg et al. (2007) provide evidence that the pro-fibrotic growth factor, TGF-β1, induces adult mouse PCs to undergo phenotypic and functional changes typical of EMT. They perform lineage-tracing experiments using AlbCre; R26RstoplacZ double transgenic mice to demonstrate that PCs which undergo EMT contribute substantially to the population of fibroblast specific protein-1 (FSP1)-positive fibroblasts in CCL_4-induced liver fibrosis. Furthermore, it is demonstrated that bone morphogenic protein-7 (BMP7), a member of the TGF-β superfamily, which is known to antagonize TGF-β signaling, significantly inhibits progression of liver fibrosis in these mice. BMP7 treatment abolishes EMT-derived fibroblasts, suggesting that the therapeutic effect of BMP7 was at least partially due to the inhibition of EMT. These results provide direct evidence for the functional involvement of adult PCs in the accumulation of activated fibroblasts in the fibrotic liver. Furthermore, these findings suggest that EMT is a promising therapeutic target for the attenuation of liver fibrosis.

8.2. Reversal of Liver Cirrhosis

Cirrhosis is associated with significant and life-threatening complications and is a major cause of morbidity and mortality worldwide.

Liver fibrosis and its end stage sequelae cirrhosis represent a major worldwide health problem. By definition progressive fibrosis occurs when the rate of matrix synthesis exceeds matrix degradation. Considerable evidence suggests that the HSC is central to the fibrotic process (see section 8.1). During liver injury these cells transform from a "quiescent" retinoid filled phenotype to a proliferative myofibroblast-like cell. In this "activated" phenotype the HSC is the major source of the interstitial collagens which characterize fibrosis. However, what was previously held as inconceivable – that cirrhosis does not inevitably lead to liver transplantation or death – is now a realistic hope. Mounting clinical and experimental evidence has demonstrated that even advanced fibrosis and cirrhosis are reversible. Reversibility of advanced liver fibrosis in patients has been recently documented, which has stimulated researchers to develop antifibrotic drugs. Emerging antifibrotic therapies are aimed at inhibiting the accumulation of fibrogenic cells and/or preventing the deposition of ECM protein. (Bataller and Brenner 2005).

At present, the only curative treatment for end stage cirrhosis is transplantation, but even in the developed world, the number of donor organs available and the clinical condition of the potential recipient limit the applicability of this technique. The alternative clinical course is one familiar to gastroenterologists that of a progressive damage limitation exercise in which the complications of fibrosis and cirrhosis are treated with greater or lesser success. There is a considerable imperative to develop antifibrotic strategies that are applicable to liver fibrosis. Such an approach is attractive precisely because it is aimed at the final common pathological pathway of chronic liver disease, regardless of etiology. However, because fibrotic liver disease may not present clinically until an advanced or cirrhotic stage, the possibility of reversing the fibrosis is an essential issue for developing therapeutic approaches.

With the advent of effective antiviral therapies, biopsy documented examples of improvements in fibrosis and in some examples resolution, including that of cirrhotic change, are accumulating in the literature. To utilize these observations and establish the attributes required of an effective antifibrotic therapy, we need to understand the nature and origin of the fibrotic ECM, the methods by which the ECM is degraded and the essential processes which occur when fibrosis undergoes recovery with restoration of the normal liver architecture (Benyon and Iredale 2000).

Cirrhosis can be defined as the end stage consequence of fibrosis of the hepatic parenchyma resulting in nodule formation and altered hepatic function. As discussed in section 8.1, a notable omission from this contemporary definition is that cirrhosis is irreversible, since ample evidence now demonstrates that reversal of cirrhosis is often possible. Fibrosis and cirrhosis represent the consequences of a sustained wound healing response to chronic liver injury from a variety of causes including viral, autoimmune, drug induced, cholestatic, and metabolic diseases.

Models of liver fibrosis, which include cell culture models, explanted and biopsied human material, and experimental animal models, have demonstrated that liver fibrosis is a highly dynamic example of solid organ wound healing. Recent work in human and animal models has shown that liver fibrosis is potentially reversible and, in specific circumstances, demonstrates resolution with a restoration of near normal architecture (Iredale 2007).

A model of spontaneous recovery from liver fibrosis has been studied to determine the biological mechanisms mediating resolution. Livers were harvested from rats at 0, 3, 7, and 28 days of spontaneous recovery from liver fibrosis induced by 4 weeks of twice weekly intraperitoneal injections with CCl_4. A rapid decrease in expression of TIMP-1 and TIMP-2, whereas collagenase mRNA expression remained at levels comparable to peak fibrosis. Collagenase activity in liver homogenates increased through recovery. Apoptosis of activated HSC may vitally contribute to resolution of fibrosis by acting as a mechanism for removing the cell population responsible for both producing fibrotic neomatrix and protecting this matrix from degradation via their production of TIMPs.

In the acute phases of liver injury and as liver fibrosis progresses, there is increased expression of matrix MMPs and their TIMPs. Among the changes described, striking features include increased expression of gelatinase A (MMP-2) and membrane type 1-MMP (MT1-MMP; MMP-14) as well as

TIMP-1 and TIMP-2. These molecules and other family members are involved in regulating degradation of both normal and fibrotic liver matrix. MMPs and TIMPs may contribute to the progression and regression of liver fibrosis. The proposal that regression of liver fibrosis is mediated by decreased expression of TIMPs and involves degradation of fibrillar collagens by a combination of MT1-MMP and gelatinase A, in addition to interstitial collagenase, is explored (Arthur 2000).

Liver fibrosis is an important prognostic factor in patients with hepatitis C. The effect of pegylated (PEG) interferon alone or its combination with ribavirin on fibrosis has been examined. PEG-interferon and ribavirin combination significantly reduces the rate of fibrosis progression in patients with hepatitis C (Poynard et al. 2002; Arthur 2002).

Data from clinical and laboratory based research are showing that cirrhosis may be reversible. By highlighting the attributes required of an effective antifibrotic, a new dynamic model is likely to lead to the development of targeted treatment for liver cirrhosis (Iredale 2003b).

8.2.1. HSCs and Reversal of Liver Cirrhosis

The paradigms of HSC activation and apoptosis remain valuable frameworks for understanding pathways of hepatic fibrogenesis and fibrosis regression, respectively. Continued progress is essential in order to identify the determinants and dynamics of fibrosis reversibility, to discover additional targets for anti-fibrotic therapy, and to develop customized multi-drug regimens (Friedman and Bansal 2006).

The “activated” HSC is the pivotal cell type involved in the development of liver fibrosis, simultaneously secreting excessive scar proteins (collagens) and potent inhibitors of collagen degradation – TIMPs. Resolution of fibrosis is characterized by matrix degradation and is associated with HSC apoptosis and the increased activity of MMPs (Iredale et al. 1998; Fallowfield and Iredale 2003; Kisseleva and Brenner 2006, 2007).

The last two decades have witnessed a considerable progress in the understanding of the mechanisms responsible for the fibrogenic progression of chronic liver diseases. However, no drugs are approved as antifibrotic agents in humans. Considering the central role attributed to HSC in liver fibrosis, this cell type has represented and still represents a major focus of antifibrotic research. Indeed, the well-described pathway of HSC activation, subsequent fibrogenesis, with the potential for apoptosis and reversibility, provides a logical framework to define sites of intervention. Consequently, the search for effective antifibrogenic strategies is based on the knowledge gained in the area of HSC biology, including the biology of the factors (growth factors, cytokines, etc.) conditioning their pro-fibrogenic attitude (Pinzani 2004).

Pirfenidone (5 methyl-1-phenyl-2(1H)-pyridone) is a novel anti-fibrotic agent, which has been shown to decrease collagen deposition in a variety of animal models *in vivo*, and recently in hepatic fibrosis also. At cellular level, pirfenidone is able to inhibit proliferation of HSCs induced by PDGF, as well as collagen type I accumulation and $\alpha 1$(I) procollagen mRNA expression. Pirfenidone treatment to rats reduced the degree of liver injury, which was associated with reduced HSC proliferation and collagen deposition. Treatment with dimethylnitrosamine increased transcripts levels for TGF-β1, procollagen $\alpha 1$(I), TIMP-1 and MMP-2 (Sario et al. 2004).

Administration of a TIMP-1 antibody attenuated CCl_4-induced liver fibrosis and decreased HSC activation and MMP-2 activity (Parsons et al. 2004).

A novel molecular mechanism by which hepatocyte growth factor (HGF) counter represses TGF-β-stimulated profibrogenic signal transduction has been proposed (Inagaki et al. 2008). Effects of HGF on TGF-β-responsive gene transcription of type I collagen, the major matrix component of fibrotic liver, were examined by using cultured hepatic HSCs and transgenic mice harboring $\alpha 2$(I) collagen gene (COL1A2) promoter. Over expression of HGF inhibited COL1A2 transcription in cultured HSC and suppressed activation of COL1A2 promoter in liver tissue induced by CCl_4 administration. HGF accelerated nuclear export of Smad3 by enhancing its interaction with galectin-7. Transfection of cells with galectin-7 small interfering RNA inhibited nuclear export of Smad3 and abolished suppressive effect of HGF on expression of TGF-β-responsive genes such as COL1A2 and plasminogen activator inhibitor-1. On the other hand, over expression of galectin-7 suppressed TGF-β-stimulated expression of those target genes. A novel function of intracellular galectin-7 as a transcriptional regulator via its interaction with Smad3 has been demonstrated and a molecular basis has been shown for the antifibrotic effect of HGF.

Several studies have focused on the suppression of TGF-β activation and intervention of the TGF-β/Smad signalling pathways to treat liver fibrosis. However, as generalized blockade of TGF-β activity may result in the promotion of carcinogenesis and excessive immune reactions, much attention has to be paid to selective intervention of the TGF-β/Smad signal specifically in collagen-producing cells in the fibrotic tissue. TGF-β also affects the growth and differentiation of stem and progenitor cells. From this point of view, a new concept of the treatment for liver fibrosis may arise from the discipline of stem cell biology by modulating TGF-β and Smad signalling in stem/progenitor cells (Inagaki and Okazaki 2007). Autologous bone marrow cells contribute to the spontaneous regression of liver fibrosis, and their therapeutic derivation could be a new treatment strategy for intractable liver fibrosis (Higashiyama et al. 2007).

Adiponectin is an adipocyte-derived, antidiabetic, antiatherogenic adipocytokine that is present in serum as three isoforms. Decreased plasma adiponectin levels are closely associated with the severity of nonalcoholic fatty liver diseases. Adiponectin inhibits HSC proliferation via activation of AMPK. AMPK activation by AICAR or metformin inhibits HSC proliferation via suppression of ROS production and subsequent inhibition of AKT pathway. Thus, adiponectin and AMPK inhibit HSC proliferation and hepatic fibrosis via multiple molecular mechanisms (Adachi and Brenner 2008).

8.2.2. Deactivation of HSCs

Molecules that induce activated HSCs into quiescent state are vigorously investigated.

In culture-activated HSCs, interferon-γ (1,000 U/ml) significantly inhibited HSC proliferation. It also markedly reduces expression of αSMA and its messenger RNA. Inhibition of cellular activation is reversible; after interferon-γ withdrawal, mRNA levels of αSMA return to untreated control levels. The effect of interferon-γ extends to ECM gene expression, with reduction of type I collagen, type IV collagen and total fibronectin mRNAs (Rockey et al. 1992).

Cyclosporin A (CsA) is shown to inhibit collagen synthesis in cultured HSCs. CsA reduced DNA without affecting total protein synthesis of cultured HSCs. CsA reduced collagen synthesis in a dose-related manner (Ikeda and Fujiwara 1995).

IFN-α and IFN-γ inhibit proliferation as well as collagen synthesis in human myofibroblastic HSCs (Mallat et al. 1995).

The expression of MMP-2 is increased in a rat model of liver fibrosis. The precursor of MMP-2 (proMMP-2) is also activated. In human liver specimens with chronic hepatitis and liver cirrhosis have been studied the expression of

MT1-MMP, which has recently been determined to activate proMMP-2. MMP-2 expression increased in chronic hepatitis and liver cirrhosis, as compared with normal liver. MT1-MMP gene expression simultaneously increased in chronic hepatitis and liver cirrhosis.

Immunoelectron microscopic examination localized MMP-2 and MT1-MMP to the rough endoplasmic reticulum of HSCs located in the lobules and periportal areas, or to fibroblasts in the fibrous septa, suggesting that MMP-2 and MT1-MMP were produced by these cells. Increased expression of MMP-2 and MT1-MMP was detected in chronic hepatitis and liver cirrhosis, while dual over-expression was found in HSCs and fibroblasts, possibly resulting in the increase of active MMP-2 in and around these cells (Takahara et al. 1997).

HSCs are also a source of matrix degrading MMPs, indicating that, together with other cells, HSC could participate in matrix remodeling (Benyon and Arthur (2001). However, HSC activation in tissue culture models and in vivo is also associated with expression of TIMP-1 and TIMP-2. TIMP expression has also been demonstrated in fibrotic human liver disease and animal models of liver fibrosis. TIMPs 1 and 2 may therefore promote progression of hepatic fibrosis through inhibition of matrix degradation (Iredale 1997).

Endothelin-1 (ET-1), which inhibited the growth of human myofibroblastic HSC, increases the formation of two NF-κB DNA binding complexes; this effect is also observed with TNFα. NF-κB, by inducing COX-2 expression, may play an important role in the negative regulation of human myofibroblastic HSC proliferation (Gallois et al. 1998).

Failure for HSC to sustain IL-10 expression underlies pathologic progression to liver cirrhosis (Wang et al. 1998).

In animal models of fibrosis (CCl_4 plus acetone giving or bile duct ligation), during the early stages of tissue injury, pentoxifylline was able to reduce fibroproliferation and myofibroblastic differentiation and to reduce hepatocellular damage and the inflammatory response, particularly in the toxin-induced model. In culture, αSMA expression decreased in both growing and quiescent HSCs treated with pentoxifylline, indicating that pentoxifylline may also exert a direct effect on hepatic fibrogenic cells (Desmoulière et al. 1999).

Collagen I induces a dose-dependent MMP2 activation in cultured human HSCs, which was not blocked by both actinomycin and cycloheximide. Collagen VI, laminin, and Matrigel were ineffective in inducing activation. Specific antibodies against the subunits of α2β1 integrins, the major collagen I receptor, induced partial inhibition of MMP2 activation. Treatment of cells with concanavalin A resulted in a marked activation of MMP2 that correlated with the proteolytic processing of MT1-MMP. The accumulation of collagen I may specifically contribute to the remodeling of extracellular matrix in fibrotic livers by inducing MMP2 activation (Théret et al. 1999).

In transgenic rats, gene transfer of Smad7 inhibits experimental fibrogenesis *in vivo*. Studies with isolated HSC suggest that the underlying mechanisms involve inhibition of TGF-β signaling and HSC transdifferentiation (Dooley et al. 2003).

In fibroblasts, thrombin induces collagen deposition through activation of a G-protein-coupled receptor, proteinase-activated receptor 1 (PAR1). HSCs express PAR1, as well as proteinase-activated receptors 2 (PAR2) and 4 (PAR4), and that all three PARs were up regulated in response to exposure to growth factor *in vitro*. Exposure to thrombin and to SFLLRN-(SF)-NH2, a PAR1 agonist, and GYPGKF (GY)-NH2, a PAR4 agonist, triggered HSC proliferation and contraction, as well as monocyte chemotactic protein-1 (MCP-1) production and collagen I synthesis and release. These effects were inhibited by the PAR1 antagonist. Administration of this antagonist bile duct ligated rats reduced liver type I collagen mRNA expression and surface collagen, as measured by quantitative morphometric analysis. Similarly, hepatic and urinary excretion of hydroxyproline was reduced significantly by the PAR1 antagonist. PARs regulates HSC activity; development of PAR antagonists might be a feasible therapeutic strategy for protecting against fibrosis in patients with chronic liver diseases. (Fiorucci et al. 2004a).

Administration of 6-ehtyl chenodeoxycholic acid promoted liver fibrosis resolution and increased the apoptosis of NPCs. By demonstrating that a farnesoid X receptor (FXR)-small heterodimer partner (SHP) regulatory cascade promotes the development of a quiescent phenotype and increases apoptosis of HSCs, this study establishes that FXR ligands may be beneficial in treatment of liver fibrosis (Fiorucci et al. 2005a).

The 70-kDa ribosomal S6 kinase is activated by mitogens, growth factors, and hormones in a phosphatidylinositol 3-kinase-dependent manner. 70-kDa ribosomal S6 kinase plays a crucial role in HSC proliferation, collagen expression, and cell cycle control, thus representing a potential therapeutic target for liver fibrosis (Gäbele et al. 2005).

AP-1 DNA-binding complexes are induced during HSC activation and contain Jun D as the predominant Jun family protein. Jun D is therefore an important transcriptional regulator of genes responsive to Jun homo- and heterodimers in activated HSCs (Smart et al. 2001).

Halofuginone, an inhibitor of collagen synthesis, prevented and caused resolution of established hepatic fibrosis. A genomic approach *in vivo* was used to search for additional genes responsible for halofuginone mode of action. Insulin-like growth factor binding protein-1 (IGFBP-1) was one of the 13 genes differentially expressed in the fibrotic liver after halofuginone treatment. After 2 and 4 weeks, halofuginone prevented the TAA-induced down-regulation of IGFBP-1 gene expression. Halofuginone also prevented the TAA-dependent changes in IGFBP-3 gene expression. Halofuginone affected IGFBP-1 synthesis in rat PCs and cells of PC origin and caused time- and dose-dependent increases in the IGFBP-1 gene expression and synthesis by HepG2 cells. The IGFBP-1 secreted by HepG2-inhibited HSC motility. Halofuginone is an anti-fibrotic drug that inhibits collagen synthesis by HSCs and preventing alteration in the synthesis of IGFBPs by liver cells (Gnainsky et al. 2004).

Thus, candidates of HSC-deactivating, therapeutic agents have been reported, but the usefulness of these agents in clinical medicine remains to be proved.

8.2.3. Induction HSCs to Apoptosis

Derangements in apoptosis of liver cells are mechanistically important in the pathogenesis of end-stage liver disease. Vulnerable PCs can undergo apoptosis via an extrinsic, death receptor–mediated pathway, or alternatively intracellular stress can activate the intrinsic pathway of apoptosis. Both pathways converge on mitochondria, and mitochondrial dysfunction is a prerequisite for PC apoptosis. Persistent apoptosis is a feature of chronic liver diseases, and massive apoptosis is a feature of acute liver diseases. Fibrogenesis is stimulated by ongoing PC apoptosis, eventually resulting in cirrhosis of the liver in chronic liver diseases. LSEC apoptosis occurs in ischemia-reperfusion injury. Natural killer and natural killer T cells remove virus-infected PCs.

A key feature of recovery from liver fibrosis is HSC apoptosis, which serves the dual function of removing the major source of neomatrix and TIMPs thereby facilitating matrix degradation. Induction of programmed cell death is a promising approach to eliminate fibrogenic HSC (Janoschek et al. 2004). HSC represent an appealing target for antifibrotic therapy (Kisseleva and Brenner 2006, 2007). Activated HSC apoptosis leads to slowing and resolution of fibrosis (Malhi and Gores 2008).

Apoptosis has emerged as an important mechanism to reduce numbers of activated HSCs during the resolution phase of hepatic fibrosis. These observations suggest that activated HSCs may be more susceptible to apoptotic stimuli than their quiescent counterparts. Because other activated cell types are more sensitive than their quiescent phenotypes to apoptosis by tumor necrosis factor-related apoptosis-inducing ligand (TRAIL). The expression of TRAIL death receptors (DRs) and susceptibility to TRAIL cytotoxicity have been examined in HSCs undergoing progressive activation. A spontaneously immortalized human HSC line, LX-2, was analyzed during 14 days of progressive activation following plating, during which time - αSMA and αBcrystallin (markers of HSC activation) mRNA increased. HSCs show activation-dependent TRAIL-R2/DR5 expression and TRAIL-mediated apoptosis. Because TRAIL-R2/DR5 is not expressed by PCs, TRAIL/DR5 agonists may be useful in reducing fibrosis by inducing HSC apoptosis (Taimr et al. 2003).

NGF is expressed during fibrotic liver injury and may regulate number of activated HSCs via induction of apoptosis (Oakley et al. 2003).

Resolution of liver fibrosis is associated with clearance of hepatic myofibroblasts by apoptosis. An inhibitor of κB kinase suppresser sulfasalazine stimulates hepatic myofibroblast apoptosis and recovery from fibrosis. Inhibition of the inhibitor of κB kinase/nuclear factor-κB pathway is sufficient to increase the rate at which activated HSCs undergo apoptosis both *in vitro* and *in vivo*, and drugs that selectively target inhibitor of κB kinase have potential as antifibrotics (Oakley et al. 2005).

Proteasome inhibitors induce apoptosis in transformed cells, especially those cells dependent upon NF-κB activation. The immortalized human HSC line, LX-2, and primary rat HSCs were treated with the proteasome inhibitors. These proteasome inhibitors induce HSC apoptosis. Proteasome inhibition is a potential therapeutic strategy for inducing HSC apoptosis and inhibiting liver fibrogenesis (Anan et al. 2006)

Compared with HSCs plated on normal collagen I, those plated on a collagenase-resistant form of collagen I (r/r collagen) had reduced thymidine incorporation and proliferating cell nuclear antigen expression but increased p21 expression. Collagen I was shown to be rendered resistant to MMPs by artificial cross-linking *in vitro* using tissue transglutaminase exerted similar antiproliferative effects on HSCs to r/r collagen. Proliferation of HSCs is promoted by pericellular collagen I proteolysis acting via v3 integrin. Cross-linking of collagen I by tissue transglutaminase, a process known to occur in chronic liver fibrosis, might not only increase its resistance to MMPs thereby inhibiting resolution of fibrosis but also functions to constrain the fibroproliferative process (Zhou et al. 2006).

Apoptosis of HSC is promoted by active MMP-2 via the cleavage of N-cadherin (Hartland et al. 2009).

Hammel et al. (2001) describe a group of patients with liver fibrosis who underwent surgical decompression of an obstructed biliary system. Liver-biopsy specimens obtained before and after surgery were compared. In some patients, the liver fibrosis significantly regressed after decompression. The implication of this study is that the fibrosis caused by biliary obstruction is reversible in some instances (Bonis et al. 2001). To test the hypothesis that HSC apoptosis is critical to recovery from biliary fibrosis and that soluble growth factors may regulate HSC survival and apoptosis. Rats (n=15) were subjected to bile duct ligation for 21 days, after which biliodigestive anastomosis was undertaken (n=13). Livers were harvested at fixed time points of recovery for periods of up to 42 days. Following biliodigestive anastomosis after 21 days of bile duct ligation, rat liver demonstrated a progressive resolution of biliary fibrosis over 42 days, associated with a fivefold decrease in activated HSC determined by αSMA staining. TUNEL staining indicated that loss of activated HSC resulted from an increase in the rate of apoptosis during the first two days post biliodigestive anastomosis. Serum deprivation and culture in the presence of cycloheximide was associated with an increase in HSC apoptosis which was significantly inhibited by addition of IGF-1, respectively ($0.05>p$, n=5). In contrast, TGF-1 caused a significant increase in HSC apoptosis compared with serum free controls. PDGF and IGF-2 were neutral with respect to their effect on HSC apoptosis. HSC apoptosis plays a critical role in the spontaneous recovery from biliary fibrosis. Both survival and apoptosis of HSC are regulated by growth factors expressed during fibrotic liver injury (Issa et al. 2001).

Vitamin A–coupled liposomes was used to deliver small interfering RNA (siRNA) against gp46, the rat homolog of human heat shock protein 47, to HSCs (Sato et al. 2008). Five treatments with the siRNA-bearing vitamin A–coupled liposomes almost completely resolved liver fibrosis and prolonged survival in rats with otherwise lethal dimethylnitrosamine-induced liver cirrhosis in a dose- and duration-dependent manner. Receptor-specific siRNA delivery was similarly effective in suppressing collagen secretion and treating fibrosis induced by CCl_4 or bile duct ligation. The efficacy of the approach using both acute and chronic models of liver fibrosis suggests its therapeutic potential for reversing human liver cirrhosis. However, the effectiveness of this method in clinical medicine remains to be testified.

8.3. Alcohol and HSCs

Alcohol and HSCs is the commonest cause of cirrhosis in the Western world, currently one of the ten most common causes of death (Stewart and Day 2003). Deaths from cirrhosis rose with per capita alcohol consumption from the 1950s to the 1970s in many Western countries, but have since declined out of proportion to the minor decrease in intake. While this may be partly explained by changes in the age and ethnic background of these populations, it also seems likely to reflect advances in the management of patients with both alcohol and non-alcohol-related advanced liver disease. Clearly, any improvement in the management of the general complications of liver disease will have a beneficial effect on the management of patients with advanced ALD.

Acetaldehyde, the first metabolite of ethanol, can upregulate transcription of collagen I directly as well as indirectly by upregulating the synthesis of TGF-β1. Reactive oxygen species (ROS) generated in PCs or hepatocytes by alcohol metabolism can activate collagen production in HSCs in a paracrine manner. Alcohol-induced PC apoptotic bodies can be phagocytosed by HSCs and KCs and result in increased expression of TGF–β1 and subsequent HSC activation. KCs may contribute to the activation of HSCs by releasing ROS and TGF-β1. Innate immunity may suppress hepatic fibrosis by killing activated HSCs and blocking TGF-β1 signaling. In patients infected with hepatitis C virus (HCV), alcohol may promote hepatic fibrosis by suppressing innate immunity. HCV core and non-structural proteins contribute to HCV-induced hepatic fibrosis. Alcohol and HCV together may promote hepatic fibrosis through increased oxidative stress and upregulation of fibrogenic cytokines. The inactive aldehyde dehydrogenase (ALDH2) and the super-active alcohol dehydrogenase (ADH2) alleles may promote hepatic fibrosis through increased accumulation of acetaldehyde in the liver. Hepatic fibrosis can be reversed by inducing selective apoptosis or necrosis of activated HSCs, or by reverse trans-differentiation of activated HSCs into the quiescent phenotype (Purohit and Brenner 2006).

The ability of the HSCs to oxidize ethanol and the inhibitory effect of ethanol on retinol oxidation may be important in the pathogenesis of alcoholic liver disease (Yamauchi et al. 1988). The formation of acetaldehyde adducts with the carboxyl-terminal propeptide of procollagen may account, at least in part, for the stimulatory effect of acetaldehyde on collagen synthesis by HSCs and may lead to collagen accumulation through a decrease of the normal feedback regulation of collagen synthesis by the propeptide (Ma et al. 1997).

Ethanol and arachidonic acid (AA) are able to be inducers of oxidative stress and key factors in alcoholic liver disease. A time- and dose-dependent induction in COL1A2 mRNA by ethanol or AA in HSCs was observed that was prevented by diallylsulfide, an ethanol-inducible cytochrome P-4502E1 (CYP2E1) inhibitor (Nieto et al. 2000). CYP2E1 activates cyclooxygenase-2 (COX-2) expression, and the oxidation of AA by COX-2 is responsible for the increase in COL1A2. CYP2E1-dependent oxidative stress to induction of COX-2 and the actions of ethanol and AA on activation of collagen gene expression in HSCs have been liked.

Deficiencies in zinc and vitamin A may play a role in the night blindness and hypogonadism of some chronic alcoholics; abstinence and zinc and vitamin A therapy may be of some benefit in these processes (McClain et al. 2008).

Alcohol-induced fatty liver, a major cause of morbidity, has been attributed to enhanced hepatic lipogenesis and decreased fat clearance of unknown mechanism. The steatosis induced in mice by a low-fat, liquid ethanol diet is attenuated by concurrent blockade of cannabinoid CB1 receptors. Global or PC-specific CB1 knockout mice are resistant to ethanol-induced steatosis and increases in lipogenic gene expression and have increased carnitine palmitoyltransferase 1 activity, which, unlike in controls, is not reduced by ethanol treatment. Ethanol feeding increases the hepatic expression of CB1 receptors and upregulates the endocannabinoid 2-arachidonoylglycerol (2-AG) and its biosynthetic enzyme diacylglycerol lipase b selectively in HSCs. In control but not CB1 receptor-deficient PCs, coculture with HSCs from ethanol-fed mice results in upregulation of CB1 receptors and lipogenic gene expression. The paracrine activation of hepatic CB1 receptors by HSC-derived 2-AG mediates ethanol-induced steatosis through increasing lipogenesis and decreasing fatty acid oxidation (Jeong et al. 2008).

Alcoholic fatty liver is a potentially pathologic condition which can progress to steatohepatitis, fibrosis, and cirrhosis if alcohol consumption is continued. Alcohol exposure may induce fatty liver by increasing NADH/NAD+ ratio, increasing sterol regulatory element-binding protein-1 (SREBP-1) activity, decreasing PPAR-γ activity, and increasing complement C3 hepatic levels. Alcohol may increase SREBP-1 activity by decreasing the activities of AMP-activated protein kinase and sirtuin-1. TNF-α produced in response to alcohol exposure may cause fatty liver by up regulating SREBP-1 activity, whereas betaine and pioglitazone may attenuate fatty liver by down-regulating SREBP-1 activity. PPAR-γ agonists have potentials to attenuate alcoholic fatty liver. Adiponectin and interleukin-6 may attenuate alcoholic fatty liver by up regulating PPAR-γ and insulin signaling pathways while down-regulating SREBP-1 activity and suppressing TNF-α production. Recent studies show that paracrine activation of hepatic cannabinoid receptor 1 by HSC-derived endocannabinoids also contributes to the development of alcoholic fatty liver. Furthermore, oxidative modifications and inactivation of the enzymes involved in the mitochondrial and/or peroxisomal β-oxidation of fatty acids could contribute to fat accumulation in the liver (Purohit et al. 2009).

A diet high in polyunsaturated fat is key for induction of experimental alcoholic liver fibrosis. Myofibroblastic activation of HSCs is evident in rats given a high-fat diet and ethanol but not in the low-fat-ethanol rats. Vitamin A depletion of HSCs is the early and general effect of chronic ethanol intake but does not necessarily predict subsequent myofibroblastic activation. Reduced CRBP level is more closely associated with the subsequent cellular activation seen under the high-fat-ethanol regimen (Tsukamoto et al. 1996).

NAFLD

Nonalcoholic fatty liver disease (NAFLD) is the most common chronic liver disease in the United States, and its prevalence is increasing worldwide. It currently affects approximately 30% of adults and 10% of children in the United States. NAFLD represents a wide spectrum of conditions ranging from simple fatty liver which in general follows a benign nonprogressive clinical course, to nonalcoholic steatohepatitis (NASH), which is a more serious form of NAFLD that may progress to cirrhosis and end-stage liver disease (Wieckowska et al. 2007). HSCs have been recognized as responsible cells for NAFLD and NASH.

8.4. Biliary Atresia and Apoptosis

Extrahepatic biliary atresia is a severe neonatal liver disease resulting from a sclerosing cholangiopathy of unknown etiology. Although biliary obstruction may be surgically corrected by "Kasai" hepatoportoenterostomy, most patients still develop progressive hepatic fibrosis. The role of HSCs has been investigated and assessed the source of TGF-β production in hepatic fibrogenesis in patients with biliary atresia (Ramm et al. 1998). Procollagen α1(I) mRNA was colocalized to αSMA-positive HSCs within the region of increased collagen protein deposition in fibrotic septa and surrounding hyperplastic bile ducts. TGF-β1 mRNA expression was demonstrated in bile duct epithelial cells and activated HSCs and in PCs in close proximity to fibrotic septa. Active TGF-β1 protein was demonstrated in bile duct epithelial cells and activated HSCs. Thus, activated HSCs are responsible for increased collagen production in patients with biliary atresia and therefore play a definitive role in the fibrogenic process.

HSC apoptosis is critical to recovery from biliary fibrosis and that soluble growth factors may regulate HSC survival and apoptosis. Rats were subjected to bile duct ligation for 21 days, after which biliodigestive anastomosis was undertaken (Issa et al. 2001). Livers were harvested at fixed time points of recovery for periods of up to 42 days. Numbers of activated HSCs were quantified after αSMA staining and HSC apoptosis was detected by terminal UDP-nick end labelling (TUNEL) staining and quantified at each time point. HSC apoptosis was quantified in vitro in the presence or absence of insulin-like growth factor (IGF)-1 and TGF-β1. Following biliodigestive anastomosis after 21 days of bile duct ligation, rat liver demonstrated a progressive resolution of biliary fibrosis over 42 days, associated with a fivefold decrease in activated HSC determined by αSMA staining. TUNEL staining indicated that loss of activated HSC resulted from an increase in the rate of apoptosis during the first two days post biliodigestive anastomosis. Serum deprivation and culture in the presence of cycloheximide was associated with an increase in HSC apoptosis which was significantly inhibited by addition of IGF-1. In contrast, TGF-1 caused a significant increase in HSC apoptosis compared with serum free controls. HSC apoptosis plays a critical role in the spontaneous recovery from biliary fibrosis. Both survival and apoptosis of HSC are regulated by growth factors expressed during fibrotic liver injury.

The lamprey can be a model system for studying human biliary atresia, because the entire bile-transport apparatus is completely lost during metamorphosis (Youson et al. 1978).

Morii et al. (2010, 2011) investigated the biliary atresia of lampreys. Lampreys are unique vertebrates in that they lose the biliary tree entirely during metamorphosis. Despite the biliary atresia that occurs in lampreys, neither cholestasis nor cirrhosis develops. This study aimed to evaluate this organism as a model system of human biliary atresia.

A total of 34 lamprey specimens were investigated. Five-μm serial sections were made from livers of larval, adult, and metamorphosing lampreys and examined under light microscopy. In larval and metamorphosing lampreys, several sections were stained using TUNEL system and anti-active caspase 3 antibody. Caspase 3 is a key regulator of the apoptotic cascade that is activated in the early phase of apoptosis before DNA fragmentation.

The entire bile-transport apparatus in lamprey larvae is similar to that in humans. In the metamorphosing period, fibrous connective tissue surrounding the bile ducts is increased and biliary epithelial cells degenerate. In the early metamorphosing stage, TUNEL-positive biliary epithelial cells were present within the cystic duct and porta hepatis, despite being negative for active caspase-3 staining. Instead, biliary epithelial cells from intrahepatic bile ducts showed positive results for active caspase-3 staining. Bile canaliculi were dilated and displayed features resembling canaliculi in cholestasis. In adult lampreys, biliary epithelial cells were absent, with only fibrous connective tissue seen near the portal vein. We could not identify any bile canaliculi between PCs.

Our observation that, in the lamprey, apoptosis of biliary epithelial cells of the cystic duct and porta hepatis precedes degeneration of intrahepatic bile ducts and subsequent cholestasis indicates a similarity between human and lamprey biliary atresia, and suggests the possibility of using the lamprey as a model for human biliary atresia. Moreover, the fact that lampreys can improve cholestasis by another metabolic pathway of bile juice indicates that further study could yield new insights into biliary atresia that could be invaluable for the treatment of biliary atresia.

We have recently discovered that the degeneration of bile ducts depends on the apoptosis of biliary epithelial cells (Morii et al. 2010, 2011). The apoptosis starts in the cystic duct. Obstruction of the cystic duct and the largest intrahepatic bile duct precedes degeneration of smaller intrahepatic bile ducts. Subsequent cholestasis observed in lamprey indicates the similarity between human and lamprey biliary atresia. In spite of this biliary atresia and intrahepatic cholestasis, the lampreys never develop biliary cirrhosis. Recently, there are several reports stating that biliary apoptosis may play an important role in obstructive cholangiopathy (Erickson et al., 2008; Harada et al., 2008). Revealing the mechanism for the apoptosis of lamprey biliary epithelia may help reveal the etiology and pathogenesis of human biliary atresia.

Chapter 9

Immunity and HSCs

The liver not only has various excretory, detoxifying, and metabolic functions: it is an intrinsic lymphoid organ (Mackay 2002).

The complement system belongs to the innate immunity and consists of about 20 interacting soluble proteins that are made by the liver and circulate in the blood and extracellular fluid (Alberts et al. 2008). The system is activated by antibody-antigen complexes or by microorganisms. The complement system helps to eliminate pathogenic microorganisms by directly causing their lysis or by promoting their phagocytosis. The early complement components are activated first. There are three sets of these, belonging to three distinct pathways of components activation—the classic pathway, the lectin pathway, and the alternative pathway. The early components of all three pathways act locally to activate C3, which is pivotal component of complement. C4 exist in both of classical pathway and lectin pathway. C4 protein was demonstrated in rat HSCs (Fimmel et al. 1996). Rats were fed with dietary supplementation for a long period to identify HSC genes that are expressed during chronic hepatic iron overload. A rat isoform of C4 protein gene was strongly induced in this model. Cultured HSCs were demonstrated to synthesize C4 precursor protein and secrete its subunits into the culture medium. Thus HSCs have been shown to synthesize and secrete at least one of the complement components.

The liver appears an excellent priming site for naïve CD8+ T cells (Klein and Crispe 2006).

Cultured human HSCs were demonstrated to express membrane proteins involved in antigen presentation, including members of the HLA family (HLA-I and HLA-II), lipid-presenting molecules (CD1b and CD1c), and factors involved in T-cell activation (CD40 and CD80) (Viñas et al. 2003).

Exposure of HSCs to proinflammatory cytokines markedly up regulates these molecules. HSCs freshly isolated from human cirrhotic livers (*in vivo* activated HSCs) highly express HLA-II and CD40, suggesting that HSCs can act as antigen-presenting cells (APCs) in human fibrogenesis. HSCs were also demonstrated to be able to process efficiently exogeneous antigens. Activated HSCs internalize low- and high-molecular-weight dextran and transferrin, indicating that they can perform fluid-phase and receptor-mediated endocytosis. Moreover, HSCs can perform phagocytosis of macromolecules because they internalize latex particles as well as bacteria. Both culture–activated and *in vivo*-activated HSCs express high levels of CD68, a protein involved in antigen trafficking. Furthermore, cytokine-stimulated HSCs stimulate the allogeneic T-lymphocyte response in an HLA-II-dependent manner. Thus, HSCs are suggested to play a role in immune function of the liver.

Activated HSCs express major histocompatibility complex class I, and produce a variety of cytokines such as IL-6 and TGF-β (Yu et al. 2004). Stimulation by IFN-γ or activated T cells enhanced expression of these molecules. Addition of the activated (but not quiescent) HSCs suppresses thymidine uptake by T cells that are stimulated by alloantigens or by anti-CD3-mediated T-cell receptor ligation in a dose-dependent manner. The HSC-induced T-cell hyporesponsiveness was associated with enhanced T-cell apoptosis. Activation of HSCs was associated with markedly enhanced expression of B7-H1 (a recently identified member of the B7 family that negatively regulates T-cell responses). Blockade of B7-H1/PD-1 (PD-1 is a receprtor for B7-H1 and can be induced on T cells and B cells on activation) ligation significantly reduced HSC immunomodulatory activity, suggesting an important role of B7-H1 (Yu et al. 2004).

HSCs have been proposed to be liver-resident antigen-presenting cells for activating T cell responsiveness (Winau F al 2007). HSCs efficiently presented antigens to CD1-, major histocomapatibility complex (MHC)-1- and MHC-II restricted T cells. HSCs presented lipid antigens to CD1-restricted T lymphocytes such as natural killer cells (NKT cells) and promote homeostatic proliferation of liver NKT cells through interleukin-15. Moreover, HSCs present antigenic peptides to CD8+ and CD4+ T cells and mediate crosspriming of CD8+ T cells. Peptide-specific T cells are activated by transgenic HSCs presenting endogenous neoantigen. Upon bacterial infection, HSCs elicit antigen-specific T cells and mediate protection. HSCs have been suggested to be a professional intrahepatic APCs activating T cells and eliciting a multitude of T cell responses specific for protein and lipid antigens.

Perisinusoidal space (space of Disse), in where HSCs localize, is an active site for the immune responses, receiving portal blood containing foreign particles, because the barrier (namely, basement membrane) between the sinusoid and this space is imperfect. Roles of HSCs in immunity will be clarified further in the near future.

Toll-Like Receptor

Toll-like receptors (TLR) are homologues of the toll protein first described in Drosophila. In Drosophila, the toll protein regulates dorsal-ventral polarity but interestingly is also critical to the adult fruit flies' response to fungal pathogens. TLRs have evolved to signal the recognition of conserved pathogen-associated molecular patterns (PAMP). In humans, the TLR family consists of members, each of which are involved in the recognition of pathogen-derived material. TLR-2 and TLR-4, regulate the induction of innate immunity to bacterial, mycobacterial, fungal, and protozoal products. Furthermore, increasing evidence points to a role for these receptors in a variety of systemic diseases. For example, TLR-4 has recently been shown to be upregulated in response to oxidized low-density lipoprotein leading to the suggestion that these receptors may mediate inflammation in atherosclerosis. TLR-2 responds to cell wall components from predominantly gram-positive bacteria, such as peptidoglycan, lipoteichoic acid, and bacterial lipoprotein. In contrast, TLR-4 has been shown to be critical for LPS and endotoxin signaling. Recently, it has been shown that TLRs may also respond to host material released during necrosis, such as heat shock proteins. Structurally the TLRs show some sequence homology with the interleukin 1 receptor (Iredale 2003).

Culture-activated HSCs and HSCs isolated from patients with hepatitis C virus-induced cirrhosis express LPS-associated signaling molecules, including CD14, TLR4, and MD2. Stimulation of culture-activated HSCs with LPS results in a rapid and marked activation of NF-κB. Lipid A induces NF-kB activation in a similar manner. Both LPS- and lipid A-induced NF-κB activation is blocked by preincubation with either anti-TLR4 blocking antibody or Polymyxin B. Lipid A induces NF-κB activation in HSCs from TLR4-sufficient mice but not from TLR4-deficient mice. LPS also activates c-Jun N-terminal kinase (JNK), as assessed by *in vitro* kinase assays. LPS upregulates IL-8 and MCP-1 gene expression and secretion. LPS-induced IL-8 secretion is completely inhibited by the IB super repressor and partially inhibited by a specific JNK inhibitor. LPS also up regulates cell surface expression of ICAM-1 and VCAM-1. Human activated HSCs utilize components of TLR4 signal transduction cascade to stimulate NF-κB and JNK and up regulate chemokines and adhesion molecules. Thus, HSCs are a potential mediator of LPS-induced liver injury (Paik et al. 2003).

Activation of macrophages by endotoxin is assumed responsible for increased circulating TNF-α and soluble TNF receptor (sTNFR) levels in cirrhosis. Relevant to this is expression of TLR4 and TLR2, which is critically involved in production of TNF-α in response to endotoxin and Gram-positive microbial stimuli, respectively. In cirrhotic patients, (1) circulating endotoxin, TNF-α, and sTNFR levels; (2) peripheral blood mononuclear cell (PBMC) expression of TLR4 and TLR2, and (3) *in vitro* TNF-α production by PBMCs stimulated with endotoxin or Staphylococcus aureus enterotoxin B (SEB), have been measured (Riordan et al. 2003). Upregulation of PBMC expression of TLR2 but not TLR4 occurs in cirrhosis, which implies, contrary to previous assumptions, an important stimulatory role for Gram-positive microbial components but not endotoxin. TLR2 likely contributes to increased circulating TNF-α and sTNFR levels in cirrhosis.

Several studies have highlighted the potential role of bacterial cell wall products absorbed from the gut in both the induction and perpetuation of inflammation in the context of liver injury (Iredale 2003). Considerable evidence suggests that endotoxin derived from Gram-negative bacteria and components of endotoxin such as lipopolysaccharide (LPS) may play a key role in the genesis of hepatic inflammation, particularly in alcohol-induced injury. Moreover, in several studies, levels of endotoxin have been shown to be raised in cirrhosis, regardless of etiology. A more direct role for LPS has been shown in experimental animal studies of hepatic injury. The current model suggests that bacterial cell wall products absorbed from the gut are cleared by KCs during passage through the hepatic circulation. However, in the context of liver injury and, in particular, as a result of excess alcohol consumption, levels of bacterial cell wall products rise and it has been suggested that these may precipitate and promote hepatic injury via induction of KC activation with release of TNF-α and other inflammatory mediators. Our understanding of this area is incomplete and several apparent paradoxes exist (Iredale 2003).

TLRs recognize pathogen-associated molecular patterns and are crucially involved in the regulation of innate immune responses. Despite chronic exposure to a high load of bacterial products, the normal liver shows no activation of TLR-signaling pathways. However, under pathologic conditions, TLRs promote proinflammatory signaling such as the NF-κB, c-Jun-N-terminal kinase (JNK), p38, and interferon pathways in the liver and regulate antiviral and antibacterial responses, hepatic injury, and wound healing.

TLRs are a group of highly conserved molecules that allow the immune system to sense molecules that are present in most classes of pathogens, but not the host, and to coordinate defense mechanisms against these pathogens. The recognition of pathogen-associated molecular patterns (PAMPs) by TLRs is a cornerstone of innate immunity and provides a quick and highly efficient response to pathogens in both vertebrate and invertebrate species. In addition, there is accumulating evidence that TLRs contribute significantly to activation of adaptive immune responses such as dendritic cell maturation and T- and B-cell responses (Schwabe et al. 2006).

Because of its anatomic links to the gut, the liver is constantly exposed to gut-derived bacterial products and functions as a major filter organ and a first line of defense. Eighty percent of intravenously injected endotoxin is detected in the liver within 20–30 minutes, and KCs are able to take up efficiently endotoxin and phagocytose bacteria carried through portal vein blood and are considered to play a major role in the clearance of systemic bacterial infection. Despite the constant exposure to low levels of gut-derived bacteria and bacterial products, there are no signs of ongoing inflammation in the normal liver. This lacking response is to some extent explained by very specific immunologic properties of the liver. The healthy liver contains low mRNA levels of TLRs such as TLR1, TLR2, TLR4, TLR6, TLR7, TLR8, TLR9, and TLR10 and signaling molecules such as MD-2 and MyD88 in comparison with other organs. However, under pathologic conditions, TLRs activate inflammatory-signaling pathways in the liver and are actively involved in the pathophysiology in a large number of hepatic diseases (Schwabe et al. 2006).

The human TLR family consists of currently 10 members, which are structurally characterized by the presence of a leucine-rich repeat (LRR) domain in their extracellular domain and a Toll/interleukin (IL)-1 receptor (TIR) domain in their intracellular domain. The existence of a large number of TLRs enables the innate immune system to discriminate between PAMPs that are characteristic of different microbial classes and launch specific defense mechanisms.

After liver injury, HSCs undergo an activation process and become the predominant ECM-producing cell type in the liver. Activated human HSCs express TLR4 and CD14 and respond to LPS with the activation of IκB kinase(IKK)/NF-κB and JNK as well as the secretion of proinflammatory cytokines. Activated mouse HSCs express TLR4 and CD14 as well as low levels of TLR2 and respond to LPS, lipoteichoic acid, and N-acetyl muramyl peptide with an up regulation of Erk phosphorylation and IL-6, TGF-β1, and MCP-1 secretion. In quiescent rat HSCs, LPS stimulates the synthesis of TNF-α, IL-6, and IL-1 but not of TGF-β. Thus, LPS and other TLR ligands may enhance fibrogenic responses in the liver through direct effects on HSCs (Schwabe et al. 2006).

Intestinal bacterial microflora and a functional TLR4, but not TLR2, are required for hepatic fibrogenesis. In quiescent HSCs, TLR4 activation not only up regulates chemokine secretion and induces chemotaxis of KCs, but also down regulates the TGF-pseudoreceptor Bambi to sensitize HSCs to TGF-β–induced signals and allow for unrestricted activation by KCs. LPS-induced Bambi down regulation and sensitization to TGF-β is mediated by a MyD88–NF-κB–dependent pathway. Accordingly, Myd88-deficient mice have decreased hepatic fibrosis. Thus, modulation of TGF-β signaling by a TLR4-MyD88–NF-κB axis provides a novel link between proinflammatory and profibrogenic signals (Seki et al. 2007).

Chapter 10

Epigenetics of HSCs

Cells of a multicellular organism are genetically homogeneous but structurally and functionally heterogeneous owing to the differential expression of genes. Many of these differences in gene expression arise during development and are subsequently retained through mitosis. Stable alterations of this kind are said to be 'epigenetic', because they are heritable in the short term but do not involve mutations of the DNA itself. Research over the past few years has focused on two molecular mechanisms that mediate epigenetic phenomena: DNA methylation and histone modifications (Jaenisch and Bird 2003).

Epigenetic effects by means of DNA methylation have an important role in development but can also arise stochastically as animals age. Identification of proteins that mediate these effects has provided insight into this complex process and diseases that occur when it is perturbed. External influences on epigenetic processes are seen in the effects of diet on long-term diseases such as cancer. Thus, epigenetic mechanisms seem to allow an organism to respond to the environment through changes in gene expression. The extent to which environmental effects can provoke epigenetic responses represents an exciting area of future research (Jaenisch and Bird 2003). Developmental stages in multicellular organisms proceed according to a temporally and spatially precise pattern of gene expression. It has become evident that changes within the chromatin structure brought about by covalent modifications of histones are of crucial importance in determining many biological processe, including development. Numerous studies have provided evidence that the enzymes responsible for the modifications of histones function in a coordinated pattern to control gene expression in the short term and, through the transferral of these modifications by inheritance to their progeny in the long term (Margueron et al. 2005).

Myofibroblasts are critical cellular elements of wound healing generated at sites of injury by transdifferentiation of resident cells. A paradigm for this process is conversion of HSCs into hepatic myofibroblasts. Treatment of HSC with DNA methylation inhibitor 5-aza-2'-deoxycytidine (5-azadC) blocked transdifferentiation. 5-azadC also prevented loss of IκBα and PPAR expression that occurs during transdifferentiation to allow acquisition of proinflammatory and profibrogenic characteristics. Chromatin immunoprecipitation assay analysis revealed IB promoter is associated with transcriptionally repressed chromatin that converts to an active state with 5-azadC treatment. The methyl-CpG-binding protein MeCP2 which promotes repressed chromatin structure is selectively detected in myofibroblasts of diseased liver. siRNA knockdown of MeCP2 elevated IB promoter activity, mRNA and protein expression in myofibroblasts. MeCP2 interacts with IκBα promoter via a methyl-CpG-dependent mechanism and recruitment into a transcriptional repressor RBP-J (CBF1) corepression complex. MeCP2 and DNA methylation exert epigenetic control over hepatic wound healing and fibrogenesis (Mann et al. 2007).

Epigenetics is a promising and intriguing research area for HSC study.

Chapter 11

Artificial Organs and HSCs

Whole organ transplantation is the only clinically effective method of treating fulminant hepatic failure and chronic liver failure due to specific genetic, hepatocellular, and anatomic defects of liver function. However, wider application of liver transplantation is limited by shortage of organ donors, high cost, a relatively high morbidity rate, and need for life long immunotherapy. As a result, investigators have attempted to develop alternative methods to treat liver insufficiency. These ranged from use of plasma exchange to use of detoxification columns and extracorporeal devices loaded with various liver tissue preparations. Several liver support systems were developed in the 1950s and 1960s, but it was not until recently that advances in PC isolation and culture, improved understanding of liver cells-matrix interactions, availability of new biomaterials, improved hollow fiber technology, and better understanding of flow and mass transport across semipermeable membranes resulted in the development of a new generation of liver assist devices. Some of these devices are being tested in the clinical setting (Rozga and Demetriou 1995).

Stimulation of Proliferation of HSCs and Tissue Formation of the Liver by a Long-Acting Vitamin C Derivative

A long-acting vitamin C derivative, L-ascorbic acid 2-phosphate (Asc 2-P), was found to stimulate cell proliferation, collagen accumulation, and tissue formation (Hata and Senoo 1989; Kurata et al. 1993). On the basis of this discovery, Asc 2-P was added to the medium in which HSCs were cultured (Senoo and Hata 1994a). The cells in the medium supplemented with Asc 2-P stretched better than the cells in the control medium. Asc 2-P stimulated cell proliferation and collagen synthesis of the HSCs, and formation of the liver tissue-like structure in coculture of PCs and fibroblasts. We named the liver tissue-like structure the mini-liver (Senoo et al. 1989).

PCs were grown in chemically defined hepatocyte growth medium (HGM) containing HGF and EGF on collagen-coated polystyrene beads in roller bottle cultures, forming clusters of beads, and proliferating PCs and NPCs, including fenestrated endothelium forming vascular structures (Michalopoulos et al. 1999). Desmin-positive cells surrounded PCs. Collagen I and III were deposited in a diffuse manner whereas collagen IV surrounded the clusters of the epithelial cells, forming a basement membrane. When the mixed cell clusters were implanted in Matrigel, PCs grew in three dimensions, forming plates and ducts. Many single, long plates of PCs were seen, suggesting progressive linear assembly guided by PC specific structural parameters. HGF, EGF, and TGF-α enhance these phenomena. HGF plus EGF elicited maximal response. TGF-β1 suppressed formation of the ducts and plates. Within three months in Matrigel, the cultures established monolayers composed of plates, ducts, and a well-delineated canalicular network. The mixed cultures expressed albumin, A1AT, α-fetoprotein (AFP), transferrin, and CYPIIB1. Following implantation of the cell clusters in Matrigel, there was decreased expression of c-met, urokinase, urokinase receptor, and TGF-β1. Electron microscopy showed differentiated PCs with nearly normal ultrastructure. The proliferating cell nuclear antigen (PCNA) labeling index was high (more than 80%) whereas the bromo-deoxyaridine labeling index of ongoing DNA synthesis varied from 10% to 15%. These results show that the mixed cultures of proliferating PCs and NPCs can reproduce the hallmark structures of hepatic histological architecture while maintaining differentiation and the capacity to proliferate (Michalopoulos et al. 1999).

Liver cells isolated from an adult rat liver, consisting of small PCs (SPCs), mature PCs (MPCs), liver epithelial cells (LECs), KCs, LSECs, and HSCs, were cultured in a medium supplemented with 10% fetal bovine serum, nicotinamide, Asc 2-P, EGF, and dimethyl sulfoxide. The SPCs rapidly proliferated and formed a colony. About 10% of cytokeratin 8 (CK8)-positive cells formed SH colonies. All SPCs at day 10 immunocytochemically showed positivity for albumin, transferrin, CK8, and CK18, which are markers for PCs. In contrast, AFP-, CK14-, OC2-, and glutathione S-transferase placental type (GST-P)-positive cells, which are thought to be markers for hepatic immature cells, were rarely observed. At day 20 some cells in the colonies were positive for AFP, CK7, CK19, and GST-P. LECs and HSCs proliferated and surrounded the colonies. About 2 weeks after plating, piled up cells were often observed on the SH colonies. In those colonies LECs and HSCs invaded under the colonies. The invasion of the cells and gradual deposits of ECM such as type I collagen, type IV collagen, and laminin induced alteration of the shape of the SPCs from relatively flat to cuboidal or rectangular (Mitaka et al. 1999)

Since the first PC isolation methodologies were published almost 30 years ago, investigators have striven to reproduce conditions *in vitro* whereby the responses of cells would mimic those found *in vivo* (Strain 1999). Although early systems were useful for examining the mitogenic response of primary PCs, their value was limited by an unstable phenotype. Epithelial cell polarity was lost, and all but a few PC-specific functions deteriorated within a relatively short time span. Many means were devised to prolong the longevity of primary PCs. ECM, including Matrigel, or double collagen gels resulted in some restoration of cell polarity and three-dimensional architecture. Spheroid aggregates, coculture with other (liver) cell types, or addition of dimethyl sulfoxide, phenobarbitone, or butyrate to the culture medium also improved functional stability. However, with all of these methods there was a trade-off: A culture environment optimized for phenotypic stability was nonpermissive for growth in response to mitogens.

Around the same time, Mitaka et al. (1992) reported a population of PCs that could expand clonally in an enriched culture medium. They used the term "small hepatocytes" to describe the cells that were proliferating and that retained a PC phenotype. This finding was confirmed and extended by Tateno et al. (1996) who showed additionally that small PCs were bipotential, that is, capable of differentiating along either the PCs or biliary cell lineages. These observations were extended by Block et al. (1996) whose PC growth medium was further enriched and included EGF and HGF. Attention has turned now to the question of hepatic morphogenesis and reconstituting the complex cellular structure of the liver in culture. The reasoning is that the correct mix of cells and ECM components may result in spontaneous formation of hepatic acinar/sinusoidal architecture.

Cells are cultured as monolayers yielding proliferating colonies of small PCs that are surrounded by NPCs, principally HSCs, which themselves proliferate and begin to synthesize matrix proteins. In turn, the colonies form three-dimensional acinar or cyst-like structures, which exhibit canalicular function. In the second article, Michalopoulos et al. (1999) take a different approach, with similar results. Their PC preparation is conventional with an estimated 3% NPC mix. PCs are attached to collagen-coated polystyrene beads and maintained in roller bottles in the presence of hepatocyte growth medium. After 2 to 3 weeks, both PCs and NPCs grow and migrate, and the beads aggregate as a mass held together by cells and ECM. The bead aggregates are implanted into Matrigel, which fosters the migration firstly of NPCs (again thought to be principally HSCs) followed by PCs in a budding process. The morphogenetic response culminates in formation of acinar-like plates of PCs with a structure resembling a canaliculus along the length of the plates. Interestingly, this acinar/ductular formation occurs in areas of the substratum that are largely free of other cell types. The whole process appears to depend on soluble factors, including both HGF and EGF, and, as seen in the study (Mitaka et al. 1999), ECM. The latter presumably derives from HSCs, suggesting that these cells play a central role.

Can the present series of observations be exploited to improve current bioartificial liver (BAL) systems? These are difficult questions to resolve but nonetheless important because of the exciting possibility that these current approaches can be used to provide a pool of stable human liver cells. The goal of generating large numbers of differentiated, and therefore, fully functional human PCs has enormous potential. Clinically relevant initiatives where progress is hampered by lack of sufficient good quality primary human PCs include BAL (discussed later), cell transplantation, and the evaluation of drug toxicology, and pharmacokinetics. Despite widespread efforts with primary human PCs and human cell lines and several recent reports of putative human liver epithelial progenitor cells, no one has yet succeeded in generating a safe, fully functional clonal, immortalized, or genetically engineered human cell model that can substitute for primary PCs in these various applications.

It remains to be seen how phenotypic stability can be achieved. One possibility might be to investigate more carefully the role of NPCs other than KCs and LSECs, which clearly are present in both studies. Rather than relying on the chance presence of contaminating cells in the starting PC preparations, for example, one way forward may be to purify (as far as is possible) individual NPC populations and to add them back in controlled ratios to PC cultures. The translation of these findings to BAL systems remains a significant challenge. All of the current BAL designs incorporate cell supports consisting of hollow-fiber capillaries or similar material, collagen-coated beads, or collagen gels. Materials with promise but still largely unproven with PCs include a biodegradable matrix that can be spun into a scaffold on which cells are then seeded. However, none of the current BAL designs incorporate NPCs, which could contribute endogenous matrix, and none deal with the question of biliary excretion by the system. Clearly the question of what happens to bile pigments, bile salts, conjugated intermediates, and potentially toxic waste products cannot be ignored. Is a ductular component actually necessary to the design? Or, in a flow-through and, therefore, fluid replenishing system, is it sufficient to wash away potentially harmful products? It is possible that the lack of a biliary excretory mechanism shortens the lifetime or reduces the efficiency of current BAL systems. In conclusion, these studies represent significant advances in hepatic tissue biology. They reinforce the importance of NPCs (in particular, HSCs) and matrix biology in control of morphogenesis and pave the way for the development of a truly stable *ex vivo* system with the capability of providing efficient artificial liver support (Strain 1999).

As mentioned above, vigorous investigations trying to make an artificial liver using PCs and NPCs have been performed, and now iPS (induced pluripotent stem) cells are available (Takahashi and Yamanaka 2006) for the development of BAL. In the near future, iPS cells will be useful tools for making BAL.

Recently, liver-like structure has been reported to be made by using iPS cells (Rashid et al. 2010).

Chapter 12

Global Climate Change and HSCs

HSCs of Arctic Animals

More than 50 years ago, Rodahl reported that animals (polar bears and seals) in the arctic area were able to store a large amount of vitamin A in the liver (Rodahl 1949a, 1949b; Rodahl and Moore 1943). To investigate the cellular and molecular mechanisms in transport and storage of vitamin A and the influence of the global climate change to the mechanisms in these arctic animals, we performed a study in Greenland and the Svalbard archipelago (situated at 80° N, 15° E) (Higashi and Senoo 2003; Senoo et al. 1999, 2012). After getting permission to hunt the animals from the district governor, 13 polar bears (*Ursus maritimus*), 11 arctic foxes (*Alopex lagopus*), 14 bearded seals (*Erignathus barbatus*), 22 glaucous gulls (*Larus hyperboreus*), 5 fulmars (*Fulmarus glacialis*), 4 Brünnich's guillemots (*Uria lomvia*), 6 ringed seals (*Phoca hispida*), 5 hooded seals (*Cystophora cristata*), 6 puffins (*Fratercula arctica*), 5 Svalbard ptarmigans (*Lagopus mutus hyperboreus*) and 7 Svalbard reindeers (*Rangifer tarandus platyrhynchus*) were caught in the period from August 1996 to March 2008. Three polar bears were shot in self-defense at Svalbard February and August 1998 in Ny Ålesund and Hornsund. We also obtained 13 brown bears (*Ursus arctos*) from Jämtland, Gävleborg and Dalarna, 4 red foxes (*Vulpes vulpes*) from Västergötaland, and 8 grey gulls (*Larus argentatus*) from Skåne, Sweden.

Fresh organs, namely, the liver, kidney, spleen, lung, and jejunum were examined by morphological methods and high-performance liquid chromatography (HPLC). Serum from each animal was analyzed with HPLC.

The arctic animals stored vitamin A in HSCs (Figs. 2-4, Fig. 10). Only a small amount of vitamin A existed within other organs such as kidney, spleen, lung, and jejunum. Top predators among arctic animals stored 6-23 μmole retinyl ester per g liver which 20-100 times the levels normally found in other animals including humans, rats, and mice. These results indicate that the HSCs in these animals have high ability for uptake and enough capacity for storage of vitamin A.

The existence of a gradient of vitamin A-storing capacity in the liver was reported and it was found to be independent on the vitamin A amount in the organ (Higashi and Senoo, 2003). This gradient was expressed as a symmetrical biphasic distribution starting at the periportal zone, peaking at the middle zone, and sloping down toward the central zone in the liver lobule.

Xenobiotics (such as PCBs and dioxins) may reduce the threshold of vitamin A-toxicity (Nilsson et al. 1999) and both vitamin A and fat-soluble xenobiotics have a tendency to accumulate in the food chain (Barrie et al. 1992; Dewailly et al. 1989; Holden 1998; Jarman et al. 1992; Muir et al. 1998; Skaare et al. 2001; Wiig al. 1998). Kidney total vitamin A, which may be used as a biomarker for retinoid-related toxicity or excess, in polar bear and bearded seal was below 1% of their liver value, which is in the normal range for most animals (Senoo et al. 2004). Arctic fox and glaucous gull, however, had kidney levels of about 9 and 42% of the liver values, respectively. This increased kidney concentrations and decreased capacity for storage in HSCs of total vitamin A in arctic fox and glaucous gull are most likely signs of vitamin A-toxicity that deserve attention. Nuclear deviation has been reported in PCs on sinusoidal surface in arctic animals (Sato et al. 2001a). These data are alarming and have not been observed previously in free-living animals.

Vitamin A storage in HSCs in polar animals reflects the environmental and climate changes in the arctic area.

The development of such an efficient vitamin A-storing mechanism in HSCs may have contributed to the survival of top predators in the extreme environment of the arctic. These animals demonstrated no signs of hypervitaminosis A. The HSC that has capacity of taking up and storing a large amount of vitamin A plays pivotal roles in maintenance of food web, food chain, biodiversity, and eventually ecology of the arctic (Senoo et al. 2012).

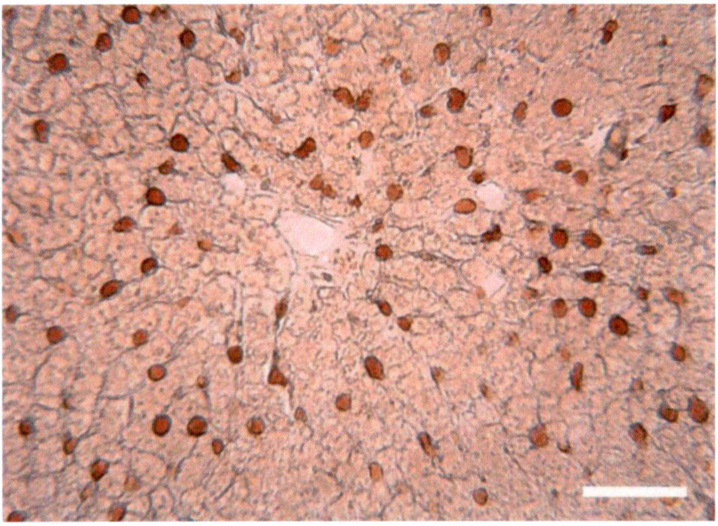

Figure 10. Sudan III lipid staining of polar bear liver. Scale bar: 100μm. Senoo, H., Imai, K., Mezaki, Y., Miura, M., Morii, M., Fujiwara, M., Blomhoff, R. (2012) Accumulation of vitamin A in the hepatic stellate cell of arctic top predators. Anat Rec. 295, 1660-1668, Wiley-Liss, Inc.

Chapter 13

Conclusion

After the re-discovery of the HSCs, the research of HSCs has developed vigorously. Especially relevant to clinical medicine, the research has advanced rapidly as described in this monograph. In the standard textbook of internal medicine, Harrison's Principles of Internal Medicine, 17th ed. (Mailliard and Sorrell 2008), HSCs have been described as a key player in hepatic fibrogenesis. Clinically, HSCs are now targets to the therapy of organ fibrosis such as liver and pancreas. However, in the standard textbook of cell biology, Molecular Biology of the Cell, 5th ed. (Alberts et al. 2008), the description on SCs is still lacking. As we introduced in this monograph, HSCs are intriguing from many directions of basic research. The authors hope more basic researchers join to the SC research.

Acknowledgment

Acknowledgment is to Drs Kenjiro Wake and late Hajime Mannen (Emeritus professors of Tokyo Medical and Dental University) who have introduced Haruki Senoo into the basic medical research and are encouraging the authors continuously.

The authors also thank Dr. Mitsuru Sato and Mr. Naosuke Kojima of this laboratory for their valuable discussion and significant techniques.

References

Adachi M, Brenner DA (2008) High molecular weight adiponectin inhibits proliferation of hepatic stellate cells via activation of adenosine monophosphate-activated protein kinase. *Hepatology* 47: 677-685.

Adachi E, Hayashi T, Hashimoto PH (1991) A comparison of the immunofluorescent localization of collagen types I, III, and V with the distribution of reticular fibers on the same liver sections of the snow monkey (*Macaca fuscata*). *Cell Tiss Res* 264: 1-8.

Adachi M, Osawa Y, Uchinami H, Kitamura T, Accili D, Brenner DA (2007) The forkhead transcription factor FoxO1 regulates proliferation and transdifferentiation of hepatic stellate cells. *Gastroenterology,* 132: 1434-1446.

Aimed Q, Hines JE, Harrison D, Burt AD (1991) Expression of muscle-associated cytoskeletal proteins by human sinusoidal liver cells. In Wisse E, Knook DL, McCuskey RS (eds) Cells Hepatic Sinusoid, vol 3, *Kupffer Cell Foundation, Leiden,* pp 203-206.

Akhmeteli KT, Ekaladze EN, Jaliashvli ZV, Medoidze TD, Melikishvili ZG, Merkviladze NZ, Papava MB, Tushurashvili PR (2008) Study of vitamin A distribution in rats by laser induced fluorescence spectroscopy. *Laser Phys Lett* 5: 471-475.

Alberts B, Johnson A, Lewis J, Raff M, Roberts K, Walter P (2008) *Molecular Biology of the Cell, 5th edn Garland Science,* New York.

Anan A, Baskin-Bey ES, Bronk SF, Werneburg NW, Shah VH, Gores GJ (2006) Proteasome inhibition induces hepatic stellate cell apoptosis. *Hepatology* 43: 335-344.

Andersen KB, Nilsson A, Blomhoff HK, Øyen TB, Gabrielsen OS, Norum KR, Blomhoff R (1992) Direct mobilization of retinol from hepatic perisinusoidal stellate cells to plasma. *J Biol Chem* 267: 1340-1344.

Andrade CMB, Trindade VMT, Cardoso CCA, Ziulkoski AL, Trugo LC, Guaragna RM, Borojevic R, Guma FCR (2003) Changes of sphingolipid species in the phenotype conversion from myofibroblasts to lipocytes in hepatic stellate cells. *J Cell Biochem* 88: 533-544.

Ankoma-Sey V, Wang Y, Dai Z (2000) Hypoxic stimulation of vascular endothelial growth factor expression in activated rat hepatic stellate cell. *Hepatology* 31: 141-148.

Antoine M, Wirz W, Tag CG, Gressner AM, Marvituna M, Wycislo M, Hellerbrand C, Kiefer P (2007) Expression and function of fibroblast growth factor (FGF) 9 in hepatic stellate cells and its role in toxic liver injury. *Biochem Biophys Res Commun* 361: 335-341.

Aoki H, Ohnishi H, Hama K, Ishijima T, Satoh Y, Hanatsuka K, Ohashi A, Wada S, Miyata T, Kita H, Yamamoto H, Osawa H, Sato K, Tamada K, Yasuda H, Mashima H, Sugano K (2006) Autocrine loop between TGF-1 and IL-1 through Smad3- and ERK-dependent pathways in rat pancreatic stellate cells. *Am J Physiol Cell Physiol* 290: C1100-C1108.

Aoki H, Ohnishi H, Hama K, Shinozaki S, Kita H, Osawa H, Yamamoto H, Sato K, Tamada K, Sugano K (2007) Cyclooxygenase-2 is required for activated pancreatic stellate cells to respond to proinflammatory cytokines. *Am J Physiol Cell Physiol* 292: C259-C268.

Apte MV, Haber PS, Applegate TL, Norton ID, McCaughan GW, Korsten MA, Pirola RC, Wilson JS (1998) Periacinar stellate shaped cells in rat pancreas: identification, isolation, and culture. *Gut* 43:128-133.

Apte MV, Haber PS, Darby SJ, Rodgers SC, McCaughan GW, Korsten MA, Pirola RC, Wilson JS (1999) Pancreatic stellate cells are activated by proinflammatory cytokines: implications for pancreatic fibrogenesis. *Gut* 44: 534-541.

Arber N, Zajicek G, Ariel I (1988) The streaming liver II. hepatocyte life history. *Liver* 8: 80-87.

Arber N, Zajicek G, Shamir R, Kenet G, Raanani P, Nordenberg J, Sidi Y (1992) Bromobenzene accelerates hepatocyte streaming in rats. *Hepatology* 103: 1273-1276.

Armendariz-Borunda J, Greenwel P, Rojkind M (1989) Kupffer cells from CCl_4-treated rat livers induce skin fibroblast and liver fat-storing cell proliferation in culture. *Matrix* 9: 150-158.

Arriza JL, Weinberger C, Cerelli G, Glaser TM, Handelin BL, Housman DE, Evans RM (1987) Cloning of human mineralocorticoid receptor complementary DNA: structural and functional kinship with the glucocorticoid receptor. *Science* 237:268-275.

Arthur MJP (2000) Fibrogenesis II. Metalloproteinases and their inhibitors in liver fibrosis. Am J Physiol Gastrointest Liver Physiol 279: G245-G249.

Arthur MJP (2002) Reversibility of liver fibrosis and cirrhosis following treatment for hepatitis C. *Gastroenterology* 122: 1525-1528.

Asahina K, Zhou B, Pu WT, Tsukamoto H (2011) Septum tansversum-derived mesothelium gives rise to hepatic stellate cells and perivascular mesenchymal cells in developing mouse liver. *Hepatology* 53: 983-995.

Athari A, Hänecke K, Jungermann K (1994) Prostaglandin F2 and D2 release from primary ito cell cultures after stimulation with noradrenaline and ATP but not adenosine. *Hepatology* 20: 142-148.

Baba S, Fujii H, Hirose T, Yasuchika K, Azuma H, Hoppo T, Naito M, Machimoto T, Ikai I (2004) Commitment of bone marrow cells to hepatic stellate cells in mouse. *J Hepatol* 40: 255–260.

Bachem MG, Riess U, Melchior R, Sell K-M, Gressner AM (1989) Transforming growth factors (TGFα and TGFβ1) stimulate chondroitin sulfate and hyaluronate synthesis in cultured rat liver fat storing cells. *FEBS Lett* 257: 134-137.

Bachem MG, Schneider E, Groß H, Weidenbach H, Schmid RM, Menke A, Siech M, Beger H, Grünert A, Adler G (1998) Identification, culture, and characterization of pancreatic stellate cells in rats and humans. *Gastroenterology* 115:421-432.

Bahr MJ, Vincent KJ, Arthur MJP, Fowler AV, Smart DE, Wright MC, Clark IM, Benyon RC, Iredale JP, Mann DA (1999) Control of the tissue inhibitor of metalloproteinases-1 promoter in culture-activated rat hepatic stellate cells: Regulation by activator protein-1 DNA binding proteins. *Hepatology* 29: 839-848.

Balabaud C, Bioulac-Sage P, Desmoulière A (2004) The role of hepatic stellate cells in liver regenration. *J Hepatol* 40: 1023-1026.

Ballardini G, Groff P, de Glorgi LB, Schuppan D, Bianchi FB (1994) Ito cell heterogeneity: Desmin negative Ito cells in normal rat liver. *Hepatology* 19: 440-446.

Balmer JE, Blomhoff R (2002) Gene expression regulation by retinoic acid. *J Lipid Res* 43:1773-1808.

Banchereau J, Steinman RM (1998) Dendritic cells and the control of immunity. *Nature* 392: 245-252.

Barrie LA, Gregor D, Hargrave B, Lake R, Muir D, Shearer R, Tracey B, Bidleman T (1992) Arctic contaminants: sources, occurrence and pathways. *Sci Total Environ* 122: 1-74.

Bastien J, Rochette-Egly C (2004) Nuclear retinoid receptors and the transcription of retinoid-target genes. *Gene* 328:1-16.

Bataller R, Brenner DA (2005) Liver fibrosis. J Clin Invest 115: 209-218.

Bataller R, Paik Y-H, Lindquist JH, Lemasters JJ, Brenner DA (2004) Hepatitis C virus core and nonstructural proteins induce fibrogenic effects in hepatic stellate cells. *Gastroenterology* 126: 529-540.

Batten ML, Imanishi Y, Maeda T, Tu DC, Moise AR, Bronson D, Possin D, Van Gelder RN, Baehr W, Palczewski K (2004) Lecithin-retinol acyltransferase is essential for accumulation of all-*trans*-retinyl esters in the eye and in the liver. *J Biol Chem* 279: 10422-10432.

Bauer M, Schuppan D (2001) TGFβ1 in liver fibrosis: time to change paradigms? *FEBS Lett* 502: 1-3.

Beno DWA, Espinal R, Edelstein BM, Davis BH (1993) Administration of prostaglandin E1 analog reduces rat hepatic and ito cell collagen gene expression and collagen accumulation after bile duct ligation injury. *Hepatology* 17: 707-714.

Beno DWA, Rapp UR, Davis BH (1994) Prostaglandin E suppression of platelet-derived-growth-factor-induced Ito cell mitogenesis occurs independent of raf perinuclear translocation and nuclear proto-oncogene expression. *Biochim Biophys Acta Mol Cell Res* 1222: 292-300.

Benyon RC, Arthur MJP (2001) Extracellular matrix degradation and the role of hepatic stellate cells. *Semin Liver Dis* 21: 373-384.

Benyon RC, Iredale JP (2000) Is liver fibrosis reversible? *Gut* 46:443-446.

Biesalski HK, Frank J, Beck SC, Heinrich F, Illek B, Reifen R, Gollnick H, Seeliger MW, Wissinger B, Zrenner E (1999) Biochemical but not clinical vitamin A deficiency results from mutations in the gene for retinol binding protein. *Am J Clin Nutr* 69: 931-936.

Bioulac-Sage P, Lafon ME, Saric J,. Balabaud C (1990) Nerves and perisinusoidal cells in human liver. *J Hepatol* 10: 105-112.

Blanchette-Mackie EJ, Dwyer NK, Barber T, Coxey RA, Takeda T, Rondinone CM, Theodorakis JL, Greenberg AS, Londos C (1995) Perilipin is located on the surface layer of intracellular lipid droplets in adipocytes. *J Lipid Res* 36:1211-1226.

Blaner WS (1989) Retinol-binding protein: the serum transport protein for vitamin A. *End Rev* 10: 308-316.

Blaner WS (2007) STRA6, a cell-surface receptor for retinol-binding protein: The plot thickens. *Cell Metab* 5: 164-166.

Blaner WS, Dixon JL, Moriwaki H, Martino RA, Stein O, Stein Y, Goodman DS (1987) Studies on the *in vivo* transfer of retinoids from parenchymal to stellate cells in rat liver. *Eur J Biochem* 164: 301-307.

Blaner WS, Hendriks HF, Brouwer A, de Leeuw AM, Knook DL, Goodman DS (1985) Retinoids, retinoid-binding proteins, and retinyl palmitate hydrolase distributions in different types of rat liver cells. *J Lipid Res* 26: 1241-1251.

Blaner WS, O'Byrne SM, Wongsiriroj N, Kluwe J, D'Ambrosio DM, Jiang H, Schwabe RF, Hillman EMC, Piantedosi R, Libien J (2009) Hepatic stellate cell lipid droplets: A specialized lipid droplet for retinoid storage. *Biochim Biophys Acta Mol Cell Biol Lipids* 1791: 467-473.

Blaner WS, van Bennekum AM, Brouwer A, Hendriks HFJ (1990) Distribution of lecithin-retinol acyltransferase activity in different types of rat liver cells and subcellular fractions. *FEBS Lett* 274: 89-92.

Block GD, Locker J, Bowen WC, Peterson BE, Katyal S, Strom SC, Riley T, Howard TA, Michalopoulos GK (1996) Population expansion, clonal division, and specific differentiation patterns in primary cultures of hepatocytes by HGF/SF, EGF, and TGFα in a chemically defined (HGM) medium. *J Cell Biol.* 132: 1133-1149.

Blomhoff R (1987) Hepatic retinol metabolism: Role of the various cell types. *Nutr Rev* 45: 257-263.

Blomhoff R (1994) Vitamin A in Health and Disease. *Marcel Dekker Inc,* New York.

Blomhoff R, Berg T (1990) Isolation and cultivation of rat liver stellate cells. *Methods Enzymol* 190: 58-71.

Blomhoff R, Berg T, Norum KR (1988a) Newly administered [^{3}H]retinol is transferred from hepatocytes to stellate cells in liver for storage. *Exp Cell Res* 150: 186-193.

Blomhoff R, Berg T, Norum KR (1988b) Distribution of retinol in rat liver cells: effect of age, sex and nutritional status. *British J Nutr* 60: 233-239.

Blomhoff R, Berg T, Norum KR (1988c) Transfer of retinol from parenchymal to stellate cells in liver is mediated by retinol-binding protein. *Proc Natl Acad Sci USA* 85: 3455-3458.

Blomhoff R, Blomhoff HK (2006) Overview of retinoid metabolism and function. *J Neurobiol* 66:606-630.

Blomhoff R, Green MH, Berg T, Norum KR (1990) Transport and storage of vitamin A. *Science* 250: 399-404.

Blomhoff R, Green MH, Green JB, Berg T, Norum KR (1991) Vitamin A metabolism: New perspectives on absorption, transport, and storage. *Physiol Rev* 71: 951-990.

Blomhoff R, Green MH, Norum KR (1992a) Vitamin A: Physiological and biochemical processing. *Annu Rev Nutr* 12: 37-57.

Blomhoff R, Helgerud P, Rasmussen M, Berg T, Norum KR (1982) *In vivo* uptake of chylomicron [^{3}H]retinyl ester by rat liver: evidence for retinol transfer from parenchymal to nonparenchymal cells. *Proc Ntl Acad Sci USA* 79: 7326-7330.

Blomhoff R, Holte K, Naess L, Berg T (1984a) Newly administered [^{3}H]retinol is transferred from hepatocytes to stellate cells in liver for storage. *Exp Cell Res* 150: 186-193.

Blomhoff R, Norum KR, Berg T (1985b) Hepatic uptake of [^{3}H]retinol bound to the serum retinol binding protein involves both parenchymal and perisinusoidal stellate cells. *J Biol Chem* 260: 13571-13575.

Blomhoff R, Rasmussen M, Nilsson A, Norum KR, Berg T, Blaner WS, Kato M, Mertz JR, DS Goodman DS, Eriksson U (1985a) Hepatic retinol metabolism. Distribution of retinoids, enzymes, and binding proteins in isolated rat liver cells. *J Biol Chem* 260: 13560-13565.

Blomhoff R, Senoo H, Smeland S, Bjerknes T, Norum KR (1992b) Cellular uptake of vitamin A. *J Nutr Sci Vitam* 38: 327-330.

Blomhoff R, Smedsrød B, Eskild W, Granum PE, Berg T (1984b) Preparation of isolated liver endothelial cells and Kupffer cells in high yield by means of an enterotoxin. *Exp Cell Res* 150: 194-204.

Blomhoff R, Wake K (1991) Perisinusoidal stellate cells of the liver: important roles in retinol metabolism and fibrosis. *FASEB J* 5:271-277.

Bloom W, Fawcett DW (1994) A Textbook of Histology, 12th edn *Chapman & Hall*, New York.

Blüher M, Tönjes A, Stumvoll M (2008) Does retinol-binding protein 4 cause or reflect fatty liver disease? *Hepatology* 48: 4-6.

Bonis PAL, Friedman SL, Kaplan MM (2001) Is liver fibrosis reversible? *New Engl J Med* 344: 452-454.

Braet F, Luo D, Spector I, Vermijlen D, Wisse E (2001) Endothelial and pit cells. In: Arias IM, Boyer JL, Chisari FV, Fausto N, Schachter D, Shafritz DA (eds) The Liver Biology and Pathobiology, 4th edn *Lippincott Williams & Wilkins,* Philadelphia, pp 437-453.

Brasaemle DL, Barber T, Wolins NE, Serrero G, Blanchette-Mackie EJ, Londos C (1997) Adipose differentiation-related protein is an ubiquitously expressed lipid storage droplet-associated protein. *J Lipid Res* 38:2249-2263.

Bronfenmajer S, Schaffner F, Popper H (1966) Fat-storing cells (lipocytes) in human liver. *Arch Pathol* 82: 447-453.

Brouwer A, Barelds RJ, de Leeuw AM, Blauw E, Plas A, Yap SH, van den Broek AMWC, Knook DL (1988a) Isolation and culture of Kupffer cells from human liver. Ultrastrucure, endocytosis and prostaglandin synthesis. *J Hepatol* 6: 36-49.

Brouwer A, Wisse E, Knook DL (1988b) Sinusoidal endothelial cells and perisinusoidal fat-storing cells. In: Arias IM, Jakoby WB, Popper H, Schachter D, Sgfritz DA (eds) The Liver: *Biology and Pahtobiology 2nd edn Raven Press,* New York, pp 665-682.

Brown DA (2001) Lipid droplets: proteins floating on a pool of fat. *Curr Biol* 11:R446-R449.

Bucala R, Spiegel LA, Chesney J, Hogan M, Cerami A (1994) Circulating fibrocytes define a new leucocyte subpopulation that mediate tissue repair. *Mol Med* 1: 71-81.

Buniatian G, Gebhardt R, Schrenk D, Hamprecht B (1996) Colocalization of three types of intermediate filament proteins in perisinusopidal stellate cells: glial fibrillary acidic protein as a new cellular marker. *Eur J Cell Biol* 70: 23-32.

Burgess HA, Daugherty LE, Thatcher TH, Lakatos HF, Ray DFM, Redonett M, Phipps RP, Sime PJ (2005) PPAR□ agonists inhibit TGF-β induced pulmonary myofibroblast differentiation and collagen production: implications for thertapy of lung fibrosis. *Am J Physiol Lung Cell Mol Physiol* 288: L1146-L1153.

Burkel WE, Low FN (1966) The fine structure of rat liver sinusoids, space of Dissé and associated tissue space. *Am J Anat* 118: 769-784.

Båvik CO, Busch C, Eriksson U (1992) Characterization of a plasma retinol-binding protein membrane receptor expressed in the retinal pigment epithelium. *J Biol Chem* 267: 23035-23042.

Båvik CO, Eriksson U, Allen RA, Peterson PA (1991) Identification and partial characterization of a retinal pigment epithelial membrane receptor for plasma retinol-binding protein. *J Biol Chem* 266: 14978-14985.

Båvik CO, Levy F, Hellman U, Wernstedt C, Eriksson U (1993) The retinal pigment epithelial membrane receptor for plasma retinol-binding protein. *J Biol Chem* 268: 20540-20546.

Calvo M, Tebar F, Lopez-Iglesias I, Enrich C (2001) Morphologic and functional characterization of caveolae in rat liver hepatocytes. *Hepatology* 33: 1259-1269.

Canbay A, Taimr P, Torok N, Higuchi H, Friedman S, Gores GJ (2003) Apoptotic body engulfment by a human stellate cell line is profibrogenic. *Lab Invest* 83:655–663.

Carloni V, Ramanelli RG, Pinzani M, Laffi G, Gentilini P (1996) Expression and function of integrin receptors for collagen and laminin in cultured human hepatic stelate cells. *Gastroenterology* 110: 1127-1136.

Carlson BM (1999) Human Embryology & Developmental Biology 2nd edn Mosby, St.Louis.

Cases S, Smith SJ, Zheng YW, Myers HM, Lear SR, Sande E, Novak S, Collins C, Welch CB, Lusis AJ, Erickson SK, Farese RV Jr! (1998) Identification of a gene encoding an acyl CoA: diacylglycerol acyltransferase, a key enzyme in triacylglycerol synthesis. *Proc Natl Acad Sci USA* 95:13018-13023.

Casini A, Ceni E, Salzano R, Schuppan D, Milani S, Pellegrini G, Surrenti C (1994) Regulation of undulin synthesis and gene expression in human fat-storing cells by acetaldehyde and transforming growth factor-β1: Comparison with fibronectin. *Biochem Biophys Res Commun* 199: 1019-1026.

Cassiman D, Barlow A, Borght SV, Libbrecht L, Pachnis V (2006) Hepatic stellate cells do not derive from the neural crest. *J Hepatol* 44: 1098-1104.

Cassiman D, Denef C, Desmet VJ, Roskams T (2001a) Human and rat hepatic stellate cells express neurotrophions and neurotrophin receptors. *Hepatology* 33: 148-158.

Cassiman D, Libbrecht L, Desmet V, Denef C, Roskams T (2002) Hepatic stellate cell/myofibroblast subpopulations in fibrotic human and rat livers. *J Hepatol* 36: 200-209.

Cassiman D, Roskams T (2002) Beauty is in the eye of the beholder: emerging concepts and pitfalls in hepatic stellate cell research. *J Hepatol* 37: 527-535.

Cassiman D, Roskams T, van Pelt J, Libbrecht L, Aertsen P, Crabbé T, Vankelecom H, Denef C (2001b) Alpha B-crystallin expression in human and rat hepatic stellate cells. *J Hepatol* 35: 200-207.

Cassiman D, van Pelt J, De Vos R, Van Lommel F, Desmet V, Yap S-H, Roskams T (1999) Synaptophysin: A novel marker for human and rat hepatic stellate cells. *Am J Pathol* 155: 1831-1839.

Chang CS, Kokontis J, Liao ST (1988) Molecular cloning of human and rat complementary DNA encoding androgen receptors. *Science* 240:324-326.

Chawla A, Repa JJ, Evans RM, Mangelsdorf DJ (2001) Nuclear receptors and lipid physiology: Opening the X-files. *Science* 294: 1866-1870.

Chen A, Davis BH (2000) The DNA binding protein BTEB mediates acetaldehyde-induced, jun N-terminal kinase-dependent α(I) collagen gene expression in rat hepatic stellate cells. *Mol Cell Biol* 20:2818-2826.

Chen PS, Zhai WR, Zhou XM, Zhang JS, Zhang YE, Ling YQ, Gu YH (2001) Effects of hypoxia, hyperoxia on the regulation of expression and activity of matrix metalloproteinase-2 in hepatic stellate cells. *World J Gastroenterol* 7:647-651.

Chen C, Zhang J, Li J, Huang J, Yang C, Huang G, Shi J (2004) Hydrodynamic-based in vivo transfection of retinoic X receptor-α gene can enhance vitamin A-induced attenuation of liver fibrosis in mice. *Liver Int* 24: 679-686.

Chiang JY (2002) Bile acid regulation of gene expression: roles of nuclear hormone receptors. *Endocr Rev* 23:443-463.

Cho YM, Youn B-S, Lee H, Lee N, Min S-S, Kwak SH, Lee HK, Park KS (2006) Plasma retinol-binding protein-4 concentrations are elevated in human subjects with impaired glucose tolerance and type 2 diabetes. *Diabetes Care* 29:2457-2461.

Choi SH, Lee YJ, Park YJ, Kim KW, Lee EJ, Lim S, Park DJ, Kim SE, Park KS, Jang HC, Cho BY (2008) Retinol binding protein-4 elevation is associated with serum thyroid-stimulating hormone level independently of obesity in elderly subjects with normal glucose tolerance. *J Clin Endocr Metabol* 93: 2313-2318.

Chytil F (1992) The lungs and vitamin A. *Am J Physiol Lung Cell Mol Physiol* 262: L517-L527.

Clark EA, Brugge JS (1995) Integrins and signal transduction pathways: the road taken. *Science* 268: 1995.

Clement B, Grimaud JA, Campion JP, Deugnier Y, Guillouzo A (1986) Cell type involved in collagen and fibronectin production in normal and fibrotic human liver. *Hepatology* 6: 225-234.

Cogger VC, Warren A, Fraser R, Ngu M, McLean AJ, Le Couteur DG (2003) Hepatic sinusoidal pseudocapillarization with aging in the non-human primate. *Exp Gerontol* 38: 1101-1107.

Collardeau-Frachon S, Scoazec J-Y (2008) Vascular development and differentiation during human liver organogenesis. *Anat Rec* 291: 614-627.

Conneely OM, Sullivan WP, Toft DO, Birnbaumer M, Cook RG, Maxwell BL, Zarucki-Schulz T, Greene GL, Schrader WT, O'Malley BW (1986) Molecular cloning of the chicken progesterone receptor. *Science* 233:767-770.

Corpechot C, Barbu V, Wendum D, Kinnman N, Rey C, Poupon R, Housset C, Rosmorduc O (2002) Hypoxia-induced VEGF and collagen I expressions are associated with angiogenesis and fibrogenesis in experimental cirrhosis. *Hepatology* 35: 1010-1021.

Critchley DR (2000) Focal adhesions-the cytoskeletal connection. *Curr Opin Cell Biol* 12: 133-139.

Cukierman E, Pankov R, Stevens DR, Yamada KM (2001) Taking cell-matrix adhesion to the third dimension. *Science* 294: 1708-1712.

Da Silva Morais A, Abarca-Quinones J, Horsmans Y, Starkel P, Leclercq IA (2007) Peroxisome proliferated-activated receptor γ ligand, Pioglitazone, does not prevent hepatic fibrosis in mice. *Int J Mol Med* 19:105-112.

Dack CL, Day CO, Johnson SJ, Burt AD (1997) Population kinetics of GFAP-positive cells following experimental acute liver injury. In: Wisse E, Knook DL, Balabaud C (eds) Cells Hepatic Sinusoid, vol 6. *Kupffer Cell Foundation, Leiden,* pp 59-61.

Davis BH (1988) Transforming growth factor β responsiveness is modulated by extracellular collagen matrix during hepatic Ito cell culture. *J Cell Physiol* 136: 547-553.

Davis BH, Chen A, Beno DWA (1996) Raf and mitogen-activated protein kinase regulate stellate cell collagen gene expression. *J Biol Chem* 271: 11039-11042.

Davis BH, Pratt BM, Madri JA (1987) Retinol and extracellular collagen matrices modulate hepatic Ito cell collagen phenotype and cellular retinol binding protein levels. *J Biol Chem* 262: 10280-10286.

Davis BH, Vucic A (1988) The effect of retinol on ito cell proliferation in vitro. *Hepatology* 8: 788-793.

Davis BH, Vucic A (1989) Modulation of vitamin A metabolism during hepatic and intestinal culture. *Biochem Biophys Acta* 1010: 318-324.

de Leeuw AM, Barelds RJ, de Zanger R, Knook DL (1982) Primary culture of endothelial cells of the rat liver. A model for ultrastructural and functional studies. *Cell Tiss Res* 223: 201-215.

de Leeuw AM, McCarthy SP, Geerts A, Knook DL (1984) Purified rat liver fat-storing cells in culture divide and contain collagen. *Hepatology* 4: 392-403.

De Minicis S, Brenner DA (2007) NOX in liver fibrosis. *Archiv Biochem Biophys,* 462: 266-272.

Desmoulière A (2007) Hepatic stellate cells: The only cells involved in liver fibrogenesis? A dogma challenged. *Gastroenterology* 132: 2059-2062.

Desmoulière A, Darby IA, Gabbiani G (2003) Normal and pathologic soft tissue remodeling: Role of the myofibroblast, with special emphasis on liver and kidney fibrosis. *Lab Invest* 83:1689–1707.

Desmoulière A, Xu G, Costa AMA, Yousef IM, Gabbiani G, Tuchweber B (1999) Effect of pentoxifylline on early proliferation and phenotypic modulation of fibrogenic cells in two rat models of liver fibrosis and on cultured hepatic stellate cells. *J Hepatol* 30: 621-631.

Dewailly E, Nantel A, Weber J-P, Meyer F (1989) High levels of PCBs in breast milk of Inuit women from arctic Quebec. *Bull Environ Contam Toxicol* 43: 641-646.

Dirami G, Massaro GD, Clerch LB, Ryan US, Reczek PR, Massaro D (2004) Lung retinol storing cells synthesize and secrete retinoic acid, an inducer of alveolus formation. *Am J Physiol Cell Mol Physiol* 286: L249-L256.

Dong D, Ruuska SE, Levinthal DJ, Noy N (1999) Distinct roles for cellular retinoic acid-binding proteins I and II in regulating signaling by retinoic acid. *J Biol Chem* 274: 23695-23698.

Dooley S, Hamzavi J, Breitkopf K, Wiercinska E, Said HM, Lorenzen J, Dijke PT, Gressner AM (2003) Smad7 prevents activation of hepatic stellate cells and liver fibrosis in rats. *Gastroenterology* 125: 178-191.

Drummond JC, Bell ME (1935) Observation of the absorption of carotene and vitamin A. *British Med J* 1:1208-1210.

Du Bois AM (1968) The embryonic liver. In: Rouiller CH (ed) The Liver, vol 1, *Academic Press,* New York, pp 1-39.

Duffield JS, Forbes SJ, Constandinou CM, Clay S, Partolina M, Vuthoori S, Wu S, Lang R, Iredale JP (2005) Selective depletion of macrophages reveals distinct, opposing roles during liver injury and repair. *J Clin Invest* 115: 56-65.

During A, Harrison EH (2007) Mechanisms of provitamin A (carotenoid) and vitamin A (retinol) transport into and out of intestinal Caco-2 cells. *J Lipid Res* 48: 2283-2294.

Elias H (1955) Origin and early development of the liver in various vertebrates. *Acta Hepatologica* 3: 1-56.

Elices MJ, Hemler ME (1989) The human integrin VLA-2 is a collagen receptor on some cells and a collagen/laminin receptor on others. *Proc Natl Acad Sci USA* 86: 9906-9910.

Elsharkawy AM, Wright MC, Hay RT, Arthur MJ, Hughes T, Bahr MJ, Degitz K, Mann DA (1999) Persistent activation of nuclear factor-B in cultured rat hepatic stellate cells involves the induction of potentially novel rel-like factors and prolonged changes in the expression of IB family proteins. *Hepatology* 30: 761-769.

Emsley J, Knight CG, Farndale RW, Barnes MJ, Liddington RC (2000) Structural basis of collagen recognition by integrin α2β1. *Cell* 101: 47-56.

Enzan H, Himeno H, Hiroi M, Kiyoku H, Saibara T, Onishi S (1997) Development of hepatic sinusoidal structure with special reference to the Ito cells. *Micros Res Tech* 39: 336-349.

Enzan H, Himeno H, Iwamura S, Onishi S, Saibara T, Yamamoto Y, Hara H (1994a) α-Smooth muscle actin-positive perisinusoidal stromal cells in human hepatocellular carcinoma. *Hepatology* 19: 895-903.

Enzan H, Himeno H, Iwamura S, Saibara T, Onishi S, Yamamoto Y, Hara H (1994b) Immunohistochemical identification of Ito cells and their myofibroblastic transformation in adult human liver. *Virchows Arch* 424:249-256.

Eriksson U, Das K, Busch C, Nordlinder H, Rask L, Sundelin J, Sallstrom J, Peterson PA (1984) Cellular retinol-binding protein. Quantitation and distribution. *J Biol Chem* 259: 13464-13470.

Erickson N, Mohanty SK, Shivakumar P, Sabla G, Chakraborty R, Bezerra JA (2008) Temporal-spatial activation of apoptosis and epithelial injury in murine experimental biliary atresia. *Hepatology* 47:1567-1577.

Everett L, Galli A, Crabb D (2000) The role of hepatic peroxisome proliferator-activated receptors (PPARs) in health and disease. *Liver* 20:191-199.

Fallowfield JA, Iredale JP (2003) Reversal of liver fibrosis and cirrhosis – an emerging reality. *Scottish Med* J 49: 3-6.

Fawcett DW (1986) Bloom and Fawcett A Textbook of Histology, 11th edn *W. S. Saunders,* Philadelphia.

Febbraio M, Hajjar DP, Silverstein RL (2001) CD36: a class B scavenger receptor involved in angiogenesis, atherosclerosis, inflammation, and lipid metabolism. *J Clin Invest* 108:785–791.

Fennekohl A, Schieferdecker HL, Jungermann K, Püschel GP (1999) Differential expression of prostanoid receptors in hepatocytes, Kupffer cells, sinusoidal endothelial cells and stellate cells of rat liver. *J Hepatol* 30: 38-47.

Fimmel CJ, Brown KE, O'Neill R, Kladney RD (1996) Complement C4 protein expression by rat hepatic stellate cells. *J Immunol* 157: 2601-2609.

Fiorucci S, Antonelli E, Distrutti E, Severino B, Fiorentina R, Baldoni M, Caliendo G, Santagada V, Morelli A, Cirino G (2004a) PAR1 antagonism protects against experimental liver fibrosis. Role of proteinase receptors in stellate cell activation. *Hepatology* 39: 365-375.

Fiorucci S, Antonelli E, Rizzo G, Renga B, Mencarelli A, Riccardi L, Orlandi S, Pellicciari R, Morelli A (2004b) The nuclear receptor SHP mediates inhibition of hepatic stellate cells by FXR and protects against liver fibrosis. *Gastroenterology* 127:1497-1512.

Fiorucci S, Rizzo G, Antonelli E, Renga B, Mencarelli A, Riccardi L, Morelli A, Pruzanski M, Pellicciari R (2005a) Cross-talk between farnesoid-X-receptor (FXR) and peroxisome proliferator-activated receptor γ contributes to the antifibrotic activity of FXR ligands in rodent models of liver cirrhosis. *J Pharmacol Exp Ther* 315:58-68.

Fiorucci S, Rizzo G, Antonelli E, Renga B, Mencarelli A, Riccardi L, Orlandi S, Pruzanski M, Morelli A, Pellicciari R (2005b) A farnesoid x receptor-small heterodimer partner regulatory cascade modulates tissue metalloproteinase inhibitor-1 and matrix metalloprotease expression in hepatic stellate cells and promotes resolution of liver fibrosis. *J Pharmacol Exp Ther* 314:584-595.

Fischer R, Cariers A, Reinehr R, Håussinger D (2002) Caspase 9-dependent killing of hepatic stellate cells by activated Kupffer cells. *Gastroenterology* 123: 845-861.

Fischer R, Reinehr R, Lu TP, Schönicke A, Warskulat U, Dienes HP, Häussinger D (2005) Intercellular communication via gap junctions in activated rat hepatic stellate cells. *Gastroenterology* 128: 433-448.

Fortuna VA, Trugo LC, Borojevic R (2001) Acyl-CoA: retinol acyltransferase (ARAT) and lecithin:retinol acyltransferase (LRAT) activation during the lipocyte phenotype induction in hepatic stellate cells. *J Nutr Biochem* 12: 610-621.

Friedman SL (1993) The cellular basis of hepatic fibrosis -- Mechanisms and treatment strategies. *New Engl J Med* 328:1828-1835.

Friedman SL (2000) Molecular regulation of hepatic fibrosis, an integrated cellular response to tissue injury. *J Biol Chem* 275: 2247-2250.

Friedman SL (2003) Liver fibrosis – from bench to bedside. *J Hepatol* 38: S38-S53.

Friedman SL (2004) Stellate cells: A moving target in hepatic fibrogenesis. *Hepatology* 40: 1041-1043.

Friedman SL (2006) Transcriptional regulation of stellate cell activation. *J Gastroenterol Hepatol* 21: S79-S83.

Friedman SL (2008a) Mechanisms of hepatic fibrogenesis. *Gastroenterology* 134: 1655-1669.

Friedman SL (2008b) Hepatic stellate cells: protean, multifunctional, and enigmatic cells of the liver. *Physiol Rev* 88:125-172.

Friedamn SL, Arthur MJP (1989) Activation of cultured rat hepatic lipocytes by Kupffer cell conditioned medium. J Clin Invest 84: 1780-1785.

Friedman SL, Arthur MJP (2002) Reversing hepatic fibrosis. *Science & Medicine* 8: 194-205.

Friedman SL, Bansal MB (2006) Reversal of hepatic fibrosis - Fact or fantasy? *Hepatology* 43: S82 - S88.

Friedman SL, Rockey DC, Bissell DM (2007) Hepatic fibrosis 2006: Report of the third AASLD Single Topic Conference. *Hepatology* 45: 242-249.

Friedamn SL, Rockey DC, McGuire RF, Maher JJ, Boyles JK, Yamasaki G (1992) Isolated hepatic lipocytes and Kupffer cells from normal human liver: Morphological and functional characteristics in primary culture. *Hepatology* 15: 234.

Friedman SL, Roll FJ, Bissell DM (1989b) Autocrine regulation of lipocyte matrix production: Activation by extracellular matrix. In: Wisse E, Knook DL, Decker K (eds) *Cells Hepatic Sinusoid vol 2, Kupffer Cell Foundation, Rijswijk,* pp 61-63.

Friedamn SL, Roll FJ, Boyles J, Arenson DM, Bissell DM (1989a) Maintenance of differentiated phenotype of cultured rat hepatic lipocytes by basement membrane matrix. *J Biol Chem* 264: 10756-10762.

Friedman SL, Roll FJ, Boyles J, Bissell DM (1985) Hepatic lipocytes: The principal collagen-producing cells of normal rat liver. *Proc Natl Acad Sci USA* 82: 8681-8685.

Friedman SL, Wei S, Blaner WS (1993) Retinol release by activated rat hepatic lipocytes: regulation by Kupffer cell-conditioned medium and PDGF. *Am J Physiol Gastrointest Liver Physiol* 264: G947-G952.

Fuja TJ, Prost-Fuja MN, Titze IR (2005) Transdifferentiation of vocal-fold stellate cells and all-*trans* retinol-induced deactivation. *Cell Tiss Res* 322: 417-424.

Fuja TJ, Probst-Fuja MN, Titze IR (2006) Changes in expression of extracellular matrix genes, fibrogenic factors, and actin cytoskeletal organization in retinol treated and untreated vocal fold stellate cells. *Matrix Biology* 25: 59-67.

Fujimoto T, Ohsaki Y (2006) Cytoplasmic lipid droplets: rediscovery of an old structure as a unique platform. *Ann NY Acad Sci* 1086:104-115.

Fujimoto T, Ohsaki Y, Cheng J, Suzuki M, Shinohara Y (2008) Lipid droplets: a classic organelle with new outfits. *Histochem Cell Biol* 130:263-279.

Fujisawa G, Muto S, Okada K, Kusano E, Ishibashi S (2006) Mineralocorticoid receptor antagonist spironolactone prevents pig serum-induced hepatic fibrosis in rats. *Transl Res* 148:149-156.

Fukuda-Taira S (1981) Hepatic induction in the avian embryo: Specificity of reactive endoderm and inductive mesoderm. *J Embryol Exp Morphol* 63: 111-125.

Fukushima M, Enjoji M, Kohjima M, Sugimoto R, Ohta S, Kotoh K, Kuniyoshi M, Kobayashi K, Imamura M, Inoguchi T, Nakamuta M, Nawata H (2005) Adipose differentiation related protein induces lipid accumulation and lipid droplet formation in hepatic stellate cells. *In Vitro Cell Dev Biol Anim* 41:321-324.

Galli A, Crabb DW, Ceni E, Salzano R, Mello T, Svegliati-Baroni G, Ridolfi F, Trozzi L, Surrenti C, Casini A (2002) Antidiabetic thiazolidinediones inhibit collagen synthesis and hepatic stellate cell activation in vivo and in vitro. *Gastroenterology* 122:1924-1940.

Galli A, Crabb D, Price D, Ceni E, Salzano R, Surrenti C, Casini A (2000) Peroxisome proliferator-activated receptor γ transcriptional regulation is involved in platelet-derived growth factor-induced proliferation of human hepatic stellate cells. *Hepatology* 31:101-108.

Gallois C, Habib A, Tao J, Moulin S, Maclouf J, Mallat A, Lotersztajn S (1998) Role of NFκB in the antiproliferative effect of endothelin-1 and tumor necrosis factor-α in human hepatic stellate cells. *J Biol Chem* 273: 23183-23190.

Gao JG, Simon M (2006) Molecular screening for GS2 lipase regulators: inhibition of keratinocyte retinylester hydrolysis by TIP47. *J Invest Dermatol* 126:2087-2095.

Gard AL, White FP, Dutton GR (1985) Extra-neural glial fibrillary acidic protein (GFAP) immunoreactivity in perisinusoidal stellate cells of rat liver. *J Neuroimmunol* 8:359-375.

Gascon-Barre M, Demers C, Mirshahi A, Neron S, Zalzal S, Nanci A (2003) The normal liver harbors the vitamin D nuclear receptor in nonparenchymal and biliary epithelial cells. *Hepatology* 37:1034-1042.

Geerts A (2004) On the origin of stellate cells: mesodermal, endodermal or neuro-ectodermal? *J Hepatol,* 40: 331-334.

Geerts A, Bleser PD, Hautekeete ML, Niki T, Wisse E (1994) Fat-storing (Ito) cell biology. In: Arias IA, Boyer JL, Fausto N, Jakoby WB, Schachter

DA, Shafritz DA (eds) *The Liver: Biology and Pathobiology, Raven Press,* New York, pp 819-838.

Geerts A, Bouwens L, Wisse E (1990) Ultrastructure and function of hepatic fat-storing and pit cells. *J Electron Microsc Tech* 14:247-256.

Geerts A, Geuze HJ, Slot JW, Voss B, Schuppan D, Schellinck P, Wisse E (1986) Immunogold localization of procollagen III, fibronectin and heparan sulfate proteoglycan on ultrathin frozen sections of the normal rat liver. *Histochemistry* 84: 355-362.

Geerts A, Schuppan D, Lazeroms S, De Zanger R, Wisse E (1990) Collagen type I and III occur together in hybrid fibrils in the space of Disse of normal rat liver. *Hepatology* 12: 233-241.

Ghyselinck NB, Båvik C, Sapin V, Mark M, Bonnier D, Hindelang C, Dierich A, Nilsson CB, Håkansson H, Sauvant P, Azaïs-Braesco V, Frasson M, Picaud S, Chambon P (1999) Cellular retinol-binding protein I is essential for vitamin A homeostasis. *EMBO J* 18: 4903–4914.

Giancotti FG (2000) Complexity and specificity of integrin signaling. *Nature Cell Biol* 2: E13-14.

Giancotti FG, Ruoslahti E (1999) Integrin signaling. *Science* 285: 1028-1032.

Gjøen T, Bjerkelund T, Blomhoff HK, Norum KR, Berg T, Blomhoff R (1987) Liver takes up retinol-binding protein from plasma. *J Biol Chem* 262: 10926-10930.

Gnainsky Y, Spira G, Paizi M, Bruck R, Nagler A, Abu-Amara SN, Geiger B, Genina O, Monsonego-Ornan E, Pines M (2004) Halofuginone, an inhibitor of collagen synthesis by rat stellate cells, stimulates insulin-like growth factor binding protein-1 synthesis by hepatocytes. *J Hepatol* 40: 269-277.

Goodman DW (1984) Plasma retinol-binding protein. In: Sporn MB, Roberts AB, Goodman DS (eds) *The Retinoids vol 2, Academic Press,* New York, pp 41-88.

Goodman DS, Blomstrand R, Werner B, Huang HS, Shiratori T (1966) The intestinal absorption and metabolism of vitamin A and β-carotene in man. *J Clin Invest* 45: 1615-162.

Grab B, Miles AJ, Furcht LT, Fields GB (1996) Promotion of fibroblast adhesion by triple-helical peptide models of type I collagen-derived sequences. *J Biol Chem* 271: 12234-12240.

Graham TE, Yang Q, Blüher M, Hammarstedt A, Ciaraldi TP, Henry RR, Wason CJ, Oberbach A, Jansson P-A, Smith U, Kahn BB (2006) Retinol-binding protein 4 and insulin resistance in lean, obese, and diabetic subjects. *New Eng J Med* 354:2552-2563.

Green S, Walter P, Kumar V, Krust A, Bornert JM, Argos P, Chambon P (1986) Human oestrogen receptor cDNA: sequence, expression and homology to v-erb-A. *Nature* 320:134-139.

Greenberg AS, Egan JJ, Wek SA, Garty NB, Blanchette-Mackie EJ, Londos C (1991) Perilipin, a major hormonally regulated adipocyte-specific phosphoprotein associated with the periphery of lipid storage droplets. *J Biol Chem* 266:11341-11346.

Greenberg AS, Egan JJ, Wek SA, Moos MC Jr, Londos C, Kimmel AR (1993) Isolation of cDNAs for perilipins A and B: sequence and expression of lipid droplet-associated proteins of adipocytes. *Proc Natl Acad Sci USA* 90:12035-12039.

Greene GL, Gilna P, Waterfield M, Baker A, Hort Y, Shine J (1986) Sequence and expression of human estrogen receptor complementary DNA. *Science* 231:1150-1154.

Greenwel P, Geerts A, Ogata I, Solis-Herruzo JA, Rojkind M (1994) Liver fibrosis. In: Arias IA, Boyer JL, Fausto N, Jakoby WB, Schachter DA, Shafritz DA (eds) The Liver: Biology and Pathobiology, *Raven Press,* New York, pp 1367-1380.

Greenwel P, Rubin J, Schwartz M, Hertzberg EL, Rojkind M (1993) Liver fat-storing cell clones obtained from a CCl_4-cirrhotic rat are heterogeneous with regard to proliferation, expression of extracellular matrix components, interleulin-6, and connexin 43. *Lab Invest* 69: 210-216.

Gressner AM, Bachem MG (1990) Cellular sources of noncollagenous matrix proteins: role of fat-storing cells in fibrogenesis. *Semin Liver Dis* 10: 30-46.

Gressner AM, Bachem MG (1995) Molecular mechanisms of liver fibrogenesis-A homage to the role of activated fat-storing cells. *Digestion* 56: 335-346.

Gressner AM, Krul N, Bachem MG (1994) Regulation of proteoglycan expression in fibrotic liver and cultured fat-storing cells. *Pathol Res Prac* 190: 864-882.

Grinnell F, Ho CH, Tamariz E, Lee DJ, Skuta G (2003) Dendritic fibroblasts in three-dimensional collagen matrices. *Mol Biol Cell* 14: 384-395.

Grizzi F, Francescini B, Gagliano N, Moscheni C, Annoni G, Vdrgani C, Hermonat PL, Chiriva-Internati M, Dioguardi N (2003) Mast cell density, hepatic stellate cell activation and TGF-β 1 transcripts in the aging Sprague-Dawley rat during early acute liver injury. *Toxicol Pathol* 31: 173-178.

Guimarães ELM, Franceschi MFS, Andrade CBM, Guaragna RM, Borojevic R, Margis R, Bernard EA, Guma FCR (2007) Hepatic stellate cell line modulates lipogenic transcription factors. *Liver Int* 27: 1255-1264.

Guo YT, Leng XS, Li T, Peng JR, Song SH, Xiong LF, Qin ZZ (2005) Effect of ligand of peroxisome proliferator-activated receptor on the biological characters of hepatic stellate cells. *World J Gastroenterol* 11:4735-4739.

Guyot C, Lepreux S, Combe C, Doudnikoff E, Bioulac-Sage P, Balabaud C, Desmoulière A (2006) Hepatic fibrosis and cirrhosis: The (myo)fibroblastic cell subpopulations involved. *Int J Biochem Cell Biol* 38: 135-151.

Gäbele E, Reif S, Tsukada S, Bataller R, Yata Y, Morris T, Schrum LW, Brenner DA, Rippe RA (2005) The role of p70S6K in hepatic stellate cell collagen gene expression and cell proliferation. *J Biol Chem* 280: 13374-13382.

Haber PS, Keogh GW, Apte MV, Moran CS, Stewart NL, Crawford DHG, Pirola RC, McCaughan GW, Ramm GA, Wilson JS (1999) Activation of pancreatic stellate cells in human and experimental pancreatic fibrosis. *Am J Pathol* 155:1087-109.

Hammel P, Couvelard A, O'Toole D, Ratouis A, Sauvanet A, Flejou JF, Degott C, Belghiti J, Bernades P, Valla D, Ruszniewski P, Levy P (2001) Regression of liver fibrosis after biliary drainage in patients with chronic pancreatitis and stenosis of the common bile duct. *New Engl J Med* 344:418-423.

Hamy F, Verwaerde P, Helbecque N, Formstecher P, Henichart JP (1991) Nuclear targeting of a viral-cointernalized protein by a short signal sequence from human retinoic acid receptors. *Bioconjug Chem* 2:375-378.

Harada K, Sato Y, Isse K, Ikeda H, Nakanuma Y (2008) Induction of innate immune response and absence of subsequent tolerance to dsRNA in biliary epithelial cells relate to the pathogenesis of biliary atresia. *Liver Int* 28:614-621.

Hartland SN, Murphy F, Aucott RL, Abergel A, Zhou X, Waung J, Patel N, Bradshaw C, Collins J, Mann D, Benyon RC, Iredale JP (2009) Active matrix metalloproteinase-2 promotes apoptosis of hepatic stellate cells via the cleavage of cellular N-cadherin. *Liver Int* 29: 966-978.

Hata R (1996) Where am I? How a cell recognizes its positional information during morphogenesis. *Cell Biol Int* 20: 59-65.

Hata R, Nagai Y (1980) Differentiation of hepatocytes into type I collagen producing cells during primary culture in the presence of aphidicolin (inhibitor of DNA polymerase alpha). *Biochem Int* 1: 567-573.

Hata R, Ninomiya Y (1984) Hepatocytes (hepatic parenchymal cells) produce a major part of liver collagen in vivo. *Biochem Int* 8: 181-186.

Hata R, Ninomiya Y, Nagai Y, Sakakibara K, Tsukada Y (1978) Active synthesis of collagen by albumin-producing liver parenchymal cell clones in culture. *Proc Japan Acad* 54 Ser B: 391-396.

Hata R, Ninomiya Y, Nagai Y, Tsukada Y (1980) Biosynthesis of interstitial type of collagen by albumin-producing rat liver parenchymal cell (hepatocyte) clones in culture. *Biochemistry* 19: 169-176.

Hata R, Senoo H (1989) L-Ascorbic acid 2-phosphate stimulates collagen accumulation, cell proliferation, and formation of a three-dimensional tissuelike substance by skin fibroblast. *J Cell Physiol* 138: 8-16.

Hata R, Senoo H (1992) Extracellular matrix system regulates cell growth, tissue formation, and cellular functions. *Tiss Cult Res Commun* 11: 337-343.

Haughton EL, Tucker SJ, Marek CJ, Durward E, Leel V, Bascal Z, Monaghan T, Koruth M, Collie-Duguid E, Mann DA, Trim JE, Wright MC (2006) Pregnane X receptor activators inhibit human hepatic stellate cell transdifferentiation in vitro. *Gastroenterology* 131:194-209.

Hazra S, Xiong S, Wang J, Rippe RA, Krishna V, Chatterjee K, Tsukamoto H (2004) Peroxisome proliferator-activated receptor γ induces a phenotypic switch from activated to quiescent hepatic stellate cells. *J Biol Chem* 279:11392-11401.

Heid HW, Moll R, Schwetlick I, Rackwitz HR, Keenan TW (1998) Adipophilin is a specific marker of lipid accumulation in diverse cell types and diseases. *Cell Tiss Res* 294:309-321.

Hellemans K, Grinko I, Rombouts K, Schuppan D, Geerts A (1999) All-*trans* and 9-*cis* retinoic acid alter rat hepatic stellate cell phenotype differentially. *Gut* 45:134-142.

Hellemans K, Michalik L, Dittie A, Knorr A, Rombouts K, De Jong J, Heirman C, Quartier E, Schuit F, Wahli W, Geerts A (2003a) Peroxisome proliferator-activated receptor-β signaling contributes to enhanced proliferation of hepatic stellate cells. *Gastroenterology* 124:184-201.

Hellemans K, Rombouts K, Quartier E, Dittie AS, Knorr A, Michalik L, Rogiers V, Schuit F, Wahli W, Geerts A (2003b) PPARβ regulates vitamin A metabolism-related gene expression in hepatic stellate cells undergoing activation. *J Lipid Res* 44:280-295.

Hellemans K, Verbuyst P, Quartier E, Schuit F, Rombouts K, Chandraratna RA, Schuppan D, Geerts A (2004) Differential modulation of rat hepatic stellate phenotype by natural and synthetic retinoids. *Hepatology* 39:97-108.

Hellerbrand C, Jobin C, Licato LL, Sartor RB, Brenner DA (1998) Cytokines induce NF-κB in activated but not in quiescent rat hepatic stellate cells. *Am J Physiol Gastrointest Liver Physiol* 275: G269-G278.

Hellerbrand C, Wang S C, Tsukamoto H, Brenner DA, Rippe R (1996) Expression of intercellular adhesion molecule 1 by activated hepatic stellate cells. *Hapatology* 24: 670-676.

Hendriks HFJ, Blaner WS, Wennekers HM, Piantedosi R, Brouwer A, de Leeuw AM, Goodman DS, Knook DL (1988) Distribution of retinoids, retinoid-binding proteins and related parameters in different types of liver cells isolated from young and old rats. *Eur J Biochem* 171: 237-244.

Hendriks HFJ, Brouwer A, Knook DL (1987) The role of hepatic fat-storing (stellate) cells in retinoid metabolism. *Hepatology* 7: 1368-1371.

Hendriks HFJ, Brouwer A, Knook DL (1990) Isolation, purification, and characterization of liver cell types. *Methods Enzymol* 190: 49-58.

Hendriks HFJ, Verhoofstad WAMM, Brouwer A, de Leeuw AM, Knook DL (1985) Perisinusoidal fat-storing cells are the main vitamin A storing sites in rat liver. *Exp Cell Res* 160: 138-149.

Hepatic stellate cell nomenclature [letter] (1996) *Hepatology* 23: 193.

Hiagashi N, Kojima N, Miura M, Imai K, Sato M, Senoo H (2004) Cell-cell junctions between mammalian (human and rat) hepatic stellate cells. *Cell Tiss Res* 317: 35-43.

Higashi N, Sato M, Kojima N, Irie T, Kawamura K, Mabuchi A, Senoo H (2005a) Vitamin A storage in hepatic stellate cells in the regenerating rat liver --with special reference to zonal heterogeneity--. *Anat Rec* 286A: 899-907.

Higashi N, Senoo H (2003) Distribution of vitamin A-storing lipid droplets in hepatic stellate cells in liver lobules-A comparative study-. *Anat Rec* Part A 271: 240-248.

Higashi N, Wake K, Sato M, Kojima N, Imai K, Senoo H (2005b) Degradation of extracellular matrix by extrahepatic stellate cells in the intestine of the lamprey, *Lampetra japonica*. *Anat Rec* 285A: 668-675.

Higashiyama R, Inagaki Y, Hong YY, Kushida M, Nakao S, Niioka M, Watanabe T, Okano H, Matsuzaki Y, Shiota G, Okazaki I (2007) Bone marrow-derived cells express matrix metalloproteinases and contribute to regression of liver fibrosis in mice. *Hepatology* 45: 213-222.

Hirosawa K (1977) A note on autoradiography; An introduction of vitamin A-storing cells. *Acta Histochem Cytochem* 10: 253-259.

Hirosawa K, Kokubo Y, Kitamura M, Shiraishi T (1988) Fine structure of intestinal fibroblasts: Autoradiographic and three-dimensional studies. *J Electron Microsc* 37: 219-228.

Hirosawa K, Yamada E (1973) The localization of the vitamin A in the mouse liver as revealed by electron microscope radioautography. *J Electron Microsc* 22: 337-346.

Holden C (1998) Polar bears and PCBs. *Science* 280: 2053.

Hollander D, Muralidhara KS (1977) Vitamin A1 intestinal absorption in vivo: influence of luminal factors on transport. *Am J Physiol* 232:F471-F477.

Hollenberg SM, Weinberger C, Ong ES, Cerelli G, Oro A, Lebo R, Thompson EB, Rosenfeld MG, Evans RM (1985) Primary structure and expression of a functional human glucocorticoid receptor cDNA. *Nature* 318:635-641.

Hong F, Tuyama A, Lee TF, Loke J, Agarwal R, Cheng X, Garg A, Fiel MI, Schwartz M, Walewski J, Branch A, Schecter AD, Bansal MB (2009) Hepatic stellate cells express functional CXCR4: Role in stromsl cell-derived factor-1a-mediated stellate cell activation. *Hepatology* 49: 2055-2067.

Hynes RO (1992) Integrins: Versatility, modulation, and signaling in cell adhesion. *Cell* 69: 11-25.

Igarashi M, Yogiashi Y, Mihara M, Takada I, Kitagawa H, Kato S (2007) Vitamin K induces osteoblast differentiation through pregnane X receptor-mediated transcriptional control of the Msx2 gene. *Mol Cell Biol* 27:7947-7954.

Ikeda H, Fujiwara K (1995) Cyclosporin A and FK-506 in inhibition of rat ito cell activation in vitro. *Hepatology* 21: 1161-1166.

Ikejima K, Takei Y, Honda H, Hirose M, Yoshikawa M, Zhang Y-J, Lang T, Fukuda T, Yamashina S, Kitamura T, Sato N (2002) Leptin receptor-mediated signaling regulates hepatic fibrogenesis and remodeling of extracellular matrix in the rat. *Gastroenterology* 122: 1399-1410.

Imai K, Sato M, Kojima N, Miura M, Matano Y, Senoo H (1997) Three-dimensional morphological changes in cultured hepatic stellate cells by type I collagen fibers. In: Wisse E, Knook DL, Balabaud C, (eds) Cells of the Hepatic Sinusoid, vol 6, *Kupffer Cell Foundation,* Leiden, pp 105-106.

Imai K, Sato M, Kojima N, Miura M, Sato T, Sugiyama T, Enomoto K, Senoo H (2000a) Storage of lipid droplets in and production of extracellular matrix by hepatic stellate cells (vitamin A-storing cells) in Long-Evans cinnamon-like colored (LEC) rats. *Anat Rec* 258: 338-348.

Imai K, Sato T, Senoo H (2000b) Adhesion between cells and exracellular matrix with special reference to hepatic stellate cell adhesion to three-dimensional collagen fibers. *Cell Struct Func* 25: 329-336.

Imai K, Senoo H (1998) Morphology of sites of adhesion between hepatic stellate cells (vitamin A-storing cells) and a three-dimensional extracellular matrix. *Anat Rec* 250: 430-437.

Imai K, Senoo H (2000) Morphology of sites of adhesion between extracellular matrix and hepatic stellate cells. *Connective Tissue* 32: 395-400.

Imanishi Y, Batten ML, Piston DW, Baehr W, Palczewski K (2004) Noninvasive two-photon imaging reveals retinyl ester storage structures in the eye. *J Cell Biol* 164:373-383.

Inagaki Y, Higashi K, Kushida M, Hong YY, Nakao S, Higashiyama R, Moro T, Itoh J, Mikami T, Kimura T, Shiota G, Kuwabara I, Okazaki I (2008) Hepatocyte growth factor suppresses profibrogenic signal transduction via nuclear export of Smad3 with galectin-7. *Gastroenterology* 134: 1180-1190.

Inagaki Y, Okazaki I (2007) Emerging insights into transforming growth factor β Smad signal in hepatic fibrogenesis. *Gut* 56: 284-292.

Ip E, Farrell G, Hall P, Robertson G, Leclercq I (2004) Administration of the potent PPARα agonist, Wy-14,643, reverses nutritional fibrosis and steatohepatitis in mice. *Hepatology* 39:1286-1296.

Iredale JP (1997) Tissue inhibitors of metalloproteinases in liver fibrosis. *Int J Biochem Cell Biol* 29: 43-54.

Iredale JP (2003a) Regulating hepatic inflammation: Pathogen-associated molecular patterns take their toll. *Hepatology* 37: 979-982.

Iredale JP (2003b) Cirrhosis: new research provides a basis for rational and targeted treatments. *British Med J* 327:143-147.

Iredale JP (2007) Models of liver fibrosis: exploring the dynamic nature of inflammation and repair in a solid organ. *J Clin Invest* 117: 539-548.

Iredale JP, Benyon RC, Pickering J, McCullen M, Northrop M, Pawley S, Hovell C, Arthur MJ (1998) Mechanisms of spontaneous resolution of rat liver fibrosis. Hepatic stellate cell apoptosis and reduced hepatic expression of metalloproteinase inhibitors. *J Clin Invest* 102: 538-549.

Irie T, Kajiwara S, Kojima N, Senoo H, Seki T (2004) Retinal is the essential form of retinoid for storage and transport in the adults of the ascidian *Halocynthia roretzi*. *Comp Biochem Physiol Part B* 139: 597-606.

Issa R, Williams E, Trim N, Kendall T, Arthur MJP, Reichen J, Benyon RC, Iredale JP (2001) Apoptosis of hepatic stellate cells: involvement in resolution of biliary fibrosis and regulation by soluble growth factors. *Gut* 48:548-557.

Itagaki T, Shimizu I, Cheng X, Yuan Y, Oshio A, Tamaki K, Fukuno H, Honda H, Okamura Y, Ito S (2005) Opposing effects of oestradiol and progesterone on intracellular pathways and activation processes in the oxidative stress induced activation of cultured rat hepatic stellate cells. *Gut* 54:1782-1789.

Ito T (1951) Cytological studies on stellate cells of Kupffer and fat-storing cells in the capillary wall of the human liver. *Acta Anat Nippon* 26: 42.

Ito Y, Sørensen KK, Bethea NW, Svistounov D, McCuskey MK, Smedsrød B, McCuskey RS (2007) Age-related changes in the hepatic microcirculation of mice. *Exp Gerontol* 42: 789-797.

Izumi N, Mizuguchi S, Inagaki Y, Saika S, Kawada N, Nakajima Y, Inoue K, Suehiro S, Friedman SL, Ikeda K (2006) BMP-7 oppose TGF-β1-mediated collagen induction in mouse pulmonary myofibroblasts through Id2. *Am J Physiol Lung Cell Mol Physiol* 290: L120-L126.

Jaenisch R, Bird A (2003) Epigenetic regulation of gene expression: how the genome integrates intrinsic and environmental signals. *Nature Genet* 33: 245-254.

Janoschek N, van de Leur E, Gressner AM, Weiskirchen R (2004) Induction of cell death in activated hepatic stellate cells by targeted gene expression of the thymidine kinase/ganciclovir system. *Biochem Biophys Res Commun* 316: 1107-1115.

Jarman WM, Simon M, Norstrom RJ, Burns SA, Bacon CA, Simoneit BRT, Risebrough RW (1992) Global distribution of Tris(4-chlorophenyl) methanol in high trophic level birds and mammals. *Environ Sci Technol* 26: 1770-1774.

Jeong W, Osei-Hyiaman D, Park O, Liu J, Bátkai S, Mukhopadhyay P, Horiguchi N, Harvey-White J, Marsicano G, Lutz B, Gao B, Kunos G (2008) Paracrine activation of hepatic CB_1 receptors by stellate cell-derived endocannabinoids mediates alcoholic fatty liver. *Cell Metabol* 7: 227-235.

Jiang F, Parsons CJ, Tefanovic B (2006) Gene expression profile of quiescent and activated rat hepatic stellate cells implicates Wnt signaling pathway inactivation. *J Hepatol* 45: 401-409.

Jiang HP, Serrero G (1992) Isolation and characterization of a full-length cDNA coding for an adipose differentiation-related protein. *Proc Natl Acad Sci USA* 89:7856-7860.

Jones PL, Schmidhauser C, Bissell MJ (1993) Regulation of gene expression and cell function by extracellular matrix. *Crit Rev Eukar Gene Express* 3: 137-154.

Kalinchenko VV, Bhattacharyya D, Zhou Y, Gussarova GA, Kim W, Shin B, Costa RH (2003) Foxf +/- mice exhibit defective stellate cell activation and abnormal liver regeneration following CCl_4 injury. *Hepatology* 37: 107-117.

Kalluri R, Neilson EG (2003) Epithelial-mesenchymal transition and its implications for fibrosis. *J Clin Invest* 112: 1776-1784.

Kanai M, Raz A, Goodman DW (1968) Retinol-binding protein: the transport protein for vitamin A in human plasma. *J Clin Invest* 47: 2025-2044.

Kanaka-Gantenbein C, Margeli A, Pervanidou P, Sakka S, Mastorakos G, Chrousos GP, Papassotiriou I (2008) Retinol-binding protein 4 and lipocalin-2 in childhood and adolescent obesity: When children are not just "small adults". *Clin Chem* 54:1176-1182.

Kapanci Y, Ribaux C, Chaponnier C, Gabbiani G (1992) Cytoskeletal features of alveolar myofibroblasts and pericytes in normal human and rat lung. *J Histochem Cytochem* 40: 1955-1963.

Kato M, Kato K, Goodman DS (1984) Immunocytochemical studies on the localization of plasma and of cellular retinol-binding proteins and of transthyretin (prealbumin) in rat liver and kidney. *J Cell Biol* 98: 1696-1704.

Kawada N, Klein H, Decker K (1992) Eicosanoid-mediated contractility of hepatic stellate cells. *Biochem J* 285: 367–371.

Kawada N, Klein H, Decker K (1993a) Contraction and relaxation of hepatic stellate cells in culture. In: Knook DL, Wisse E (eds) Cells of the Hepatic Sinusoid, vol 4, *Kupffer Cell Foundation,* Leiden, pp 161-164.

Kawada N, Kristensen DB, Asahina K, Nakatani K, Minamiyama Y, Seki S, Yoshizato K (2001) Characterization of a stellate cell activation-associated protein (STAP) with peroxidase activity found in rat hepatic stellate cells. *J Biol Chem* 276, 25318-25323.

Kawada N, Tran-Thi T-A, Klein H, Decker K (1993b) The contraction of hepatic stellate (Ito) cells stimulated with vasoactive substances Possible involvement of endothelin 1 and nitric oxide in the regulation of the sinusoidal tonus. *Eur J Biochem* 213: 815-823.

Kawaguchi R, Yu J, Honda J, Hu J, Whitelegge J, Ping P, Wiita P, Bok D, Sun H (2007) A membrane receptor for retinol binding protein mediates cellular uptake of vitamin A. *Science* 315: 820-825.

Kida Y, Asahina K, Inoue K, Kawada N, Yoshizato K, Wake K, Sato T (2007) Characterization of vitamin A-storing cells in mouse fibrous kidneys using cygb/STAP as a marker of activated stellate cells. *Arch Histol Cytol* 70: 95-106.

Kidd M, Modlin IM, Shapiro MD, Camp RL, Mane SM, Usinger W, Murren JR (2007) CTGF, intestinal stellate cells and carcinoid fibrogenesis. *World J Gastroenterol* 13: 5208-5216.

Kisseleva T, Brenner DA (2006) Hepatic stellate cells and the reversal of fibrosis. *J Gastroenterol Hepatol* 21: S84-S87.

Kisseleva T, Brenner DA (2007) Role of hepatic stellate cells in fibrogenesis and the reversal of fibrosis. *J Gastroenterol Hepatol* 22: S73-S78.

Kisseleva T, Uchinami H, Feirt N, Quintana-Bustamante O, Segovia JC, Schwabe RF, Brenner DA (2006) Bone marrow-derived fibrocytes participate in pathogenesis of liver fibrosis. *J Hepatol* 45: 429-438.

Klein I, Crispe IN (2006) Complete differentiation of CD8+ T cells activated locally within the transplanted liver. *J Exp Med* 203: 437-447.

Kleinman HK, McGarvey ML, Hassell JR, Star VL, Cannon FB, Laurie GW, Martin GR (1986) Basement membrane complexes with biological activity. *Biochemistry* 25: 312-318.

Knight V, Tchongue J, Lourensz D, Tipping P, Sievert W (2012) Protease-activated receptor 2 promotes experimental liver fibrosis in mice and activates human hepatic stellate cells. *Hepatology* 55: 879-887.

Knittel T, Aurisch S, Neubauer K, Eichhorst S, Ramadori G (1996) Cell-type-specific expression of neural cell adhesion molecule (N-CAM) in Ito cells of rat liver. Upregulation during in vitro activation and in hepatic tissue repair. *Am J Pathol* 149: 449-462.

Knittel T, Kobold D, Saile B, Grundmann A, Neubauer K, Piscaglia F, Ramadori G (1999) Rat liver myofibroblasts and hepatic stellate cells: Different cell populations of the fibroblast lineage with fibrogenic potential. *Gastroenterology* 117: 1205-1221.

Knook DL, Blansjaar N, Sleyster EC (1977) Isolation and characterization of Kupffer and endothelial cells from the rat liver. *Exp Cell Res* 109: 317-329.

Knook DL, Seffelaar AM, de Leeuw AM (1982) Fat-storing cells of the rat liver. Their isolation and purification. Preliminary notes. *Exp Cell Res* 139: 468-471.

Kobayashi K, Takahashi Y (1971) Effect of the administration of large dose of vitamin A on the fine structure of rat liver with special reference to changes in the fat-storing cell. *Arch Histol Jap* 33: 421-443.

Kobayashi K, Takahashi Y, Shibasaki S (1973) Cytological studies of fat-storing cells in the liver of rats given large doses of vitamin A. *Nature New Biol* 243: 186-188.

Koda H, Okuno M, Imai S, Moriwaki H, Muto Y, Kawada N, Kojima S (1996) Retinoic acid-stimulated liver stellate cells suppress the production of albumin from parenchymal cells via TGF-β. *Biochem Biophys Res Commun* 221: 565-569.

Kojima N, Miura M, Matano Y, Imai K, Sato M, Senoo H, Hata R (1997) Reversible regulation of hepatic stellate cell functions by three-dimensional structure of extracellular matrix. In: Wisse E, Knook DL, Balabaud C (eds) Cells of the Hepatic Sinusoid, Vol 6, *Kupffer Cell Foundation, Leiden,* pp 107-109.

Kojima N, Sato M, Imai K, Miura M, Senoo H (1998) Hepatic stellate cells (vitamin A-storing cells) change their cytoskeleton structure by extracellular matrix through signal transduction system. *Histochem Cell Biol* 110: 121-128.

Kojima N, Sato M, Miura M, Imai K, Senoo H (1999) Alteration in distribution of focal adhesion components by signaling inhibitors in hepatic stellate cells and fibroblasts cultured on type I collagen gel. In: Wisse E, Knook DL, de Zanger R, Fraser R (eds) Cells Hepatic Sinusoid vol 7, *Kupffer Cell Foundation, Leiden*, pp 24-25.

Kojima N, Sato M, Suzuki A, Sato T, Satoh S, Kato T, Senoo H (2001) Enhanced expression of B7-1, B7-2, and intercellular adhesion molecule 1 in sinusoidal endothelial cells by warm ischemia/reperfusion injury in rat liver. *Hepatology* 34: 751-757.

Kon K, Ikejima K, Hirose M, Yoshikawa M, Enomoto N, Kitamura T, Takei Y, Sato N (2002) Pioglitazone prevents early-phase hepatic fibrogenesis caused by carbon tetrachloride. *Biochem Biophys Res Commun* 291:55-61.

Kornberg LJ, Earp HS, Tuener CE, Prockop C, Juliano RL (1991) Signal transduction by integrins: inceased protein tyrosine-phosphorylation caused by clustering of β1 integrins. *Proc Natl Acad Sci USA* 88: 8392-8396.

Kozak M (1991) An analysis of vertebrate mRNA sequences: intimations of translational control. *J Cell Biol* 115:887-903.

Kristensen DB, Kawada N, Imamura K, Miyamoto Y, Tateno C, Seki S, Kuroki T, Yoshizato K (2000) Proteome analysis of rat hepatic stellate cells. *Hepatology* 32: 268-277.

Krizhanovsky V, Yon M, Dickins RA, Hearn S, Simon J, Miething C, Yee H, Zender L, Scott W. Lowe SW (2008) Senescence of activated stellate cells limits liver fibrosis. *Cell* 134, 657-667.

Krust A, Green S, Argos P, Kumar V, Walter P, Bornert JM, Chambon P (1986) The chicken oestrogen receptor sequence: homology with v-erbA and the human oestrogen and glucocorticoid receptors. *EMBO J* 5:891-897.

Kubota H, Yao H-L, Reid LM (2007) Identification and characterization of vitamin A-storing cells in fetal liver: Implications for functional importance of hepatic stellate cells in liver development and hematopoiesis. *Stem Cells* 25: 2339-2349.

Kupffer Cv (1876) Ueber Sternzellen der Leber. Briefliche Mitteilung an Prof. Waldeyer. *Arch mikr Anat* 12: 353-358.

Kupffer Cv (1898) Ueber Sternzellen der Leber. Verh anat Ges 12: *Versammulung in Kiel,* 80-86.

Kupffer Cv (1899) Ueber die sogenannten Sternzellen der Sugethierleber. *Arch mikr Anat* 54: 254-288.

Kurata S, Senoo H, Hata R-I (1993) Transcriptional activation of type I collagen genes by ascorbic acid 2-phosphate in human skin fibroblasts and its failure in cells from a patient with α2(I)-chain-defective Ehlers-Danlos syndrome. *Exp Cell Res* 206: 63-71.

Kusumoto Y, Fujita T (1977) Vitamin A uptake cells distributed in the liver and other organs of the rat. *Arch Histol Jpn* 40:121-136.

Lang A, Schrum LW, Schoonhoven R, Tuvia S, Solís-Herruzo JA, Tsukamoto H, Brenner DA, Rippe RA (2000) Expression of small heat shock protein B-crystallin is induced after hepatic stellate cell activation. *Am J Physiol Gastrointest Liver Physiol* 279: G1333-G1342.

Lawrence CW, Crain FD, Lotspeich FJ, Krause RF (1966) Absorption, transport, and storage of retinyl-15-^{14}C palmitate-9, 10-^{3}H in the rat. *J Lipid Res* 7: 226-229.

Leclercq IA, Sempoux C, Starkel P, Horsmans Y (2006) Limited therapeutic efficacy of pioglitazone on progression of hepatic fibrosis in rats. *Gut* 55:1020-1029.

Le Couteur DG, Warren A, Cogger VC, Smedsrød B, Sørensen KK, De Cabo R, Fraser R, McCuskey RS(2008) Old age and the hepatic sinusoid. *Anat Rec* 291: 672-683.

Leo MA, Lieber CS (1983) Hepatic fibrosis after long-term administration of ethanol and moderate vitamin A supplementation in the rat. *Hepatology* 3:1-11.

Lepreux S, Bioulac-Sage P, Gabbiani G, Sapin V, Housset C, Rosenbaum J, Balabaud C, Desmoulière A (2004) Cellular retinol-binding protein-1 expression in normal and fibrotic/cirrhotic human liver: different patterns of expression in hepatic stellate cells and (myo)fibroblast subpopulations. *J Hepatol* 40: 774-780.

Levin MS (1993) Cellular retinol-binding proteins are determinants of retinol uptake and metabolism in stably transfected Caco-2 cells. *J Biol Chem* 268: 8267-8276.

Levine D, Rockey DC, Milner TA, Breuss JM, Fallon JT, Schnapp LM (2000) Expression of the integrin α8β1. *Am J Pathol* 156: 1927-1935.

Li D, Friedman SL (2001) Hepatic stellate cells: Morphology, function, and regulation. In: Arias IM, Boyer JL, Chisari FV, Fausto N, Schachter D, Shafritz DA (eds) The Liver Biology and Pathobiology, 4th edn *Lippincott Williams & Wilkins, Philadelphia*, pp 455-468.

Li YL, Sato M, Kojima N, Miura M, Senoo H (1999) Regulatory role of extracellular matrix components in expression of matrix metalloproteases in cultured hepatic stellate cells. *Cell Struct Func* 24: 255-261.

Lin J, Chen A (2008) Activation of peroxisome proliferator-activated receptor-γ by curcumin blocks the signaling pathways for PDGF and EGF in hepatic stellate cells. *Lab Invest* 88:529-540.

Lindsay CK, Thorgeirsson UP (1995) Localization of messenger RNA for tissue inhibitor of metalloproteinases-1 and type IV collagenases /gelatinases in monkey hepatocellular carcinomas. *Clin Exp Metastasis* 13: 381-388.

Loreal O, Levavasseur F, Fromaget C, Gros D, Guillouzo A, Clement B (1993) Cooperation of Ito cells and hepatocytes in deposition of an extracellular matrix in vitro. *Am J Pathol* 143: 538-544.

Lu X, Gruia-Gray J, Copeland NG, Gilbert DJ, Jenkins NA, Londos C, Kimmel AR (2001) The murine perilipin gene: the lipid droplet-associated perilipins derive from tissue-specific, mRNA splice variants and define a gene family of ancient origin. *Mamm Genome* 12:741-749.

Lubahn DB, Joseph DR, Sullivan PM, Willard HF, French FS, Wilson EM (1988) Cloning of human androgen receptor complementary DNA and localization to the X chromosome. *Science* 240:327-330.

Ma X, Svegliati-Baroni G, Poniachik J, Baraona E, Lieber CS (1997) Collagen synthesis by liver stellate cells is released from its normal feedback regulation by acetaldehyde-induced modification of the carboxyl-terminal propeptide of procollagen. *Alcoholism Clin Exp Res* 21: 1204-1211.

Mabuchi A, Mullaney I, Sheard PA, Hessian PA, Mallard BL, Tawadrous MN, Zimmermann A, Senoo H, Wheatley AM (2004) Role of hepatic stellate cells in the early phase of liver regeneration in rat: Formation of tight adhesions to parenchymal cells. *J Hepatol* 40: 910-916.

MacDonald PN, Ong DE (1988) A lecithin:retinol acyltransferase activity in human and rat liver. *Biochem Biophys Res Commun* 156:157-163.

Mackay IR (2002) Hepatoimmunology: A perspective. *Immnunol Cell Biol* 80: 36-44.

Maeda N, Kawada N, Seki S, Arakawa T, Ikeda K, Iwao H, Okuyama H, Hirabayashi J, Kasai K, Yoshizato K (2003) Stimulation of proliferation of rat hepatic stellate cells by galectin-1 and galectin-3 through different intracellular signaling pathways. *J Biol Chem* 278: 18938-18944.

Magness ST, Bataller R, Yang L, Brenner DA (2004) A dual reporter gene transgenic mouse demonstrates heterogeneity in hepatic fibrogenic cell populations. *Hepatology* 40: 1151-1159.

Mailliard ME, Sorrell MF (2008) Alcoholic liver disease. In: Fauci AS, Braunwald E, Kasper DL, Hauser SL, Longo DL, Jameson JL, Loscalzo J (eds) *Harrison's Principles of Internal Medicine.* 17th edn pp 1969-1971.

Majno G (1979) The story of the myofibroblasts. *Am J Surg Pathol* 6: 535-542.

Maksvytis HJ, Niles RM, Simanovsky L, Minassian IA, Richardson LL, Hamosh M, Hamosh P, Brody JS (1984) In vitro characteristics of the lipid-filled interstitial cell associated with postnatal lung growth: Evidence for fibroblast heterogeneity. *J Cell Physiol* 118: 113-123.

Maksvytis HJ, Vaccaro C, Brody JS (1981) Isolation and characterization of the lipid-containing interstitial cell from the developing rat lung. *Lab Invest* 45: 248-259.

Malaba L, Smeland S, Senoo H, Norum KR, Berg T, Blomhoff R, Kindberg GM (1995) Retinol-binding protein and asialo-orosomucoid are taken up by different pathways in liver cells. *J Biol Chem* 270: 15686-15692.

Malhi H, Gores GJ (2008) Cellular and molecular mechanisms of liver injury. *Gastroenterology* 134: 1641-1654.

Mallat A, Gallois C, Tao J, Habib A, Maclouf J, Mavier P, Préaux A-M, Lotersztajn S (1998) Platelet-derived growth factor-BB and thrombin generate positive and negative signals for human hepatic stellate cell proliferation. *J Biol Chem* 273: 27300-27305.

Mallat A, Preaux A-M, Blazejewski S, Rosenbaum J, Dhumeaux D, Mavier P (1995) Interferon alfa and gamma inhibit proliferation and collagen synthesis of human ito cells in culture. *Hepatology* 21: 1003-1010.

Mann J, Oakley F, Akiboye F, Elsharkawy A, Thorne AW, Mann DA (2007) Regulation of myofibroblast transdifferentiation by DNA methylation and MeCP2: implications for wound healing and fibrogenesis. *Cell Death Different* 14: 275–285.

Mann DA, Smart DE (2002) Transcriptional regulation of hepatic stellate cell activation. *Gut* 50:891-896.

Marek CJ, Tucker SJ, Konstantinou DK, Elrick LJ, Haefner D, Sigalas C, Murray GI, Goodwin B, Wright MC (2005) Pregnenolone-16α-carbonitrile inhibits rodent liver fibrogenesis via PXR (pregnane X receptor)-dependent and PXR-independent mechanisms. *Biochem J* 387:601-608.

Margis R, Borojevic R (1989) Retinoid-mediated induction of the fat-storing phenotype in a liver connective tissue cell line (GRX). *Biochim Biophys Acta Mol Cell Res* 1011: 1-5.

Margueron R, Trojer P, Reinberg D (2005) The key to development: interpreting the histone code? *Current Opinion Genet Develop* 15: 163-176.

Marra F (2002) Leptin and liver fibrosis: A matter of fat. *Gastroenterology* 122: 1529-1532.

Marra F (2006) Thiazolidinediones and hepatic fibrosis: don't wait too long. *Gut* 55:917-919.

Marra F, Efsen E, Romanelli RG, Caligiuri A, Pastacaldi S, Batignani G, Bonacchi A, Caporale R, Laffi G, Pinzani M, Gentilini P (2000) Ligands of peroxisome proliferator-activated receptor γ modulate profibrogenic and proinflammatory actions in hepatic stellate cells. *Gastroenterology* 119:466-478.

Marra F, Pinzani M, DeFranco R, Laffi G, Gentilini P (1995) Involvement of phosphatidylinositol 3-kinase in the activation of extracellular signal-regulated kinase by PDGF in hepatic stellate cells. *FEBS Lett* 376: 141-145.

Martin G, Sewell B, Yeomans ND, Smallwood RA (1992) Ageing has no effect on the volume density of hepatocytes, reticulo-endothelial cells or the exracellular space in livers of female Sprague-Dawley rats. *Clin Exp Pharmacol Physiol* 19: 537-539.

Martinez-Hernandez A (1984) The hepatic extracellular matrix. I. Electron immunohistochemical studies in normal rat liver. *Lab Invest* 51: 57-73.

Martinez-Hernandez A, Amenta PS (1993a) The hepatic extracellular matrix. I. Components and distribution in normal liver. *Virchows Archiv A Pathol Anat* 423: 1-11.

Martinez-Hernandez A, Amenta PS (1993b) The hepatic extracellular matrix. II. Ontogenesis regeneration and cirrhosis. *Virchows Archiv A Pathol Anat* 423: 77-84.

Martinez-Hernandez A, Amenta PS (1995) The extracellular matrix in hepatic regeneration. *FASEB J* 9: 1401-1410.

Martucci EB, Ziulkoski AL, Fortuna VA, Guaragna AM, Guma FCR, Trugo LC, Borojevic R (2004) β-Carotene storage, conversion to retinoic acid, and induction of the lipocyte phenotype in hepatic stellate cells. *J Cell Biochem* 92: 414-423.

Masamune A, Kikuta K, Satoh M, Sakai Y, Satoh A, Shimosegawa T (2002) Ligands of peroxisome proliferator-activated receptor-γ block activation of pancreatic stellate cells. *J Biol Chem* 277: 141-147.

Masamune A, Kikuta K, Watanabe T, Satoh K, Hirota M, Shimosegawa T (2008) Hypoxia stimulates pancreatic stellate cells to induce fibrosis and angiogenesis in pancreatic cancer. *Am J Physiol Gastrointest Liver Physiol* 295: G709-G717.

Matano Y, Miura M, Kojima N, Sato M, Imai K, Senoo H (1999) Hepatic stellate cells and extrahepatic stellate cells (extrahepatic vitamin A-storing cells). In: Wisse E, Knook DL, de Zanger R, Fraser R (eds) Cells of the Hepatic Sinusoid, vol 7, *Kupffer Cell Foundation,* Leiden, pp 26-27.

Matsumoto E, Hirosawa K (1983) Some observations on the structure of Suncus liver with special reference to the vitamin A-storing cells. *Am J Anat* 167: 193-204.

Matsuura T, Hasumura S, Nagamori S (1999) Retinol esterification activity contributes to retinol transport in stellate cells. *Cell Struct Func* 24: 111-116.

Matsuura T, Nagamori S, Fujise K, Hasumura S, Homma S, Sujino H, Shimizu K, Niiya M, Kameda H, Hirosawa K (1989) Retinol transport in cultured fat-storing cells of rat liver. Quantitative analysis by anchored cell analysis and sorting system. *Lab Invest* 61:107-115.

Matsuura T, Nagamori S, Hasumura S, Sujino H, Shimizu K, Niiya M, Hirosawa K (1993) Retinol transport in cultured stellate cells of rat liver: studies by light and electron microscope autoradiography. *Exp Cell Res* 206:111-118.

McCarroll JA, Phillips PA, Kjumar RK, Park S, Pirola RC, Wilson JS, Apte MV (2004) Pancreatic stellate cell migration: role of the phosphatidylinositol 3-kinase (PI3-kinase) pathway. *Biochem Pharmacol* 67: 1215-1225.

McCarroll JA, Phillips PA, Santucci N, Pirola RC, Wilson JS, Apte MV (2006) Vitamin A inhibits pancreatic stellate cell activation: implications for treatment of pancreatic fibrosis. *Gut* 55: 79-89.

McClain CJ, Van Thiel DH, Parker S, Badzin LK, Gilbert H (2008) Alterations in zinc, vitamin A, and retinol-binding protein in chronic alcoholics: A possible mechanism for night blindness and hypogonadism. *Alcoholism Clin Exp Res* 3: 135-131.

McCuskey RS (2008) The hepatic microvascular system in health and its response to toxicants. *Anat Rec* 291: 661-671.

McDonnell DP, Mangelsdorf DJ, Pike JW, Haussler MR, O'Malley BW (1987) Molecular cloning of complementary DNA encoding the avian receptor for vitamin D. *Science* 235:1214-1217.

Melton AC, Datta A, Yee HF Jr (2006) $[Ca^{2+}]_i$-independent contractile force generation by rat hepatic stellate cells in response to endothelin-1. *Am J Physiol Gastrointest Liver Physiol* 290: G7-G13.

Menke A, Yamaguchi H, Gress TN, Adler G (1997) Extracellular matrix is reduced by inhibition of transforming growth factor beta1 in pancreatitis in the rat. *Gastroenterology* 113: 295-303.

Mercier I, Lechaire JP, Desmoulière A, Gaill F, Aumailley M (1996) Interactions of human skin fibroblasts with monomeric or fibrillar collagens induce different organization of cytoskeleton. *Exp Cell Res* 225: 245-256.

Messing A (1999) Nestin in the liver-Lessons from the brain. *Hepatology* 29: 602-603.

Mezaki Y, Morii M, Hebiguchi T, Yoshikawa K, Yamaguchi N, Miura M, Imai K, Yoshino H, Senoo H (2013b) Differential increases in the expression of intermediate filament proteins and concomitant morphological changes of transdifferentiating rat hepatic stellate cells observed *in vitro. Acta Histochem Cytochem in press.*

Mezaki Y, Morii M, Hebiguchi T, Yoshikawa K, Yamaguchi N, Yoshino H, Senoo H (2013a) The role of retinoic acid receptors in activated hepatic stellate cells. *Med Hypothesis* 81: 222-224.

Mezaki, M., Morii, M., Yoshikawa, K., Yamaguchi, N., Miura, M., Imai, K., Yoshino, H., Senoo, H. (2012a) Characterization of a cellular retinol binding protein from lamprey, *Lethenteron japonicum*. CBP Part B: *Biochemistry & Molecular Biology* 161, 233-239.

Mezaki Y, Morii M, Yoshikawa K, Yamaguchi N, Satoyoshi K, Miura M, Imai K, Hebuguchi T, Habuchi T, Senoo H (2012b) Elevated expression of transforming growth factor β3in carbon tetrachloride-treated rat liver and involvement of retinoid signaling. *Int J Mol Med.* 29: 18-24.

Mezaki Y, Yamaguchi N, Yoshikawa K, Miura M, Imai K, Itoh H, Senoo H (2009) Insoluble speckled cytosolic distribution of retinoic acid receptor alpha protein as a marker of hepatic stellate cell activation in vitro. *J Histochem Cytochem* 57: 687-699.

Mezaki Y, Yoshikawa K, Yamaguchi N, Miura M, Imai K, Kato S, Senoo H (2007) Rat hepatic stellate cells acquire retinoid responsiveness after activation *in vitro* by post-transcriptional regulation of retinoic acid receptor alpha gene expression. *Arch Biochem Biophys* 465:370-379.

Michalopoulos GK, Bowen WC. Zajac VF, Beer-Stolz D, Watkins S, Kostrubsky V, Strom SC (1999) Morphogenetic events in mixed cultures of rat hepatocytes and nonparenchymal cells maintained in biological matrices in the presence of hepatocyte growth factor and epidermal growth factor. *Hepatology* 29: 90-100.

Migita K, Maeda Y, Abiru S, Komori A, Yokoyama T, Takii Y, Nakamura M, Yatsuhashi H, Eguchi K, Ishibashi H (2005) Peroxynitrite-mediated matrix metalloproteinase-2 activation in human hepatic stellate cells. *FEBS Lett* 579: 3119-3125.

Minicis SD, Seki E, Uchinami H, Kluwe J, Zhang Y, Brenner DA, Schwabe R (2007) Gene expression profiles during hepatic stellate cell activation in culture and in vivo. *Gastroenterology*, 132, 1937-1946.

Mitaka T, Mikami M, Sattler GL, Pitot HC, Mochizuki Y (1992) Small cell colonies appear in the primary culture of adult rat hepatocytes in the presence of nicotinamide and epidermal growth factor. *Hepatology* 16: 440-447.

Mitaka T, Sato F, Mizuguchi T, Yokono T, Mochizuki Y (1999) Reconstruction of hepatic organoid by rat small hepatocytes and hepatic nonparenchymal cells. *Hepatology* 29: 111-125.

Miura S, Gan JW, Brzostowski J, Parisi MJ, Schultz CJ, Londos C, Oliver B, Kimmel AR (2002) Functional conservation for lipid storage droplet association among perilipin, ADRP, and TIP47 (PAT)-related proteins in mammals, *Drosophila*, and *Dictyostelium*. *J Biol Chem* 277:32253-32257.

Miura M, Sato M, Toyoshima I, Senoo H (1997) Extension of long cellular processes of hepatic stellate cells cultured on extracellular type I collagen gel by microtubule assembly: observation utilizing time-lapse video-microscopy. *Cell Struct Funct* 22: 487-492.

Miura M, Sato M, Toyoshima I, Senoo H (1999) Elongation of long, multipolar processes in hepatic stellate cell culture on type I collagen gel by microtubule assembly: Observation utilizing time-lapse video-microscopy. In: Wisse E, Knook DL, de Zanger R, Fraser R (eds) Cells Hepatic Sinusoid vol 7, *Kupffer Cell Foundation, Leiden*, pp 17-20.

Miyahara T, Schrum L, Rippe R, Xiong S, Yee Jr HF, Motomura K, Anania FA, Willson TM, Tsukamoto H (2000) Peroxisome proliferator-activated receptors and hepatic stellate cell activation. *J Biol Chem* 275:35715-35722.

Miyata E, Masuya M, Yoshida S, Nakamura S, Kato K, Sugimoto Y, Shibasaki T, Yamamura K, Ohishi K, Nishii K, Ishikawa F, Shiku H, Katayama N (2008) Hematopoietic origin of hepatic stellate cells in the adult liver. *Blood* 111: 2427-2435.

Montfort I, Pérez-Tamayo R, Alvizouri AM, Tello E (1990) Collagenase of hepatocytes and sinusoidal liver cells in the reversibility of experimental cirrhosis of the liver. *Virchows Archiv B Cell Pathol* 59: 281-289.

Moore T (1931) Vitamin A and carotene VII. The distribution of vitamin A and carotene in the body of the rat. *Biochem J* 25: 274-286.

Moore KL, Persaud TVN, Torchia MG (2008) The Developing Human Clinically Oriented Embryology, 8th edn Saunders, Philadelphia.

Morii M, Mezaki Y, Yamaguchi N, Yoshikawa K, Miura M, Imai K, Yoshino H, Hebiguchi T, Hebiguchi T, Senoo H (2010) Onset of apoptosis in cystic duct during metamorphosis of a Japanese lamprey, *Lethenteron reissneri*. *Anat Rec,* 293, 1155-1166.

Morii, M., Mezaki, Y., Yoshikawa, K., Miura, M., Imai, K., Hebuguchi, T., Watanabe, R., Asanuma, Y., Yoshino, H., Senoo, H. (2011) How do lampreys avoid cholestasis after bile duct degeneration. *Cholestasis. Ed. Tripodi V. INTECH, Rijeka,* Croatia, ISBN 979-953-307-187-8, 81-98.

Moriwaki H, Blaner WS, Piantedosi R, Goodman DS (1988) Effects of dietary retinoid and triglyceride on the lipid composition of rat liver stellate cells and stellate cell lipid droplets. *J Lipid Res* 29: 1523-1534.

Mousavi SA, Sato M, Sporstøl M, Smedsrød B, Berg T, Kojima N, Senoo H (2005) Uptake of collagen into hepatic stellate cells: Evidence of the involvement of urokinase plasminogen activator associated protein/Endo 180. *Biochem J* 387: 39-46.

Muir DCG, Wagemann R, Harrave BT, Thomas DJ, Peakall DB, Norstrom RJ (1992) Arctic marine ecosystem contamination. *Sci Total Environ* 122: 75-134.

Murakami K, Abe T, Miyazawa M, Yamaguchi M, Masuda T, Matsuura T, Nagamori S, Takeuchi K, Abe K, Kyogoku M (1995) Establishment of a new human cell line, LI90, exhibiting characteristics of hepatic Ito (fat-storing) cells. *Lab Invest* 72: 731-739.

Murphy DJ, Vance J (1999) Mechanisms of lipid-body formation. *Trends Biochem Sci* 24:109-115.

Musso O, Rehn M, Saarela J, Théret N, Liétard J, Hintikka E, Lotrian D, Campion J-P, Pihlajaniemi T, Clément B (1998) Collagen XVIII is localized in sinusoids and basement membrane zones and expressed by hepatocytes and activated stellate cells in fibrotic human liver. *Hepatology* 28: 98-107.

Muto Y, Shidoji Y, Kanda Y (1982) Isolation and characterization of serum retinol-binding protein. In: Parker L (ed) *Methods Enzymol* vol 81, pp 840-852.

Nagatsuma K, Hayashi Y, Hano H, Sagara H, Murakami K, Saito M, Masaki T, Lu T, Tanaka M, Enzan H, Aizawa Y, Tajiri H, Matsuura T (2009) Lecithin:retinol acyltransferase protein is distributed in both hepatic stellate cells and endothelial cells of normal rodent and human liver. *Liver Int* 29:47-54.

Nagy NE, Holven KB, Roos N, Senoo H, Kojima N, Norum KR, Blomhoff R (1997) Storage of vitamin A in extrahepatic stellate cells in normal rats. *J Lipid Res* 38: 645-658.

Nakagawa M, Nakabayashi H, Nakano H (1991) A simple method for the isolation of human Ito cells (fat-storing cells). *Acta Hepatol Japonica* 45: 169-174.

Nakatani K, Okuyama H, Shimahara Y, Saeki S, Kim D-H, Nakajima Y, Seki S, Kawada N, Yoshizato K (2004) Cytoglobin/STAP, its unique localization in splanchnic fibroblast-like cells and function in organ fibrogenesis. *Lab Invest* 84: 91-101.

Napoli JL (1993) Biosynthesis and metabolism of retinoic acid: Roles of CRBP and CRABP in retinoic acid homeostasis. *J Nutr* 123: 362-366.

Napoli JL (1999) Interactions of retinoid binding proteins and enzymes in retinoid metabolism. *Biochim Biophys Acta* 1440:139-162.

Neesse A, Wagner M, Ellenrieder V, Bachem M, Gress TM, Buchholz M (2007) Pancreatic stellate cells potentiate proinvasive effects of SERPINE2 expression in pancreatic cancer xenograft tumors. *Pancreatology* 7: 380-385.

Neubauer K, Knittel T, Aurisch S, Fellmer P, Ramadori G (1996) Glial fibrillary acidic protein—a cell type specific marker for Ito cells *in vivo* and *in vitro*. *J Hepatol* 24: 719-730.

Newcomer ME, Ong DE (1990) Purification and crystallization of a retinoic acid-binding protein from rat epididymis. *J Biol Chem* 265: 12876-12879.

Nieto N, Greenwel P, Friedman SL, Zhang F, Dannenberg AJ, Cederbaum AI (2000) Ethanol and arachidonic acid increase α 2(I) collagen expression in rat hepatic stellate cells overexpressing cytochrome P450 2E1. Role of H_2O_2 and cyclooxygenase-2. *J Biol Chem* 275: 20136-20145.

Niki T, De Bleser PJ, Xu G, Van den Berg K, Wisse E, Geerts A (1996) Comparison of glial fibrillary acidic protein and desmin staining in normal and CCl_4-induced fibrotic rat livers. *Hepatology* 23: 1538-1545.

Niki T, Penky M, Hellemans K, De Bleser P, Van den Berg K, Vaeyens F, Quartier E, Schuit F, Geerts A (1999) Class VI intermediate filament protein nestin is induced during activation of rat hepatic stellate cells. *Hepatology* 29: 520-527.

Nilsson M, Berg T (1977) Uptake and degradation of formaldehyde-treated ^{125}I-labelled human serum albumin in rat liver cells in vivo and in vitro. *Biochim Biophys Acta* 497: 171-182.

Nilsson CB, Hoegberg P, Trossvik C, Azaïs-Bræsco V, Blaner WS, Fex G, Harrison EH, Nau H, Schmidt CK, van Bennekum AM, Håkansson H (2000) 2,3,7,8-Tetrachlorodibenzo-*p*-dioxin increases serum and kidney retinoic acid levels and kidney retinol esterification in the rat. *Toxicol Applied Pharmacol* 169: 121-131.

Nilsson A, Trøen G, Petersen LB, Reppe S, Norum KR, Blomhoff R (1997) Retinyl ester storage is altered in liver stellate cells and in HL60 cells transfected with cellular retinol-binding protein type I. *Int J Biochem Cell Biol* 29: 381-378.

Nishimura T, Nakano T (2000) Immunocytochemical localization of bovine serum albumin (BSA) in the liver and testis of rats injected with testosterone-BSA, hydrocortisone-BSA or corticosterone-BSA. *Cell Struct Funct* 25:161-169.

Norum KR (1984) The name of the perisinusoidal stellate cells, fat storing cells, Ito cells, pericyte, vitamin A storing cells of the liver. *Kupffer Cell Bulletin* 5: 13.

Noy N (2000) Retinoid-binding proteins: mediators of retinoid action. *Biochem J* 348: 481–495.

Oakley F, Meso M, Iredale JP, Green K, Marek CJ, Zhou X, May MJ, Millward-Sadler H, Wright MC, Mann DA (2005) Inhibition of inhibitor of κB kinases stimulates hepatic stellate cell apoptosis and accelerated recovery from rat liver fibrosis. *Gastroenterology* 128: 108-120.

Oakley F, Trim N, Constandinou CM, Ye W, Gray AM, Frantz G, Hillan K, Kendall T, Benyon AC, Mann DA, Iredale JP (2003) Hepatocytes express nerve growth factor during liver injury. Evidence for paracrine regulation of hepatic stellate cell apoptosis. *Am J Pathol* 163:1849-1858.

Oben JA, Yang S, Lin H, Ono M, Mae Diehl A (2003) Norepinephrine and neuropeptide Y promote proliferation and collagen gene expression of hepatic myofibroblastic stellate cells. *Biochem Biophys Res Commun* 302: 685-690.

O'Byrne SM, Wongsiriroj N, Libien J, Vogel S, Goldberg IJ, Baehr W, Palczewski K, Blaner WS (2005) Retinoid absorption and storage is impaired in mice lacking lecithin:retinol acyltransferase (LRAT). *J Biol Chem* 280: 35647-35657.

Ohata M, Lin M, Satre M, Tsukamoto H (1997) Diminished retinoic acid signaling in hepatic stellate cells in cholestatic liver fibrosis. *Am J Physiol* 272:G589-G596.

Ohnishi N, Miyata T, Ohnishi H, Yasuda H, Tamada K, Ueda N, Mashima H, Sugano K (2003) Activin A is an autocrine activator of rat pancreatic stellate cells: potential therapeutic role of follistatin for pancreatic fibrosis. *Gut* 52:1487-1493.

Ohnishi H, Miyata T, Yasuda H, Satoh Y, Hanatsuka K, Kita H, Ohashi A, Tamada K, Makita N, Iiri T, Ueda N, Mashima H, Sugano K (2004) Distinct roles of Smad2-, Smad3-, and ERK-dependent pathways in transforming growth factor-1 regulation of pancreatic stellate cellular functions. *J Biol Chem* 279: 8873-8878.

Oide H, Thurman RG (1994) Hepatic ito cells contain calcium channels: Increases with transforming growth factor-β1. *Hepatology* 20:1009 – 1014.

Oikawa H, Masuda T, Kawaguchi J, Sato R (2002) Three-dimensional examination of hepatic stellate cells in rat liver and response to endothelin-1 using confocal laser scanning microscopy. *J Gastroenterol Hepatol* 17: 861 – 872.

Okabe T, Yorifuji H, Yamada E, Takaku F (1984) Isolation and characterization of vitamin A-storing lung cells. *Exp Cell Res* 154: 125-135.

Okuno M, Kojima S, Akita K, Matsushima-Nishiwaki R, Adachi S, Sano T, Takano Y, Takai K, Obora A, Yasuda I, Shiratori Y, Okano Y, Shimada J, Suzuki Y, Muto Y, Moriwaki H (2002) Retinoids in liver fibrosis and cancer. *Front Biosc* 7:d204-d218.

Okuno M, Moriwaki H, Imai S, Muto Y, Kawada N, Suzuki Y, Kojima S (1997) Retinoids exacerbate rat liver fibrosis by inducing the activation of latent TGF-β in liver stellate cells. *Hepatology* 26:913-921.

Okuno M, Muto Y, Moriwaki H, Kato M, Noma A, Yagaya O, Nozaki Y, Suzuki Y (1990) Inhibitory effect of acyclic (polyprenoic acid) on hepatic fibrosis in CCl_4-treated rats. *Gastroenterol Jpn* 25: 223-229.

Okuno M, Sato T, Kitamoto T, Imai S, Kawada N, Suzuki Y, Yoshimura H, Moriwaki H, Onuki K, Masushige S, Muto Y, Friedman SL, Kato S, Kojima S (1999) Increased 9,13-di-*cis*-retinoic acid in rat hepatic fibrosis: implication for a potential link between retinoid loss and TGF-β mediated fibrogenesis *in vivo*. *J Hepatol* 30:1073-1080.

Olaso E, Ikeda K, Eng FJ, Xu L, Wang L-H, Lin HC, Friedman SL (2001) DDR2 receptor promotes MMP-2–mediated proliferation and invasion by hepatic stellate cells. *J Clin Invest* 108: 1369-1378.

Ong DE (1994) Absorption of vitamin A. In:Blomhoff R (ed) Vitamin A in Health and Disease. *Marcel Dekker Inc,* New York, pp 37-72.

Ong DE, MacDonald PN, Gubitosi AM (1988) Esterification of retinol in rat liver. Possible participation by cellular retinol-binding protein and cellular retinol-binding protein II. *J Biol Chem* 263:5789-5796.

Ong DE, Newcomer M, Lareyre J-J, Orgebin-Crist M-C (2000) Epididymal retinoic acid-binding protein. *Biochim Biophys Acta Prot Struct Mol Enzymol* 1482: 209-217.

Orland MD, Anwar K, Cromley D, Chu CH, Chen L, Billheimer JT, Hussain MM, Cheng D (2005) Acyl coenzyme A dependent retinol esterification by acyl coenzyme A:diacylglycerol acyltransferase 1. *Biochim Biophys Acta* 1737:76-82.

Paik Y-H, Schwabe RF, Bataller R, Russo MP, Jobin C, Brenner DA (2003) Toll-Like receptor 4 mediates inflammatory signaling by bacterial lipopolysaccharide in human hepatic stellate cells. *Hepatology* 37: 1043–1055.

Paik J, Vogel S, Quadro L, Piantedosi R, Gottesman M, Lai K, Hamberger L, de Morais Vieira M, Blaner WS (2004) Vitamin A: overlapping delivery pathways to tissues from the circulation. *J Nutr* 134:276S-280S.

Paradis V, Dargere D, Bonvoust F, Vidaud M, Segarini P, Bedossa P (2002) Effects and regulation of connective tissue growth factor on hepatic stellate cells. *Lab Invest* 82:767–774.

Parsons CJ, Bradford BU, Pan CQ, Cheung E, Schauer M, Knorr A, Krebs B, Kraft S, Zahn S, Brocks B, Feirt N, Mei B, Cho M-S, Ramamoorthi R, Roldan G, Ng P, Lum P, Hirth-Dietrich C, Tomkinson A, Brenner DA

(2004) Antifibrotic effects of a tissue inhibitor of metalloproteinase-1 antibody on established liver fibrosis in rats. *Hepatology* 40: 1106-1115.

Parsons CJ, Takashima M, Rippe RA (2007) Molecular mechanisms of hepatic fibrogenesis. *J Gastroenterol Hepatol* 22: S79 - S84.

Pasutto F, Sticht H, Hammersen G, Gillessen-Kaesbach G, FitzPatrick DR, Nürnberg G, Brasch F, Schirmer-Zimmermann H, Tolmie JL, Chitayat D, Houge G, Fernández-Martínez L, Keating S, Mortier G, Hennekam RCM, von der Wense A, Slavotinek A, Meinecke P, Bitoun P, Becker C, Nürnberg P, Reis A, Rauch A (2007) Mutations in STRA6 cause a broad spectrum of malformations including anophthalmia, congenital heart defects, diaphragmatic hernia, alveolar capillary dysplasia, lung hypoplasia, and mental retardation. *Am J Human Genetics* 80: 550-560.

Pérez-Pomares JM, Carmona R, González-Iriarte M, Macías D, Guadix JA, Muñoz-Chápuli R (2004) Contribution of mesothelium-derived cells to liver sinusoids in avian embryos. *Develop Dynam* 229:465-474.

Petkovich M, Brand NJ, Krust A, Chambon P (1987) A human retinoic acid receptor which belongs to the family of nuclear receptors. *Nature* 330:444-450.

Petta S, Cammà C, Di Marco V, Alessi N, Barbaria F, Cabibi D, Caldarella R, Ciminnisi S, Licata A, Massenti MF, Mazzola A, Tarantino G, Marchesini G, Craxì A (2008) Retinol-binding protein 4: A new marker of virus-induced steatosis in patients infected with hepatitis C virus genotype. *Hepatology* 48: 28-37.

Phillips PA, McCarroll JA, Park S, Wu M-J, Pirola R, Korsten M, Wilson JS, Apte MV (2003a) Rat pancreatic stellate cells secrete matrix metalloproteinases: implications for extracellular matrix turnover. *Gut* 52: 275-282.

Phillips PA, Wu MJ, Kjumar RK, Doherty E, McCarroll JM, Park S, Pirola RC, Wilson JS, Apte MV (2003b) Cell migration: a novel aspect of pancreatic stellate cell biology. *Gut* 52: 677-682.

Picard D, Yamamoto KR (1987) Two signals mediate hormone-dependent nuclear localization of the glucocorticoid receptor. *EMBO J* 6:3333-3340.

Pinzani M (1999) New kids on the block: pancreatic stellate cells enter the fibrogenesis world. *Gut* 44: 451-452.

Pinzani M (2004) Therapies for hepatic fibrosis: real hope or just academic exercise? *Dig Liver Dis* 36: 714-716.

Pinzani M (2006) Pancreatic stellate cells: new kids become mature. *Gut* 55: 12-14.

Pinzani M, Gentilini P, Abboud HE (1992) Phenotypical modulation of liver fat-storing cells by retinoids. Influence on unstimulated and growth factor-induced cell proliferation. *J Hepatol* 14:211-220.

Pinzani M, Gesualdo L, Sabbah GM, Abboud HE (1989) Effects of platelet-derived growth factor and other polypeptide mitogens on DNA synthesis and growth of cultured rat liver fat-storing cells. *J Clin Invest* 84: 1786-1793.

Pinzani M, Marra F (2001) Cytokine receptors and signaling in hepatic stellate cells. *Semin Liver Dis* 21: 397-416.

Pinzani M, Marra F, Carloni V (1998) Signal transduction in hepatic stellate cells. *Liver* 18: 2-13.

Pinzani M, Rombouts K, Colagrande S (2005) Fibrosis in chronic liver diseases: diagnosis and management. *J Hepatol* 42: S22-S36.

Polonsky KS (2006) Retinol-binding protein 4, insulin resistance, and type 2 diabetes. *New Eng J Med* 354:2596-2598.

Popper H (1941) Histologic distribution of vitamin A in human organs under normal and under pathologic conditions. *Arch Pathol* 31: 766-802.

Popper H (1944) Distribution of vitamin A in tissue as visualized by fluorescence microscopy. *Physiol Rev* 24: 205-224.

Popper H, Steigmann F, Meyer KA, Zevin SS (1943) Relation between hepatic and plasma concentrations of vitamin A in human beings. *Arch Int Med* 72: 439-460.

Popper H, Volk BW (1944) Absorption of vitamin A in the rat. *Arch Pathol* 38: 71-75.

Porter SB, Fraker LD, Chytil F, Ong DE (1983) Localization of retinol-binding protein in several tissues. *Proc Natl Acad Sci USA* 80: 6586-6590.

Potter JJ, Womack L, Mezey E, Anania FA (1998) Transdifferentiation of rat hepatic stellate cells results in leptin expression. *Biochem Biophys Res Commun* 244: 178-182.

Poynard T, McHutchison J, Manns M, Trepo C, Lindsay K, Goodman Z, Ling M-H, Albrecht J, PEG-FIBROSIS Project Group (2002) Impact of pegylated interferon alfa-2b and ribavirin on liver fibrosis in patients with chronic hepatitis C. *Gastroenterology* 122:1303-1313.

Prickett TCR, McKenzie JL, Hart DNJ (1988) Characterization of interstitial dendritic cells in human liver. *Transplantation* 46: 754-761.

Purohit V, Brenner DA (2006) Mechanisms of alcohol-induced hepatic fibrosis: A summary of the Ron Thurman symposium. *Hepatology* 43: 872-878.

Purohit V, Gao B, Song B-J (2009) Molecular mechanisms of alcoholic fatty liver. Alcoholism *Clin Exp Res* 33: 191-205.

Purton MD (1976) Extravascular cells with in perisinusoidal space of the avian liver. *Experientia* 32: 737-740.

Püschel GP (2004) Control of hepatocyte metabolism by sympathetic and parasympathetic hepatic nerves. *Anat Rec* 280A: 854–867.

Quadro L, Blaner WS, Hamberger L, Novikoff PM, Vogel S, Piantedosi R, Gottesman ME, Colantuoni V (2004) The role of extrahepatic retinol binding protein in the mobilization of retinoid stores. *J Lipid Res* 45: 1975-1982.

Quadro L, Blaner WS, Salchow DJ, Vogel S, Piantedosi R, Gouras P, Freeman S, Cosma MP, Colantuoni V, Gottesman ME (1999) Impaired retinal function and vitamin A availability in mice lacking retinol-binding protein. *EMBO J* 18: 4633–4644.

Quadro L, Hamberger L, Colantuoni V, Gottesman ME, Blaner WS (2003) Understanding the physiological role of retinol-binding protein in vitamin A metabolism using transgenic and knockout mouse models. *Mol Aspect Med* 24: 421-430.

Quan TE, Cowper S, Wu S-P, Bockenstedt LK, Bucala R (2004) Circulating fibrocytes: collagen-secreting cells of the peripheral blood. *Int J Biochem Cell Biol* 36: 598-606.

Raddatz D, Henneken M, Armbrust T, Ramadori G (1996) Subcellular distribution of glucocorticoid receptor in cultured rat and human liver-derived cells and cell lines: influence of dexamethasone. *Hepatology* 24:928-933.

Radaeva S, Wang L, Radaev S, Jeong WI, Park O, Gao B (2007) Retinoic acid signaling sensitizes hepatic stellate cells to NK cell killing via upregulation of NK cell activating ligand RAE1. *Am J Physiol Gastrointest Liver Physiol* 293:G809-G816.

Raica N, Scott J, Lowry L, Sauberlich HE (1972) Vitamin A concentration in human tissues collected from five areas in the United States. *Am J Clin Nutr* 25: 291-298.

Ralli EP, Papper E, Paley K, Bauman E (1941) Vitamin A and carotene content of human liver in normal and in diseased subjects. *Arch Int Med* 68: 102-111.

Ramadori G (1991) The stellate cell (Ito-cell, fat-storing cell, lipocyte, perisinusoidal cell) of the liver. New insights into pathophysiology of an intriguing cell. *Virchows Archiv* [B] 61: 147-158.

Ramadori G, Knittel T, Schwogler S, Bieber F, Rieder H, Meyer zum Buschenfelde KH (1991) Dexamethasone modulates α 2-macroglobulin and apolipoprotein E gene expression in cultured rat liver fat-storing (Ito) cells. Hepatology 14:875-882.

Ramadori G, Saile B (2002) Mesenchymal cells in the liver-one cell type or two? *Liver* 22: 283-294.

Ramm GA, Britton RS, O'Neill R, Blaner WS, Bacon BR (1995) Vitamin A-poor lipocytes: a novel desmin-negative lipocyte subpopulation, which can be activated to myofibroblasts. *Am J Physiol Gastrointest Liver Physiol* 269: G532-G541.

Ramm GA, Nair VG, Bridle KR, Shepherd RW, Crawford DHG (1998) Contribution of hepatic parenchymal and nonparenchymal cells to hepatic fibrogenesis in biliary atresia. *Am J Pathol* 153:527-535.

Randolph RK, Winkler KE, Ross AC (1991) Fatty acyl CoA-dependent and -independent retinol esterification by rat liver and lactating mammary gland microsomes. *Arch Biochem Biophys* 288:500-508.

Rashid ST, Corbineau S, Hannan N, Marciniak S J, Miranda E, Alexander G, Huang-Doran I, Griffin J, Ahrlund-Richter L, Skepper J, Semple R, Weber A, Komas DA, Vaillier L (2010) Modeling inherited metabolic disorders of the liver using human induced pluripotent stem cells. *J Clin Invest* 120: 3127-3130.

Ratziu V, Lalazar A, Wong L, Dang Q, Collins C, Shaulian E, Jensen S, Friedman SL (1998) Zf9, a Kruppel-like transcription factor up-regulated *in vivo* during early hepatic fibrosis. *Proc Natl Acad Sci USA* 95: 9500-9505.

Redlich CA, Grauer JN, Van Bennekum AM, Clever SL, Ponn RB, Blaner WS (1996) Characterization of carotenoid, vitamin A, and α tocopherol–levels in human lung tissue and pulmonary macrophages. *Am J Respir Cri Care Med* 154: 1436-1443.

Reid LM, Fiorino AS, Sigal SH, Brill S, Holst PA (1992) Extracellular matrix gradients in the space of Disse: Relevance to liver biology. *Hepatology* 15: 1198-1203.

Reif S, Lang A, Lindquist JN, Yata Y, Gäbele E, Scanga A, Brenner DA, Rippe RA (2003) The role of focal adhesion kinase-phosphatidylinositol 3-kinase-Akt signaling in hepatic stellate cell proliferation and type I collagen expression. *J Biol Chem* 278: 8083-8090.

Reilly FD, McCuskey PA, McCuskey RS (1978) Intrahepatic distribution of nerves in the rat. *Anat Rec* 191: 55-67.

Reimann T, Hempel U, Krautwald S, Axmann A, Scheibe R, Seidel D, Wenzel K-W (1997) Transforming growth factor-β 1 induces activation of Ras, Raf-1, MEK and MAPK in rat hepatic stellate cells. *FEBS Lett* 403: 57-60.

Riordan SM, Skinner N, Nagree A, McCallum H, McIver CJ, Kurtovic J, Hamilton JA, Bengmark S, Williams R, Visvanathan K (2003) Peripheral blood mononuclear cell expression of toll-like receptors and relation to cytokine levels in cirrhosis. *Hepatology* 37: 1154-1164.

Rippe RA, Brenner DA (2004) From quiescence to activation: Gene regulation in hepatic stellate cells. *Gastroenterology* 127: 1260-1262.

Robenek H, Hofnagel O, Buers I, Robenek MJ, Troyer D, Severs NJ (2006) Adipophilin-enriched domains in the ER membrane are sites of lipid droplet biogenesis. *J Cell Sci* 119:4215-4224.

Rockey DC (1995) Characterization of endothelin receptors mediating rat hepatic stellate cell contraction. *Biochem Biophys Res Commun* 207: 725-731.

Rockey DC (2003) Vascular mediators in the injured liver. *Hepatology* 37: 4-12.

Rockey DC, Maher JJ, Jarnagin WR, Gabbiani G, Friedman SL (1992) Inhibition of rat hepatic lipocyte activation in culture by interferon-γ. *Hepatology* 16: 776-784.

Rockey DC, Weisiger RA (1996) Endothelin induced contractility of stellate cells from normal and cirrhotic rat liver: implications for regulation of portal pressure and resistance. *Hepatology* 24: 233-240.

Rodahl K (1949a) Toxicity of polar bear liver. Nature (London) 164: 530-531.

Rodahl K (1949b) Vitamin sources in Arctic regions. *Norsk polarinstitutt skrifter* 91: 1-64.

Rodahl K, Moore T (1943) The vitamin A content and toxicity of bear and seal liver. *Biochem J* 37: 166-168.

Rojkind M, Greenwel P (1994) The extracellular matrix of the liver. In: Arias IA, Boyer JL, Fausto N, Jakoby WB, Schachter DA, Shafritz DA (eds) *The Liver: Biology and Pathobiology, Raven Press,* New York, pp 843-868.

Rojkind M, Novikoff PM, Greenwel P, Rubin J, Rojas-Valencia L, de Carvalho AC, Stockert R, Spray D, Hertzberg EL, Wolkoff AW (1995) Characterization and functional studies on rat liver fat-storing cell line and freshly isolated hepatocyte coculture system. *Am J Pathol* 146: 1508-1519.

Rombouts K, Knittel T, Machesky L, Braet F, Wielant A, Hellemans K, De Bleser P, Gelman I, Ramadori G, Albert A (2002) Actin filament formation, reorganization and migration are impaired in hepatic stellate cells under influence of trichostatin A, a histone deacetylase inhibitor. *J Hepatol* 37: 788-796.

Rombouts K, Niki T, Wielant A, Hellemans K, Schuppan D, Kormoss N, Geerts A (2001) Effect of aldosterone on collagen steady state levels in primary and subcultured rat hepatic stellate cells. *J Hepatol* 34:230-238.

Rosales C, O'Brien V, Kornberg L, Juliano R (1995) Signal transduction by cell adhesion receptors. *Biochim Biophys Acta* 1242: 77-98.

Rosette C, Karin M (1995) Cytoskeletal control of gene expression: Depolymerization of microtubules activates NF-κB. *J Cell Biol* 128: 1111-1119.

Roskelley CD, Srebrow A, Bissell MJ (1995) A hierarchy of ECM-mediated signaling regulates tissue-specific gene expression. *Curr Opin Cell Biol* 7: 736-747.

Ross AC (1982) Retinol esterification by rat liver microsomes. *J Biol Chem* 257: 2453-2459.

Ross AC (1993) Cellular metabolism and activation of retinoids: roles of cellular retinoid-binding proteins. *FASEB* J 7: 317-327.

Ross AC (1999) Mutations in the gene encoding retinol binding protein and retinol deficiency: is there compensation by retinyl esters and retinoic acid? *Am J Clin Nutr* 69: 829-830.

Ross AC (2004) On the sources of retinoic acid in the lung: understanding the local conversion of retinol to retinoic acid. *Am J Physiol Lung Cell Mol Physiol* 286: L247-L248.

Rothe P (1882) Ueber die Sternzellen der Leber. *Inaug-Dissertation,* München.

Rozga J, Demetriou AA (1995) Artificial liver: Evolution and future perspectives. *ASAIO Journal.* 41:831-837.

Ruiz A, Winston A, Lim YH, Gilbert BA, Rando RR, Bok D (1999) Molecular and biochemical characterization of lecithin retinol acyltransferase. *J Biol Chem* 274:3834-3841.

Russo FP, Alison MR, Bigger BW, Amofah E, Florou A, Amin F, Bou-Gharios G, Jeffery R, Iredale JP, Forbes SJ (2006) The bone marrow functionally contributes to liver fibrosis. *Gastroenterology* 130: 1807-1821.

Saari JC, Bredberg L, Garwin GG (1982) Identification of the endogenous retinoids associated with three cellular retinoid-binding proteins from bovine retina and retinal pigment epithelium. *J Biol Chem* 257: 13329-13333.

Sakakibara K, Saito M, Umeda M, Enaka K, Tsukada Y (1976) Native collagen formation by liver parenchymal cells in culture. *Nature* 262: 316-318.

Sancho-Bru P, Bataller R, Colmenero J, Gasull X, Moreno M, Arroyo V, Brenner DA, Ginès P (2006) Norepinephrine induces calcium spikes and proinflammatory actions in human hepatic stellate cells. *Am J Physiol Gastrointest Liver Physiol* 291: G877-G884.

Sandgren ME, Bronnegard M, DeLuca HF (1991) Tissue distribution of the 1,25-dihydroxyvitamin D_3 receptor in the male rat. *Biochem Biophys Res Commun* 181:611-616.

Sario AD, Bendia E, Macarri G, Candelaresi C, Taffetani S, Marzioni M, Omenetti A, De Minicis S, Trozzi L, Benedetti A (2004) The anti-fibrotic effect of pirfenidone in rat liver fibrosis is mediated by downregulation of procollagen α 1(I), TIMP-1 and MMP-2. *Dig Liver Dis* 36: 744-751.

Sato M, Imai K, Kojima N, Miura M, Senoo H (1997) Long cellular processes of hepatic stellate cells cultured on or in type I collagen gel. In: Wisse E, Knook DL, Balabaud C (eds) *Cells Hepatic Sinusoid,* vol 6, Kupffer Cell Foundation, Leiden, pp 85-89.

Sato T, Kato R, Tyson CA (1995) Regulation of differentiated phenotype of rat hepatic lipocytes by retinoids in primary culture. *Exp Cell Res* 217: 72-83.

Sato M, Kojima N, Miura M, Imai K, Senoo H (1998) Induction of cellular processes containing collagenase and retinoid by integrin-binding to interstitial collagen in hepatic stellate cell culture. *Cell Biol Int* 22: 115-125.

Sato M, Kojima N, Miura M, Imai K, Senoo H (1999) Intracellular signaling for process elongation in cultured hepatic stellate cells on type I collagen gel. In: Wisse E, Knook DL, de Zanger R, Fraser R (eds) Cells Hepatic Sinusoid, vol 7, *Kupffer Cell Foundation,* Leiden, pp 32-33.

Sato M, Miura M, Kojima N, Higashi N, Imai K, Sato T, Wold HL, Moskaug JØ, Blomhoff R, Wake K, Roos N, Berg T, Norum KR, Senoo H (2001a) Nuclear deviation in hepatic parenchymal cells on sinusoidal surface in arctic animals. *Cell Struct Func* 26: 71-77.

Sato Y, Murase K, Kato J, Kobune M, Sato T, Kawano Y, Takimoto R, Takada K, Miyanishi K, Matsunaga T, Takayama T, Niitsu Y (2008) Resolution of liver cirrhosis using vitamin A-coupled liposomes to deliver siRNA against a collagen-specific chaperone. *Nature Biotechnol.* 26: 431-442.

Sato M, Sato T, Kojima N, Imai K, Higashi N, Wang DR, Senoo H (2004) Three-dimensional structure of extracellular matrix regulates gene expression in cultured stellate cells to induce process elongation. *Comp Hepatol* 3 (Suppl 1): S4.

Sato M, Sato T, Kojima N, Miura M, Imai K, Wang DR, Senoo H (2001b) Induction of cellular process elongation mediated by microtubule-associated protein 2 in hepatic stellate cells cultured on type I collagen gel. In: Wisse E, Knook DL, de Zanger R, Arthur MJP (eds) Cells Hepatic Sinusoid, vol 8, *Kupffer Cell Foundation,* Leiden, pp 205-206.

Sato M, Senoo H (1998) Morphological regulation of cultured hepatic stellate cells by extracellular matrix through intracellular signaling. *Connective Tissue* 30: 219-224.

Sato M, Suzuki S, Senoo H (2003) Hepatic stellate cells: Unique characteristics in cell biology and phenotype. *Cell Struct Func* 28: 105-112.

Sauvant P, Sapin V, Alexandre-Gouabau M-C, Dodeman I, Delpal S, Quadro L, Partier A, Abergel A, Colantuoni V, Rock E, Azaïs-Braesco V (2001) Retinol mobilization from cultured rat hepatic stellate cells does not require retinol binding protein synthesis and secretion. *Int J Biochem Cell* Biol 33: 1000-1012.

Schieferdecker HK, Pestel S, Rothermel E, Püschel GP, Götze O, Jungermann K (1998) Stimulation by anaphylatoxin C5a of glycogen phosphorylase in rat hepatocytes via prostanoid release from hepatic stellate cells but not sinusoidal endothelial cells. *FEBS Lett* 434: 245-250.

Schneider E, Schmid-Kotsas A, Zhao J, Weidenbach H, Schmid RM, Menke A, Adler G, Waltenberger J, Grünert A, Bachem MG (2001) Identification of mediators stimulating proliferation and matrix synthesis of rat pancreatic stellate cells. *Am J Physiol Cell Physiol* 281: G532-G543.

Schneiderhan W, Schmid-Kotsas A, Zhao J, Grünert A, Nüssler A, Weidenbach H, Menke A, Schmid RM, Adler G, Bachem MG (2001) Oxidized low-density lipoproteins bind to the scavenger receptor, CD36, of hepatic stellate cells and stimulate extracellular matrix synthesis. *Hepatology* 34: 729-737.

Schwabe RF, Seki E, Brenner DA (2006) Toll-like receptor signaling in the liver. *Gastroenterology* 130: 1886-1900.

Schwögler S, Odenthal M, Knittel T, Meyer zum Büschenfelde K-H, Ramadori G (1992) Fat-storing cells of the rat liver synthesize and secrete C1-esterase inhibitor; modulation by cytokines. *Hepatology* 16: 794-802.

Seeliger MW, Biesalski HK, Wissinger B, Gollnick H, Gielen S, Frank J, Beck S, Zrenner E (1999) Phenotype in retinol deficiency due to a hereditary defect in retinol binding protein synthesis. *Invest Ophthalmol Vis Sci* 40: 3-11.

Seifert WF, Bosma A, Brouwer A, Hendriks HFJ, Roholl PJM, van Leeuwen REW, van Thiel-DeRuiter GCF, Seifert-Bock I, Knook DL (1994a) Vitamin A deficiency potentiates carbon tetrachloride-induced liver fibrosis in rats. *Hepatology* 19: 193–201.

Seifert WF, Roholl PJ, Blauw B, van der Ham F, van Thiel-De Ruiter CF, Seifert-Bock I, Bosma A, Knook DL, Brouwer A (1994b) Fat-storing cells and myofibroblasts are involved in the initial phase of carbon tetrachloride-induced hepatic fibrosis in BN/BiRij rats. *Int J Exp Pathol* 75:131-146.

Seki E, De Minicis S, Österreicher CH, Kluwe J, Osawa Y, Brenner DA, Schwabe RF (2007) TLR4 enhances TGF-β signaling and hepatic fibrosis. *Nature Med* 13: 1324-1332.

Senoo H (2000) Digestion, Metabolism. In: The Digital Handbook of Experimental Laboratory Animals: The rat. Krinke GJ (ed) *Academic Press,* London, pp 359-383.

Senoo H (2004) Structure and function of hepatic stellate cells. *Med Electron Microsc* 37:3-15.

Senoo H (2007a) Stellate cell-endothelial cell interactions. In: Aird WC (ed) Endothelial Biomedicine. *Cambridge University Press,* Cambridge, pp 616-619.

Senoo H (2007b) Vitamin A-storing cell (stellate cell) system. In: Loessing IT (ed) Vitamin A: New Research. *Nova Science Publishers*, New York. pp 59-70.

Senoo H, Hata R (1993a) Tissue formation and extracellular matrix system--Cellular devices for adhesion to extracellular matrix--. *Tiss Cult Res Commun* 12: 237-245.

Senoo, H, Hata R (1993b) Isolation of perisinusoidal stellate cells (vitamin A-storing cells, fat-storing cells) of the rat liver. *Connective Tissue* 25: 129-137.

Senoo H, Hata R (1994a) Extracellular matrix regulates and L-ascorbic acid 2-phosphate further modulates morphology, proliferation, and collagen synthesis of the perisinusoidal stellate cells. *Biochem Biophys Res Commun* 200: 999-1006.

Senoo H, Hata R (1994b) Extracellular matrix regulates cell morphology, proliferation, and tissue formation. *Acta Anat Nippon* 69: 719-733.

Senoo H, Hata R (1995) Regulation of morphology, proliferation, and collagen metabolism of perisinusoidal stellate cells by extracellular matrix. In: Wisse E, Knook DL, Wake K (eds), *Cells of the Hepatic Sinusoid,* vol 5, Kupffer Cell Foundation, Leiden, pp 430-431.

Senoo H, Hata R, Nagai Y, Wake K (1984) Stellate cells (vitamin A-storing cells) are the primary site of collagen synthesis in non-parenchymal cells in the liver. *Biomed Res* 5: 451-458.

Senoo H, Hata R, Wake K, Nagai Y (1991) Isolation and serum free culture of stellate cells. In: Wisse E, Knook DL, McCuskey RS (eds) Cells of the Hepatic Sinusoid, vol 3, *Kupffer Cell Foundation,* Leiden, pp 259-262.

Senoo H, Imai K, Matano Y, Sato M (1998) Molecular mechanisms in the reversible regulation of morphology, proliferation and collagen metabolism in hepatic stellate cells by the three-dimensional structure of the extracellular matrix. *J Gastroent Hepatol* 13(Suppl.): S19-S32.

Senoo, H., Imai, K., Mezaki, Y., Miura, M., Morii, M., Fujiwara, M., Blomhoff, R (2012) Accumulation of vitamin A in the hepatic stellate cell of arctic top predators. *Anat Rec.* 295, 1660-1668.

Senoo H, Imai K, Sato M, Kojima N, Miura M, Hata R (1996) Three-dimensional structure of extracellular matrix reversibly regulates morphology, proliferation and collagen metabolism of perisinusoidal stellate cells (vitamin A-storing cells). *Cell Biol Int* 20: 501-512.

Senoo H, Imai K, Wake K, Wold HL, Moskaug JØ, Kojima N, Matano Y, Miura M, Sato M, Roos N, Berg T, Langvatn R, Norum KR, Blomhoff R (1999) Vitamin A-storing system in mammals and birds in Arctic area-A study in the Svalbard archipelago-. In: Wisse E, Knook DL, de Zanger R, Fraser R (eds) Cells Hepatic Sinusoid, vol 7, *Kupffer Cell Foundation,* Leiden, pp 34-35.

Senoo H, Kojima N, Sato M (2007) Vitamin A-storing cells (stellate cells). *Vitam Horm* 75:131-159.

Senoo H, Mezaki Y, Miura M, Sanada C, Umezono-Hanata Y, Morii M, Imai K, Fujiwara M. (2011a) Hepatic stellate cell (vitamin A-storing cell) and its relative Recent *Res. Devel. Nutrition,* 8, 129-147 ISBN: 978-81-308-0468-2, editor Shankar Pandalai.

Senoo H, Mezaki Y, Morii M, Hebiguchi T, Miura M, Imai K (2013) Uptake and storage of vitamin A as lipid droplets in the cytoplasm in cells in lamina propria mucosae of rat intestine. *Cell Biol Int* 37: 1171-1180.

Senoo H, Sato M, Imai K (1997) Hepatic stellate cells -From the viewpoint of retinoid handling and function of the extracellular matrix-. *Acta Anat Nippon* 72: 79-94.

Senoo H, Smeland S, Malaba L, Bjerknes T, Stang E, Roos N, Berg T, Norum KR, Blomhoff R (1993) Transfer of retinol-binding protein from HepG2 human hepatoma cells to cocultured rat stellate cells. *Proc Natl Acad Sci USA* 90:3616-3620.

Senoo H, Stang E, Nilsson A, Kindberg GM, Berg T, Roos N, Norum KR, Blomhoff R (1990) Internalization of retinol-binding protein in parenchymal and stellate cells of rat liver. *J Lipid Res* 31:1229-1239.

Senoo H, Tsukada Y, Sato T, Hata RI (1989) Co-culture of fibroblasts and hepatic parenchymal cells induces metabolic changes and formation of a three-dimensional structure. *Cell Biol Int Rep* 13: 197-206.

Senoo H, Wake K (1985) Suppression of experimental hepatic fibrosis by administration of vitamin A. *Lab Invest* 52:182-194.

Senoo H, Wake K (1988) Histochemical method for detection of vitamin A. *Vitamins* 59: 465-469.

Senoo H, Wake K, Wold HL, Higashi N, Imai K, Moskaug JØ, Kojima N, Miura M, Sato T, Sato M, Roos N, Berg T, Norum KR, Blomhoff R (2004) Decreased capacity for vitamin A storage in hepatic stellate cells in arctic animals. *Comp Hepatol* 3(Suppl 1): S18.

Senoo H, Yoshikawa K, Morii M, Fujiwara M, Besshi K, Mezaki Y (2011) Regulation of vitamin A homeostasis by the stellate cell (vitamin A-storing cell) system. in Vitamin A: Nutrition, Side Effects and Supplements Nutrition and Diet Research Progress Editors: Lucas P. Scott ebook *Nova Science Publishers, Inc.,* New York p 47-74.

Senoo H, Yoshikawa K, Morii M, Miura M, Imai K, Mezaki Y (2010) Hepatic stellate cell (vitamin A-storing cell) and its relative--past, present, and future. *Cell Biol Int* (editor's special 70th birthday edition) 34, 1247-1272.

Severn CB (1971) A morphological study of the development of the human liver. I. Development of the hepatic diverticulum. *Am J Anat* 131: 133-158.

Severn CB (1972) A morphological study of the development of the human liver. II. Establishment of liver parenchyma, extrahepatic ducts and associated venous channels. *Am J Anat* 133: 85-108.

Servetnick DA, Brasaemle DL, Gruia-Gray J, Kimmel AR, Wolff J, Londos C (1995) Perilipins are associated with cholesteryl ester droplets in steroidogenic adrenal cortical and Leydig cells. *J Biol Chem* 270 :16970-16973.

She H, Xiong S, Hazra S, Tsukamoto H (2005) Adipogenic transcriptional regulation of hepatic stellate cells. *J Biol Chem* 280:4959-4967.

Shidoji Y, Muto Y (1977) Vitamin A transport in plasma of the non-mammalian vertebrates: isolation and partial characterization of piscine retinol-binding protein. *J Lipid Res* 18: 679-691.

Shimada T, Ross AC, Muccio DD, Brouillette WJ, Shealy YF (1997) Regulation of hepatic lecithin:retinol acyltransferase activity by retinoic acid receptor-selective retinoids. *Arch Biochem Biophys* 344: 220-227.

Shimizu I (2003) Impact of oestrogens on the progression of liver disease. *Liver Int* 23:63-69.

Shimizu K, Kobayashi M, Tahara J, Shiratori K (2005) Cytokines and peroxisome proliferator-activated receptor γ ligand regulate phagocytosis by pancreatic stellate cells. *Gastroenterology* 128: 2105-2118.

Shimizu I, Mizobuchi Y, Yasuda M, Shiba M, Ma YR, Horie T, Liu F, Ito S (1999) Inhibitory effect of oestradiol on activation of rat hepatic stellate cells in vivo and in vitro. *Gut* 44:127-136.

Shin YC (1981) Some observations on perisinusoidal lipocyte (Ito cell) of *Carassius Auratus* liver as revealed by electron microscopy. *Acta Anat Nippon* 56: 133-144.

Shiota G, Tsuchiya H, Hoshikawa Y (2006) The liver as a target organ of retinoids. *Hepatol Res* 36:248-254.

Sigal SH, Brill S, Fiorino AS, Reid LM (1992) The liver as a stem cell and lineage system. *Am J Physiol Gastrointest Liver Physio*l 263: G139-G148.

Skaare JU, Bernhoft A, Wiig Ø, Norum KR, Haug E, Eide DM, Derocher AE (2001) Relationship between plasma levels of organochlorines, retinol and thyroid hormones from polar bears (*Ursus maritimus*) at Svalbard. *J Toxicol Environ Health* 62: 227-241.

Smart DE, Vincent KJ, Arthur MJP, Eickelberg O, Castellazzi M, Mann DA (2001) JunD regulates transcription of the tissue inhibitor of metalloproteinases-1 and interleukin-6 genes in activated hepatic stellate cells. *J Biol Chem* 276: 24414-24421.

Smedsrød B, Le Couteur D, Ikejima K, Jaeschke H, Kawada N, Naito M, Knolle P, Nagy L, Senoo H, Vidal-Vanaclocha F, Yamaguchi N (2009) Hepatic sinusoidal cells in health and disease: Update from the 14th International Symposium. *Liver Int* 29: 491-501.

Smeland S, Bjerknes T, Malaba L, Eskild W, Norum KR, Blomhoff R (1995) Tissue distribution of the receptor for plasma retinol-binding protein. *Biochem J* 305: 419-424.

Smith FR, Goodman DS (1971) The effects of diseases of the liver, thyroid, and kidneys on the transport of vitamin A in human plasma. *J Clin Invest* 50: 2426-2436.

Smith JE, Goodman DW (1979) Retinol-binding protein and the regulation of vitamin A transport. *Fed Proc* 38: 2504-2509.

Spit BJ (1983) Induction of lipid droplets in fibroblasts of the hamster lung by a diet high in vitamin A. *Exp Lung Res* 4: 247-257.

Staatz WD, Fok KF, Zutter MM, Adams SP, Rodriguez BA, Santoro SA (1991) Identification of a tetrapeptide recognition sequence for the α2β1 integrin in collagen. *J Biol Chem* 266: 7363-7367.

Stefan N, Hennige AM, Staiger H, Machann J, Schick F, Schleicher E, Fritsche A, Häring H-U (2007) High circulating retinol-binding protein 4 is associated with elevated liver fat but not with total, subcutaneous, visceral, or intramyocellular fat in humans. *Diabetes Care* 30:1173-1178.

Steffan A-M, Gendrault J-L, McCuskey RS, McCuskey PA, Kirn A (1986) Phagocytosis, an unrecognized property of murine endothelial liver cells. *Hepatology* 6: 830-836.

Steiniger B, Klempnauer J, Wonigeit K (1984) Phenotype and histological distribution of interstitial dendritic cells in the rat pancreas, liver, heart, and kidney. *Transplantation* 38: 169-175.

Stewart SF, Day CP (2003) The management of alcoholic liver disease. *J Hepatol* 38: S2-S13.

Strain AJ (1999) *Ex vivo* liver cell morphogenesis: One step nearer to the bioartificial liver? *Hepatology* 29: 288-290.

Straub BK, Stoeffel P, Heid H, Zimbelmann R, Schirmacher P (2008) Differential pattern of lipid droplet-associated proteins and de novo perilipin expression in hepatocyte steatogenesis. *Hepatology* 47:1936-1946.

Sundaram M, Sivaprasadarao A, DeSousa, MM, Findlay JBC (1998) The transfer of retinol from serum retinol-binding protein to cellular retinol-binding protein is mediated by a membrane receptor. *J Biol Chem* 273: 3336-3342.

Sung CK, She H, Xiong S, Tsukamoto H (2004) Tumor necrosis factor-α inhibits peroxisome proliferator-activated receptor γ activity at a posttranslational level in hepatic stellate cells. *Am J Physiol Gastrointest Liver Physiol* 286:G722-G729.

Suskind DL, Muench MO (2004) Searching for common stem cells of the hepatic and hematopoietic systems in the human fetal liver: $CD34^+$ cytokeratin $7/8^+$ cells express markers for stellate cells. *J Hepatol* 40: 261–268.

Suzuki K (1958) A silver impregnation method in histyology. *Takeda Pharmaceut Ind* Osaka No. 310-320.

Svegliati-Baroni G, Ridolfi F, Hannivoort R, Saccomanno S, Homan M, De Minicis S, Jansen PL, Candelaresi C, Benedetti A, Moshage H (2005) Bile acids induce hepatic stellate cell proliferation via activation of the epidermal growth factor receptor. *Gastroenterology* 128:1042-1055.

Tabb MM, Sun A, Zhou C, Grun F, Errandi J, Romero K, Pham H, Inoue S, Mallick S, Lin M, Forman BM, Blumberg B (2003) Vitamin K_2 regulation of bone homeostasis is mediated by the steroid and xenobiotic receptor SXR. *J Biol Chem* 278:43919-43927.

Tahashi Y, Matsuzaki K, Date M, Yoshida K, Furukawa F, Sugano Y, Matsushita M, Himeno Y, Inagaki Y, Inoue K (2002) Differential regulation of TGF-β signal in hepatic stellate cells between acute and chronic rat liver injury. *Hepatology* 35: 49-61.

Taimr P, Higuchi H, Kocova E, Rippe RA, Friedman SL, Gores GJ (2003) Activated stellate cells express the TRAIL receptor-2/death receptor-5 and undergo TRAIL-mediated apoptosis. *Hepagtology* 37: 87-95.

Takada Y, Wayner EA, Carter WG, Hemler ME (1988) Extracellular matrix receptors, ECMRII and ECMRI, for collagen and fibronectin correspond to VLA-2 and VLA-3 in the VLA family of heterodimers. *J Cell Biochem* 37: 385-393.

Takahara T, Furui K, Yata Y, Jin B, Zhang LP, Nambu S, Sato H, Seiki M, Watanabe A (1997) Dual expression of matrix metalloproteinase-2 and membrane-type 1-matrix metalloproteinase in fibrotic human livers. *Hepatology* 26: 1521-1529.

Takahashi K, Yamanaka S (2006) Induction of pluripotent stem cells from mouse embryonic and adult fibroblast cultures by defined factors. *Cell* 126: 663-676.

Takase S, Leo MA, Nouchi T, Lieber C (1988) Desmin distinguishes cultured fat-storing cells from myofibroblasts, smooth muscle cells and fibroblasts in the rat. *J Hepatol* 6: 267-276.

Tanaka K (1955) Histochemical studies of vitamin A. *J Kyoto Pref Med Univ* 58: 333-377.

Tateno C, Yoshizato K (1996) Long-term cultivation of adult rat hepatocytes that undergo multiple cell divisions and express normal parenchymal phenotypes. *Am J Pathol* 148: 383-392.

Tauchi-Sato K, Ozeki S, Houjou T, Taguchi R, Fujimoto T (2002) The surface of lipid droplets is a phospholipid monolayer with a unique fatty acid composition. *J Biol Chem* 277:44507-44512.

Théret N, Lehti K, Musso O, Clément B (1999) MMP2 activation by collagen I and concanavalin A in cultured human hepatic stellate cells. *Hepatology* 30: 462 - 468.

Tomasek JJ, Hay ED (1984) Analysis of the role of microfilaments and microtubules in acquisition of bipolarity and elongation of fibroblasts in hydrated collagen gels. *J Cell Biol* 99: 536-549.

Tomasek JJ, Hay ED, Fujiwara K (1982) Collagen modulates cell shape and cytoskeleton of embryonic corneal and fibroma fibroblasts: Distribution of actin, α-actinin, and myosin. *Dev Biol* 92: 107-122.

Tran-Thi T, Kawada N, Decker K (1993) Regulation of endothelin-1 action on the perfused rat liver. *FEBS Lett* 318: 353-357.

Trim N, Morgan S, Evans M, Issa R, Fine D, Afford S, Wilkins B, Iredale J (2000) Hepatic stellate cells express the low affinity nerve growth factor receptor p75 and undergo apoptosis in response to nerve growth factor stimulation. *Am J Pathol* 156: 1235-1243.

Trøen G, Nilsson A, Norum KR, Blomhoff R (1994) Characterization of liver stellate cell retinyl ester storage. *Biochem J* 300: 793–798.

Tsuiki E, Fujita A, Ohsaki Y, Cheng J, Irie T, Yoshikawa K, Senoo H, Mishima K, Kitaoka T, Fujimoto T (2007) All-*trans*-retinol generated by rhodopsin photobleaching induces rapid recruitment of TIP47 to lipid droplets in the retinal pigment epithelium. *Invest Ophthalmol Vis Sci* 48:2858-2867.

Tsukamoto H (2005) Fat paradox in liver disease. *Keio J Med* 54:190-192.

Tsukamoto H, Cheng S, Blaner WS (1996) Effects of dietary polyunsaturated fat on ethanol-induced Ito cell activation. *Am J Physiol Gastrointest Liver Physiol* 270: G581-G586.

Tsutsumi M, Takada A, Takase S (1987) Characterization of desmin-positive rat liver sinusoidal cells. *Hepatology* 7: 277-284.

Uchio K, Tuchweber B, Manabe N, Gabbiani G, Rosenbaum J, Desmoulière A (2002) Cellular retinol-binding protein-1 expression and modulation during in vivo and in vitro myofibroblastic differentiation of rat hepatic stellate cells and portal fibroblasts. *Lab Invest* 82: 619-628.

Ueno T, Bioulac-Sage P, Balabaud C, Rosenbaum J (2004) Innervation of the sinusoidal wall: Regulation of the sinusoidal diameter. *Anat Rec Part A* 280A: 868–873.

Uyama N, Shimahara Y, Kawada N, Seki S, Okuyama H, Iimuro Y, Yamaoka Y (2002) Regulation of cultured rat hepatocyte proliferation by stellate cells. *J Hepatol* 36: 590-599.

Vaccaro C, Brody JS (1978) Ultrastructure of developing alveoli. I. The role of the interstitial fibroblast. *Anat Rec* 192: 467-479.

Varela-Rey M, Montiel-Duarte C, Osés-Prieto JA, López-Zabalza MJ, Jaffrèzou JP, Rojkind M, Iraburu MJ (2002) p38 MAPK mediates the regulation of α1(I) procollagen mRNA levels by TNF-α and TGFβ in a cell line of rat hepatic stellate cells. *FEBS Lett* 528: 133-138.

Varet KS, Grompe M (2008) Generation and regeneration of cells of the liver and pancreas. *Science* 322: 1490-1494.

Vincent KJ, Jones E, Arthur MJP, Smart DE, Trim J, Wright MC, Mann DA (2001) Regulation of E-box DNA binding during in vivo and in vitro activation of rat and human hepatic stellate cells. *Gut* 49:713-719.

Vinñs O, Bataller R, Sacho-Bru P, Gines P, Berenguer C, Enrich C, Nicolás JM, Ercilla G, Gallart T, Vives J, Arroyo V, Rodés J (2003) Human hepatic stellate cells show features of antigen-presenting cells and stimulate lymophocyte proliferation. *Hepatology* 38: 919-929.

Vogel W, Gish GD, Alves F, Pawson T (1997) The discoidin domain receptor tyrosine kinases are activated by collagen. *Mol Cell* 1: 13-23.

Vogel S, Mendelsohn CL, Mertz JR, Piantedosi R, Waldburger C, Gottesman ME, Blaner WS (2001) Characterization of a new member of the fatty acid-binding protein family that binds all-*trans*-retinol. *J Biol Chem* 276: 1353-1360.

Vollmar B, Heckmann C, Richter S, Menger MD (2002a) High, but not low, dietary retinoids aggravate manifestation of rat liver fibrosis. *J Gastroenterol Hepatol* 17: 791-799.

Vollmar B, Pradrarutti S, Richter S, Menger MD (2002b) *In vivo* quantification of ageing changes in the rat liver from early juvenile to senescent life. *Liver,* 22: 330-341.

Vyalov SL, Gabbiani G, Kapanci Y (1993) Rat alveolar myofibroblasts acquire alpha-smooth muscle actin expression during bleomycin-induced pulmonary fibrosis. *Am J Pathol* 143: 1754-1765.

Wake K (1964) Distribution of vitamin A in the liver. In: Miyake M (ed) *Proc 5th Annual Meeting of Japanese Histochemical Association*, pp 103-106.

Wake K (1971) "Sternzellen" in the liver: perisinusoidal cells with special reference to storage of vitamin A. *Am J Anat* 132:429-462.

Wake K (1973) Cytochemistry of the lipid droplets containing vitamin A in the liver. In: Wisse E, Daems WTh, Molenaar I, van Duijn P (eds) Electron Microscopy and Cytochemistry, *North-Holland Publishing Company,* Amsterdam, pp 279-282.

Wake K (1974) Development of vitamin A-rich lipid droplets in multivesicular bodies of rat liver stellate cells. *J Cell Biol* 63:683-691.

Wake K (1975a) One hundred years of the stellate cells of von Kupffer. *Proceedings of 10th International Congress of Anatomists,* August 25-30.

Wake K (1975b) Lysosomes in the hypervitaminosis A rat liver, with special reference to storage of vitamin A in the perisinusoidal stellate cells. *Recent Advances in RES Research* 15: 83-92.

Wake K (1975c) The stellate cell of the liver. *Kagaku (Science)* 45: 33-42.

Wake K (1978) Kupffer's original article of the discovery of stellate cells ("Sternzellen"). *Acta Anat Nippon* 53: 368-372.

Wake K (1980a) Perisinusoidal stellate cells (fat-storing cells, interstitial cells, lipocytes), their related structure in and around the liver sinusoids, and vitamin A-storing cells in extrahepatic organs. *Int Rev Cytol* 66:303-353.

Wake K (1980b) So-called Kupffer cells and hepatic stellate cells. *Saibo (Cell)* 12: 189-198.

Wake K (1982) The Sternzellen of von Kupffer-After 106 years. In: Knook DL, Wisse E (eds) Sinusoidal Liver Cells. *Elsevier Biomed Press,* Amsterdam, pp 1-12.

Wake K (1983) Vitamin A-storing cells: Recent advances. *Vitamins* 57: 587-600.

Wake K (1993) Intralobular heterogeneity of perisinusoidal stellate cells in porcine liver. *Cell Tiss Res* 273: 227-237.

Wake K (1995) Structure of the sinusoidal wall in the liver. In: Wisse E, Knook DL, Wake K (eds) Cells of the Hepatic Sinusoid, vol 5, *Kupffer Cell Foundation, Leiden,* pp 241-246.

Wake K (1997a) Cells in and around the hepatic sinusoid: past, present and future. In: Motta PM (ed) *Recent Advances in Microscopy of Cells, Tissues and Organs.* Antonio Delfino Editore, Rome, pp 421-428.

Wake K (1997b) One hundred years of sinusoidal cells in the liver. *Acta Anatomica Nippon* 72: 407-423.

Wake K (1998) Hepatic stellate cells. *Connective Tissue* 30: 245-246.

Wake K (2006) Hepatic stellate cells: Three-dimensional structure, localization, heterogeneity and development. *Proc Japan Acad Ser* B 82: 155-164.

Wake K (2009) Browcz's phagocytic cells and Kupffer's 'so-called stellate cells'. *Acta Anat Noppon* 84: 17-21.

Wake K, Motomatsu K, Senoo H (1987) Stellate cells storing retinol in the liver of adult lamprey, *lampetra japonica*. *Cell Tiss Res* 249: 289-299.

Wake K, Motomatsu K, Senoo H, Masuda A, Adachi E (1986) Improved Kupffer's gold chloride method for demonstrating the stellate cells storing retinol (vitamin A) in the liver and extrahepatic organs of vertebrates. *Stain Technol* 61: 193-200.

Wake K, Senoo H (1986) Morphological aspects of the differentiation of stellate cell line in the vertebrates. In: Kirn A, Knook DL, Wisse E (eds) *Cells of the Hepatic Sinusoid,* vol 1, Leiden, pp 215-220.

Wang SC, Ohata M, Schrum L, Rippe RA, Tsukamoto H (1998) Expression of interleukin-10 by *in vitro* and *in vivo* activated hepatic stellate cells. *J Biol Chem* 273: 302-308.

Wang L, Potter JJ, Rennie-Tankersley L, Novitskiy G, Sipes J, Mezey E (2007) Effects of retinoic acid on the development of liver fibrosis produced by carbon tetrachloride in mice. *Biochim Biophys Acta* 1772:66-71.

Wang DR, Sato M, Li LN, Miura M, Kojima N, Senoo H (2003) Stimulation of pro-MMP-2 production and activation by native form of extracellular type I collagen in cultured hepatic stellate cells. *Cell Struct Func* 28: 505-513.

Wang X, Tang X, Gong X, Albanis E, Friedman SL, Mao Z (2004a) Regulation of hepatic stellate cell activation and growth by transcription factor myocyte enhancer factor 2. *Gastroenterology* 127: 1174-1188.

Wang L, Tankersley LR, Tang M, Potter JJ, Mezey E (2002) Regulation of the murine α_2(I) collagen promoter by retinoic acid and retinoid X receptors. *Arch Biochem Biophys* 401:262-270.

Wang L, Tankersley LR, Tang N, Potter JJ, Mezey E (2004) Regulation of α2(I) collagen expression in stellate cells by retinoic acid and retinoid X receptors through interactions with their cofactors. *Arch Biochem Biophys* 428, 92-98.

Wanless IR (1999) Physioanatomic considerations. In: Schiff ER, Sorrell MF, Maddrey WC (eds) Schiff's Diseases of the Liver. 8th edn *Lippincott-Raven Publishers,* Philadelphia, pp 3-37.

Warren A, Bertolino P, Cogger VC, McLean AJ, Fraser R, Le Couteur DG (2005) Hepatic pseudocapillarization in aged mice. *Exp Gerontol* 40: 807-812.

Weinberger C, Hollenberg SM, Ong ES, Harmon JM, Brower ST, Cidlowski J, Thompson EB, Rosenfeld MG, Evans RM (1985a) Identification of human glucocorticoid receptor complementary DNA clones by epitope selection. *Science* 228:740-742.

Weinberger C, Hollenberg SM, Rosenfeld MG, Evans RM (1985b) Domain structure of human glucocorticoid receptor and its relationship to the v-erb-A oncogene product. *Nature* 318:670-672.

Weinberger C, Thompson CC, Ong ES, Lebo R, Gruol DJ, Evans RM (1986) The c-erb-A gene encodes a thyroid hormone receptor. *Nature* 324:641-646.

Weiner FR, Blaner WS, Czaja MJ, Shah A, Geerts A (1992) Ito cell expression of a nuclear retinoic acid receptor. *Hepatology* 15:336-342.

Weiner FA, Giambrone M-A, Czaja MJ, Shah A, Annoni G, Takahashi S, Eghbali M, Zern MA (1990) Ito-cell gene expression and collagen regulation. *Hepatology* 11: 111-117.

Wells RG, Crawford J (1998) Pancreatic stellate cells. The new stars of chronic pancreatitis? *Gastroenterology* 115: 491-493.

Wickert L, Abiaka M, Bolkenius U, Gressner AM (2004) Corticosteroids stimulate selectively transforming growth factor (TGF)-β receptor type III expression in transdifferentiating hepatic stellate cells. *J Hepatol* 40:69-76.

Wieckowska A, McCullough AJ, Feldstein AE (2007) Noninvasive diagnosis and monitoring of nonalcoholic steatohepatitis: *Present and future. Hepatology* 46: 582-589.

Wiig Ø, Derocher AE, Cronin MM, Skaare JU (1998) Female pseudohermaphrodite polar bears at Svalbard. *J Wildlife Dis* 34: 792-796.

Winau F, Hegasy G, Weiskirchen R, Weber S, Cassan C, Sieling PA, Modlin RL, Liblau RS, Gressner AM, Kaufmann S (2007) Ito cells are liver-resident antigen-presenting cells for activating T cell responses. *Immunity* 26: 117-129.

Wisse E (1970) An electron microscopic study of the fenestrated endothelial lining of rat liver sinusoid. *J Ultrastruct Res* 31: 125-150.

Wisse E (1972) An ultrastructural characterization of the endothelial cell in the rat liver sinusoid under normal and various experimental conditions, as a contribution to the distinction between endothelial and Kupffer cells. *J Ultrastruct Res* 38: 528-562.

Wold HL, Wake K, Higashi N, Wang D-R, Kojima N, Imai K, Blomhoff R, Senoo H (2004) Vitamin A distribution and content in tissues of the lamprey (*Lampetra japonica*). *Anat Rec* 276A: 134-142.

Wolins NE, Brasaemle DL, Bickel PE (2006) A proposed model of fat packaging by exchangeable lipid droplet proteins. *FEBS Lett* 580:5484-5491.

Wolins NE, Rubin B, Brasaemle DL (2001) TIP47 associates with lipid droplets. *J Biol Chem* 276:5101-5108.

Wright MC (2006) The impact of pregnane X receptor activation on liver fibrosis. *Biochem Soc Trans* 34:1119-1123.

Wu H, Jia W, Bao Y, Lu J, Zhu J, Wang R, Chen Y, Xiang K (2008) Serum retinol binding protein 4 and nonalcoholic fatty liver disease in patients with type 2 diabetes mellitus. *Diabetes Res Clin Pract* 79: 185-190.

Xu J, Fu Y, Chen A (2003) Activation of peroxisome proliferator-activated receptor-γ contributes to the inhibitory effects of curcumin on rat hepatic stellate cell growth. *Am J Physiol Gastrointest Liver Physiol* 285:G20-G30.

Yagmur E, Weiskirchen R, Gressner AM, Trautwein C, Tacke F (2007) Insulin resistance in liver cirrhosis is not associated with circulating retinol-binding protein 4. *Diabetes Care* 30:1168-1172.

Yamada E (1982) Vitamin A storing cell. *Method Enzymol* 81:834-839.

Yamada M, Blaner WS, Soprano DR, Dixon JL, Kjeldbye HM, Goodman DS (1987) Biochemical characteristics of isolated rat liver stellate cells. *Hepatology* 7:1224-1229.

Yamada E, Hirosawa K (1976) The possible existence of a vitamin A-storing cell system. *Cell Struct Func* 1: 201-204.

Yamada KM, Miyamoto S (1995) Integrin transmembrane signaling and cytoskeletal control. *Curr Opin Cell Biol* 7: 681-689.

Yamaguchi K, Yang L, McCall S, Huang J, Yu XX, Pandey SK, Bhanot S, Monia BP, Li YX, Diehl AM (2008) Diacylglycerol acyltranferase 1 anti-sense oligonucleotides reduce hepatic fibrosis in mice with nonalcoholic steatohepatitis. *Hepatology* 47:625-635.

Yamamoto M, Enzan H (1975) Morphology and function of Ito cell (fat-storing cell) in the liver. *Recent Advances RES Res* 15: 54-75.

Yamamoto M, Enzan H, Hara H, Iijima S (1978) Fluorescence and electron microscopic studies on the perivascular mesenchymal cells and fibroblasts after vitamin A administration. *Acta Pathol Jap* 28: 513-521.

Yamamoto K, Ogawa K (1983) Fine structure and cytochemistry of lysosomes in the Ito cells of the rat liver. *Cell Tissue Res* 233:45-57.

Yamamoto K, Ogawa K (1984) Freeze-replica study of lipid droplets in the Ito cells of rat liver. *Anat Rec* 210:415-420.

Yamauchi M, Potter JJ, Merzey E (1988) Characteristics of alcohol dehydrogenase in fat-storing (Ito) cells of rat liver. *Gastroenterology* 94: 163-169.

Yang Q, Graham TE, Mody N, Preitner F, Peroni OD, Zabolotny JM, Kotani K, Quadro L, Kahn BB (2005) Serum retinol binding protein 4 contributes to insulin resistance in obesity and type 2 diabetes. *Nature* 436: 356-362.

Yang L, Jung Y, Omenetti A, Witek RP, Choi S, Vandongen HM, Huang J, Alpini GD, Diehl AM (2008) Fate-mapping evidence that hepatic stellate cells are epithelial progenitors in adult mouse livers. *Stem Cells* 26: 2104-2113.

Yang C, Zeisberg M, Mosterman B, Sudhakar A, Yerramalla U, Holthaus K, Xu L, Eng F, Afdhal N, Kalluri R (2003) Liver fibrosis: Insights into migration of hepatic stellate cells in response to extracellular matrix and growth factors. *Gastroenterology* 124: 147-159.

Yavrom S, Chen L, Xiong S, Wang J, Rippe RA, Tsukamoto H (2005) Peroxisome proliferator-activated receptor γ suppresses proximal α1(I) collagen promoter via inhibition of p300-facilitated NF-I binding to DNA in hepatic stellate cells. *J Biol Chem* 280:40650-40659.

Yen CL, Monetti M, Burri BJ, Farese Jr RV (2005) The triacylglycerol synthesis enzyme DGAT1 also catalyzes the synthesis of diacylglycerols, waxes, and retinyl esters. *J Lipid Res* 46:1502-1511.

Yin C, Evason KJ, Maher JJ, Stainer YR (2012) The basic helix-loop-helix transcript factor, heart and neural crest derivatives expressed transcript 2, marks hepatic stellate cells in zebrafish: Analysis of stellate cell entry into the developing liver. *Hepatology* 56: 1958-1970.

Ylikomi T, Bocquel MT, Berry M, Gronemeyer H, Chambon P (1992) Cooperation of proto-signals for nuclear accumulation of estrogen and progesterone receptors. *EMBO J* 11:3681-3694.

Yokoi Y, Namihisa T, Kuroda H, Komatsu I, Miyazaki A, Watanabe S, Usui K (1984) Immnunocytochmical detection of desmin in fat-storing cells (Ito cells). *Hepatology* 4: 709-714.

Yorifuji H, Hirosawa K, Yamada E (1980) Vitamin A storing cell in mouse urinary bladder—An autoradiographic study. *J Electron Microsc* 29: 288.

Yoshikawa K, Imai K, Seki T, Higashi-Kuwata N, Kojima N, Yuuda M, Koyasu K, Sone H, Sato M, Senoo H, Irie T (2006) Distribution of retinylester-storing stellate cells in the arrowtooth halibut, *Atheresthes evermanni*. *Comp Biochem Physiol Part A* 145: 280-286.

Youson JH, Sidon EW (1978) Lamprey biliary atresia: first model system for the human condition? *Experientia* 34:1084-1086.

Yu MC, Chen CH, Liang X, Wang L, Gandhi CR, Fubg JJ, Lu L, Qian S (2004) Inhibition of T-cell responses by hepatic stellate cells via B7-H1-mediated T-cell apoptosis in mice. *Hepatology* 40: 1312-1321.

Zajicek G, Ariel I, Arber N (1988) The streaming liver III. Littoral cells accompany the streaming hepatocyte. Liver 8: 213-218.

Zajicek G, Oren R, Weinreb Jr M (1985) The streaming liver. *Liver* 5: 293-300.

Zaret KS (2001) Embryonic development of the liver. In: Arias IM, Boyer JL, Chisari EV, Fausto N, Schachter D, Shafritz DA (eds) The Liver: Biology and Pathobiology, 4th edn *Lippincott Williams & Wilkins*, Philadelphia, pp 17-25.

Zeisberg M, Yang C, Martino M, Duncan MB, Rieder F, Tanjore H, Kalluri R (2007) Fibroblasts derive from hepatocytes in liver fibrosis via epithelial to mesenchymal transition. *J Biol Chem* 282: 23337-23347.

Zhan S-S, Jiang JX, Wu J, Halsted C, Friedman SL, Zern MA, Torok NJ (2006) Phagocytosis of apoptotic bodies by hepatic stellate cells induces NADPH oxidase and is associated with liver fibrosis *in vivo*. *Hepatology* 43: 435-443.

Zhang JX, Pegoli Jr W, Clemens MG (1994) Endothelin-1 induces direct constriction of hepatic sinusoids. *Am J Physiol Gastrointest Liver Physiol* 266: G624 - G632.

Zhao C, Chen W, Yang L, Chen L, Stimpson SA, Diehl AM (2006) PPARγ agonists prevent TGFβ1/Smad3-signaling in human hepatic stellate cells. *Biochem Biophys Res Commun* 350:385-391.

Zheng S, Chen A (2004) Activation of PPARγ is required for curcumin to induce apoptosis and to inhibit the expression of extracellular matrix genes in hepatic stellate cells *in vitro*. *Biochem J* 384:149-157.

Zheng S, Chen A (2006) Curcumin suppresses the expression of extracellular matrix genes in activated hepatic stellate cells by inhibiting gene expression of connective tissue growth factor. *Am J Physiol Gastrointest Liver Physiol* 290:G883-G893.

Zhou X, Jamil A, Nash A, Chan J, Trim N, Iredale JP, Benyon RC (2006) Impaired proteolysis of collagen I inhibits proliferation of hepatic stellate cells. Implications for regulation of liver fibrosis. *J Biol Chem* 281: 39757-39765.

Zhou Y, Shimizu I, Lu G, Itonaga M, Okamura Y, Shono M, Honda H, Inoue S, Muramatsu M, Ito S (2001) Hepatic stellate cells contain the functional estrogen receptor β but not the estrogen receptor α in male and female rats. *Biochem Biophys Res Commun* 286:1059-1065.

Zizola CF, Schwartz GJ, Vogel S (2008) Cellular retinol-binding protein type III is a PPAR target gene and plays a role in lipid metabolism. *Am J Physiol Endocrinol Metab* 295: E1358-E1368.

Index

A

access, 56, 58
accounting, 121
acetaldehyde, 86, 141, 176, 177, 196
acetone, 135
acetylcholine, 104
acidic, 8, 92, 175, 183, 203, 204
active site, 149
adenosine, 169, 171
adhesion, 8, 13, 19, 28, 29, 32, 76, 88, 123, 150, 178, 184, 189, 190, 193, 194, 210, 212, 215
adhesions, 178, 197
adipocyte, 6, 53, 59, 68, 74, 76, 134, 185
adiponectin, 53, 134, 169
adipose, 43, 51, 52, 59, 66, 191
adipose tissue, 43, 51, 53, 59
adrenal gland, 105
adulthood, 8
adults, 53, 114, 142, 190, 192
adventitia, 105
adverse effects, 47
age, vii, 2, 4, 52, 64, 110, 111, 117, 140, 153, 173, 195
agonist, 68, 96, 112, 136, 190
albumin, 101, 156, 157, 187, 194
alcohol abuse, 127
alcohol consumption, 140, 142, 150
alcoholic cirrhosis, 76
alcoholic liver disease, 77, 121, 141, 219
alcoholics, 141, 200
alcohols, 59
aldosterone, 70, 212
alpha-2-macroglobulin, 70
alveoli, 109, 111, 222
alveolus, 111, 179
amino acid(s), 15, 31, 59, 60, 67, 93
ammonium sulfate, 83
anastomosis, 139, 143
anchoring, 94
androgen, 66, 177, 196
angiogenesis, 48, 97, 108, 178, 180, 199
angiotensin II, 80, 95, 96, 129
antagonism, 181
antibody, 15, 22, 26, 29, 64, 107, 108, 111, 119, 133, 144, 147, 149, 207
antigen, 128, 139, 147, 148, 156, 222, 225
antigen-presenting cell, 128, 148, 222, 225
antioxidant, 68, 79
antisense, 39
aorta, 105
APCs, 149
apoptosis, 68, 85, 91, 101, 102, 125, 132, 133, 136, 137, 138, 139, 141, 143, 144, 148, 169, 180, 186, 190, 202, 204, 205, 220, 221, 228
arabinogalactan, 34
arteries, 127
ascorbic acid, 89, 156, 195, 215

asymptomatic, 58
atherosclerosis, 114, 149, 180
ATP, 78, 103, 112, 171
atrophy, 114
attachment, 24, 48
avian, 183, 200, 207, 209

B

bacteria, 56, 148, 149, 150, 151
bacterial infection, 148, 151
barriers, 4
basal lamina, 100
base, 110
basement membrane, 18, 19, 24, 25, 88, 94, 100, 149, 156, 182, 203
basic research, viii, 1, 165
behaviors, 25
beneficial effect, 140
benign, 142
bile, 8, 45, 46, 65, 68, 69, 71, 78, 84, 93, 126, 128, 135, 136, 139, 140, 143, 144, 159, 172, 202
bile acids, 71
bile duct, 8, 45, 65, 68, 69, 71, 78, 84, 93, 126, 128, 135, 136, 139, 140, 143, 144, 172, 202
biliary atresia, 143, 144, 145, 180, 186, 210, 228
biliary cirrhosis, 145
biliary obstruction, 139, 143
bilirubin, 52
biodiversity, viii, 162
biological activities, 24, 49
biological activity, 107, 193
biological processes, 48
biomaterials, 155
biopsy, 122, 131, 139
biosynthesis, 15, 129
birds, 191, 216
blindness, 52, 141, 200
blood, 2, 17, 37, 38, 39, 40, 41, 43, 50, 51, 52, 57, 59, 61, 64, 65, 77, 93, 95, 96, 97, 99, 100, 102, 104, 127, 147, 149, 151, 211
blood flow, 77, 95, 96, 97, 104
blood plasma, 37
blood stream, 102
bloodstream, 39, 40, 61, 65
body fluid, 17
body mass index (BMI), 53, 54
bone, 8, 97, 105, 112, 126, 129, 130, 134, 171, 212, 220
bone marrow, 8, 97, 105, 129, 134, 171, 212
brain, 56, 200
branching, 12, 18, 19, 94, 102
breast milk, 179
budding, 158

C

Ca^{2+}, 95, 96, 97, 200
calcium, 205, 213
CAM, 8, 13, 32, 193
cancer, 13, 24, 107, 108, 115, 126, 153, 205
candidates, 83, 137
capillary, 55, 100, 109, 191, 207
capsule, 8, 127
carbon, 95, 194, 201, 215, 224
carbon dioxide, 95
carbon tetrachloride, 194, 201, 215, 224
carboxyl, 141, 196
carcinogenesis, 134
carcinoid tumor, 114
cardiovascular disease, 54
cardiovascular risk, 53
carotene, 36, 41, 52, 59, 179, 184, 202, 209
carotenoids, 40, 41, 112
cascades, 29, 123
CD8+, 147, 148, 193
CD95, 102, 125
cDNA, 56, 59, 64, 66, 185, 189, 191
cecum, 9
cell biology, 35, 81, 134, 165, 183, 207, 214
cell body, 18
cell culture, 26, 35, 44, 84, 131, 171, 178, 201, 213
cell cycle, 107, 123, 137
cell death, 138, 191
cell differentiation, 66

cell division, 125, 221
cell killing, 209
cell line(s), 2, 24, 41, 43, 45, 47, 157, 158, 176, 186, 198, 203, 209, 211, 222, 224
cell signaling, 96
cell surface, viii, 2, 18, 19, 22, 23, 24, 27, 30, 31, 32, 40, 63, 81, 86, 88, 93, 99, 150
central nervous system, 32
ceramide, 47
chaperones, 73
chemical, 50
chemokines, 76, 97, 128, 150
chemotaxis, 152
chicken, 178, 195
childhood, 53, 192
children, 53, 142, 192
cholestasis, 144, 145
cholesterol, 39, 53, 71, 73
choline, 68
chondroitin sulfate, 24, 84, 171
choroid, 56, 60
cilium, 17
circulation, 40, 44, 51, 57, 64, 113, 150, 206
cirrhosis, 54, 66, 103, 121, 122, 123, 125, 126, 127, 128, 130, 131, 132, 135, 137, 140, 142, 143, 144, 149, 150, 171, 178, 180, 186, 199, 202, 211
clarity, 6
classes, 39, 49, 77, 106, 151
cleavage, 59, 69, 139, 186
climate, 162
climate change, 162
clinical presentation, 53
clinical symptoms, 52
cloning, 74, 177, 178, 200
clustering, 24, 29, 194
clusters, 100, 119, 156
coding, 69, 125, 191
coenzyme, 206
colon, 70
common bile duct, 128, 186
common signs, 55
communication, 31, 47, 104, 181
compensation, 212
complement, 125, 142, 147
complementary DNA, 171, 177, 185, 196, 200, 225
complications, 75, 114, 130, 131, 140
composition, 43, 44, 76, 94, 111, 123, 202, 221
compounds, 49, 72, 95
conditioning, 133
Congress, 3, 223
connective tissue, 5, 45, 90, 109, 127, 128, 129, 144, 198, 206, 228
consensus, 6, 122
conservation, 201
constituents, 123, 126
contamination, 202
controversial, 9, 39, 41, 44, 46, 51, 74
conviction, 125
coordination, 31
corepressor, 46
correlations, 53
cost, 155
creatine, 64
crystallization, 204
cultivation, 173, 221
culture, vii, 1, 15, 18, 19, 22, 23, 27, 31, 33, 34, 35, 37, 41, 43, 65, 68, 69, 76, 77, 81, 82, 84, 86, 87, 88, 89, 92, 93, 94, 95, 101, 102, 106, 108, 115, 127, 134, 135, 139, 143, 147, 148, 149, 155, 157, 170, 171, 175, 178, 182, 186, 187, 192, 197, 201, 211, 213, 216, 217
culture conditions, 94
culture medium, 41, 43, 101, 102, 147, 157
curcumin, 196, 226, 228
cycling, 97
cyclooxygenase, 141, 204
cyst, 158
cystic duct, 144, 202
cytochrome, 79, 80, 141, 204
cytochromes, 60
cytokine networks, 119
cytokines, 3, 76, 88, 99, 106, 123, 128, 129, 133, 140, 148, 152, 170, 215
cytoplasm, vii, 2, 3, 13, 15, 18, 27, 35, 37, 42, 50, 61, 63, 66, 69, 88, 100, 105, 110, 112, 113, 114, 120, 217

cytoskeleton, viii, 23, 27, 29, 93, 194, 200, 221
cytotoxicity, 138

D

deaths, 121
defects, 60, 155, 207
defense mechanisms, 151
deficiency, 43, 45, 51, 52, 57, 58, 172, 212, 215
degenerate, 144
degradation, 15, 22, 23, 48, 60, 86, 89, 103, 106, 107, 123, 126, 130, 132, 135, 138, 172, 204
dendritic cell, 1, 99, 151, 208, 219
deposition, 37, 44, 79, 86, 101, 122, 123, 124, 126, 128, 129, 130, 133, 136, 143, 196
deposits, 101, 157
deprivation, 139, 143
derivatives, 8, 73, 227
detectable, 7, 86, 125
detection, 11, 217, 227
detoxification, 155
deviation, 162, 213
diabetes, 39, 53
diacylglycerol, 75, 141, 176, 206
diaphragmatic hernia, 55, 207
diet, 34, 46, 52, 53, 58, 64, 68, 110, 141, 142, 153, 219
dietary fat, 71
dietary intake, 44, 52, 64
dietary supplementation, 147
diffusion, 112
digestion, 17, 34, 83
dioxin, 204
disease model, 8
disease progression, 68
diseases, 1, 81, 107, 112, 121, 122, 131, 137, 149, 151, 153, 187, 219
disposition, 49, 57
dissociation, 85
distribution, viii, 4, 9, 15, 37, 38, 42, 50, 56, 62, 63, 76, 104, 106, 113, 125, 162, 169, 180, 191, 194, 198, 201, 202, 208, 209, 210, 213, 219, 226
diversity, 24
DNA, 52, 67, 68, 71, 77, 90, 93, 101, 110, 119, 125, 134, 135, 137, 144, 153, 154, 156, 171, 177, 186, 198, 208, 222, 227
DNA polymerase, 186
dogs, 3
donors, 155
down-regulation, 94, 137
drainage, 186
Drosophila, 149, 201
drugs, 23, 122, 130, 133, 138
dysplasia, 55, 207

E

ECM degradation, 79, 122
ecology, 162
ecosystem, 202
ECs, 2, 157
Ehlers-Danlos syndrome, 195
elastin, 24, 109, 110
electron, vii, 4, 15, 16, 18, 26, 27, 28, 29, 35, 42, 43, 63, 74, 105, 110, 114, 117, 120, 126, 189, 199, 218, 225, 226
electron microscopy, vii, 4, 16, 18, 26, 27, 28, 29, 35, 42, 43, 110, 114, 218
electrophoresis, 82, 83, 92, 93
elongation, 19, 22, 23, 26, 29, 30, 76, 213, 214, 221
elucidation, 126
emphysema, 109
encoding, 57, 176, 177, 200, 212
endoderm, 8, 183
endothelial cells, vii, 1, 2, 4, 35, 93, 100, 174, 175, 178, 180, 193, 194, 198, 203, 214
endothelium, 2, 7, 95, 99, 109, 156
energy, 60
enlargement(s), 102
environment, 48, 128, 153, 157, 162
environmental effects, 153

enzyme(s), 34, 39, 42, 50, 53, 56, 57, 58, 59, 60, 63, 71, 74, 115, 141, 142, 153, 174, 176, 203, 227
epidermis, 97
epididymis, 204
epithelia, 145
epithelial cells, 66, 93, 99, 106, 112, 113, 114, 126, 143, 144, 156, 157, 183, 186
epithelium, 7, 50, 55, 56, 74, 109, 175, 213, 221
equilibrium, 51
erythrocytes, 48
ester, vii, 38, 39, 41, 42, 48, 57, 58, 59, 66, 74, 75, 106, 114, 162, 174, 190, 204, 218, 221
estrogen, 66, 70, 227, 229
ETA, 96
ethanol, 44, 140, 141, 142, 195, 221
ethnic background, 140
etiology, 79, 123, 131, 143, 145, 150
Europe, 122
evidence, 15, 48, 80, 84, 100, 103, 108, 109, 129, 130, 131, 149, 150, 151, 153, 174, 227
evolution, viii, 9, 52, 101, 125
excretion, 53, 136, 159
exercise, 130, 207
experimental condition, 33, 225
exposure, 79, 107, 136, 142, 151
extracellular matrix, vii, 2, 8, 19, 136, 182, 185, 188, 189, 190, 192, 194, 196, 198, 199, 207, 211, 214, 215, 216, 217, 227, 228
extracellular matrix (ECM), vii, 8
extracts, 41
extrahepatic stellate cells (EHSCs), vii

F

falciparum malaria, 48
families, 55
family members, 132
fantasy, 182
fat, vii, 4, 5, 6, 53, 54, 73, 76, 113, 117, 141, 142, 162, 170, 171, 175, 176, 178, 184, 185, 188, 191, 193, 194, 198, 199, 203, 204, 208, 209, 210, 211, 215, 219, 220, 223, 226, 227
fat-storing cells, vii, 4, 5, 175, 176, 178, 185, 188, 191, 194, 199, 203, 208, 215, 220, 223, 227
fatty acids, 39, 44, 48, 57, 59, 111, 142
female rat, 229
fetus, 56
fiber(s), 19, 24, 26, 27, 28, 29, 30, 88, 112, 155, 159, 169, 189, 190
fibroblast growth factor, 90, 170
fibroblast proliferation, 102
fibroblasts, vii, 19, 28, 44, 65, 66, 86, 89, 93, 105, 109, 110, 111, 112, 115, 124, 126, 127, 128, 129, 135, 136, 156, 185, 189, 194, 195, 200, 217, 219, 220, 221, 226
fibrocytes, 8, 126, 127, 175, 193, 209
filament, 94, 111, 175, 200, 204, 212
filtration, 51, 77
fish, 17, 56
fluid, 147, 148, 159
fluorescence, 4, 15, 23, 35, 42, 57, 83, 105, 113, 119, 120, 169, 208
food, 59, 162
food chain, 162
food web, 162
force, 97, 200
formaldehyde, 204
formation, 7, 31, 42, 47, 58, 59, 61, 66, 73, 74, 79, 85, 89, 94, 107, 110, 111, 122, 123, 124, 128, 129, 131, 135, 141, 156, 158, 179, 183, 187, 203, 212, 213, 215, 216, 217
functional changes, 129

G

gadolinium, 78
gel, 19, 20, 21, 22, 23, 24, 26, 27, 28, 29, 30, 82, 83, 87, 88, 89, 92, 93, 194, 201, 213, 214
gelatinase A, 132

gene expression, 8, 26, 43, 54, 68, 70, 78, 81, 83, 84, 86, 90, 92, 93, 94, 103, 123, 124, 126, 134, 135, 137, 141, 150, 153, 172, 176, 177, 178, 186, 187, 191, 192, 201, 205, 210, 212, 214, 225, 228
gene promoter, 86
gene targeting, 64
gene transfer, 136
genes, 13, 36, 47, 49, 60, 69, 78, 80, 84, 93, 133, 137, 147, 153, 172, 182, 195, 218, 228
genome, 90, 191
genotype, 207
gestation, 7
gill, 9, 114
gland, 210
global climate change, 161
glucocorticoid, 66, 70, 171, 189, 195, 207, 209, 225
glucocorticoid receptor, 66, 171, 189, 195, 207, 209, 225
glucose, 52, 53, 54, 78, 104, 177
glucose tolerance, 53, 54, 177
GLUT4, 52, 53
glutathione, 157
glycogen, 15, 78, 214
glycoproteins, vii, 24, 86, 101, 123
glycosaminoglycans, 24, 84
glycosylation, 86
governor, 161
grading, 54
granular vesicles, 104
granules, 48
growth factor, 7, 9, 22, 42, 76, 90, 101, 114, 128, 129, 133, 136, 137, 139, 143, 170, 171, 178, 183, 184, 190, 191, 197, 201, 206, 208, 211, 220, 221, 227, 228
growth hormone, 46

H

harbors, 183
healing, 96, 122, 154
health, 130, 180, 200, 218
heat shock protein, 139, 149, 195
hematopoietic system, 220
hepatic failure, 155
hepatic fibrosis, viii, 5, 44, 68, 70, 71, 75, 83, 90, 92, 97, 102, 122, 124, 125, 126, 129, 133, 134, 135, 137, 138, 140, 143, 152, 178, 181, 182, 183, 195, 198, 206, 207, 208, 210, 215, 217, 226
hepatic injury, 42, 150, 151
hepatic lobule, vii, 1, 2, 18, 104, 120
hepatitis, 52, 54, 81, 121, 122, 124, 127, 132, 135, 140, 149, 171, 207, 208
hepatocarcinogenesis, 96
hepatocellular cancer, 13
hepatocellular carcinoma, 180, 196
hepatocytes, vii, 1, 2, 40, 71, 126, 129, 140, 157, 173, 174, 176, 180, 184, 186, 196, 198, 201, 202, 203, 214, 221, 228
hepatoma, 43, 217
heterogeneity, 104, 120, 124, 125, 171, 188, 197, 223, 224
histochemistry, 11
histology, 3, 5, 119
histone(s), 94, 153, 198, 212
histone deacetylase, 94, 212
history, vii, 4, 170
HLA, 147
homeostasis, vii, 39, 41, 45, 54, 61, 65, 73, 77, 79, 100, 105, 113, 114, 120, 126, 184, 203, 217, 220
hormone(s), 49, 51, 66, 76, 136, 177, 218, 225
human condition, 228
human estrogen receptor, 185
human lung fibroblasts, 112
human skin, 195, 200
human subjects, 177
hybrid, 184
hydrocortisone, 204
hydrogen, 79
hydrogen peroxide, 79
hydrolysis, 38, 57, 183
hydroxyl, 49, 79
hypogonadism, 141, 200
hypoplasia, 207
hypothesis, 8, 54, 81, 98, 114, 139

hypothyroidism, 54
hypoxia, 96, 97, 108, 177

I

ibuprofen, 90
ICAM, 32, 150
identification, 126, 170, 180
identity, 55, 59, 60, 74
IFN, 135, 148
IL-8, 150
immune function, 49, 148
immune reaction, 134
immune response, 3, 99, 149, 151, 186
immune system, 151
immunity, 126, 140, 149, 171
immunofluorescence, 30, 34, 120, 127
immunoglobulin, 32
immunoglobulin superfamily, 32
immunohistochemistry, 80, 117
immunolocalization, 65
immunomodulatory, 148
immunoprecipitation, 154
immunoreactivity, 41, 92, 183
immunotherapy, 155
impregnation, 4, 11, 35, 220
improvements, 124, 131
in vitro, 30, 31, 32, 41, 44, 45, 47, 79, 84, 92, 93, 95, 110, 125, 127, 136, 138, 139, 143, 150, 157, 178, 183, 187, 189, 193, 196, 200, 201, 203, 204, 218, 221, 222, 224, 228
India, 3
individuals, 37
inducer, 179
induction, 22, 29, 43, 44, 47, 78, 96, 101, 105, 106, 107, 109, 138, 141, 142, 149, 150, 180, 181, 183, 191, 198, 199
inflammation, 48, 53, 67, 77, 78, 90, 102, 105, 106, 107, 126, 149, 150, 151, 180, 190
inflammatory cells, 90
inflammatory mediators, 150
ingestion, 105
inheritance, 154
inhibition, 68, 76, 80, 84, 85, 86, 107, 130, 134, 135, 136, 138, 169, 181, 183, 189, 200, 227
inhibitor, 22, 71, 86, 90, 91, 93, 94, 97, 107, 108, 111, 125, 133, 137, 138, 141, 150, 154, 171, 181, 184, 186, 196, 204, 207, 212, 215, 218
initiation, 85, 108
injections, 84, 107, 131
injury(ies), 8, 24, 48, 65, 77, 78, 79, 80, 81, 90, 95, 96, 98, 101, 103, 124, 128, 130, 131, 132, 133, 135, 138, 139, 144, 150, 152, 154, 170, 172, 178, 179, 180, 181, 185, 192, 194, 197, 205, 220
innate immunity, 140, 147, 149, 151
inoculation, 20
inositol, 22, 31
insulin, 39, 52, 53, 54, 68, 76, 142, 143, 184, 208, 227
insulin resistance, 39, 52, 53, 54, 184, 208, 227
insulin sensitivity, 53, 54
insulin signaling, 142
integrin(s), viii, 22, 24, 26, 27, 28, 29, 30, 48, 76, 89, 94, 136, 139, 176, 179, 180, 184, 194, 196, 213, 219
integrity, 94
intercellular adhesion molecule, 32, 188, 194
interface, 127
interference, 44, 46
interferon, 76, 86, 132, 134, 151, 208, 211
interleukin-8, 97
intervention, 133, 134
intestine, 3, 9, 17, 56, 57, 59, 105, 112, 113, 114, 115, 188, 217
intoxication, 77
intravenously, 38, 151
ions, 31
iron, 147
ischemia, 137, 194
isolation, vii, 1, 33, 34, 35, 37, 84, 155, 157, 170, 193, 203, 218
isomers, 59
issues, 76

IV collagenase, 196

J

Japan, 121
jejunum, 161, 162

K

keratinocyte, 183
keratinocytes, 74
kidney(s), vii, 3, 9, 51, 56, 105, 109, 114, 115, 123, 161, 162, 179, 192, 193, 204, 219
kill, 102
kinetics, 97, 178
kinship, 171

L

labeling, 156
larvae, 144
laryngeal cancer, 115
latency, 85
LDL, 48
lecithin, 15, 57, 74, 173, 181, 197, 205, 212, 218
leptin, 53, 76, 77, 129, 208
lesions, 127, 128
leucine, 151
leucocyte, 175
liberation, 57
lifetime, 159
ligand, 49, 50, 55, 57, 58, 60, 61, 63, 67, 68, 69, 71, 81, 85, 102, 125, 138, 178, 186, 209, 218
light, 35, 110, 122, 144, 199
lipases, 74
lipid metabolism, 44, 180, 229
lipid peroxidation, 48, 79, 80
lipids, 39, 73, 87
lipoproteins, 48
liposomes, 139, 213
liquid chromatography, 161
liver cancer, 121, 122
liver cells, 3, 4, 11, 33, 34, 38, 62, 63, 119, 137, 155, 158, 169, 173, 174, 188, 197, 202, 204, 219
liver cirrhosis, viii, 54, 82, 83, 92, 101, 121, 132, 135, 140, 181, 213, 226
liver damage, 77, 126
liver disease, 54, 76, 79, 81, 91, 94, 121, 122, 124, 125, 126, 131, 133, 134, 135, 136, 137, 140, 142, 143, 174, 197, 208, 218, 221, 226
liver failure, 155
liver sinusoidal endothelial cells (LSECs), vii, 1
liver transplantation, 130, 155
localization, 4, 22, 26, 67, 72, 92, 125, 169, 184, 189, 192, 196, 203, 204, 207, 224
longevity, 157
low-density lipoprotein, 48, 149, 214
lumen, 2, 15, 40, 100
luminescence, 6
lymph, 40, 105
lymph node, 105
lymphatic system, 59, 113
lymphocytes, 25, 109
lymphoid, 3, 99, 147
lymphoid organs, 3, 99
lysine, 19, 26
lysis, 147
lysosome, 17, 48, 73

M

macromolecules, 87, 148
macrophages, 2, 6, 91, 93, 99, 103, 126, 150, 179, 210
magnitude, 95
major histocompatibility complex, 148
majority, 62, 75, 111, 121, 124
malnutrition, 76
mammals, vii, 3, 9, 37, 62, 104, 191, 201, 216
man, 184
management, 126, 140, 208, 219
mapping, 227

marrow, 8, 126, 188, 193
mass, 7, 37, 53, 62, 108, 119, 155, 158
mast cells, 109
materials, 4
matrix metalloproteinase, 24, 128, 177, 186, 188, 201, 207, 220
matter, 198
maturation process, 98
MCP-1, 67, 68, 136, 150, 152
meat, 17
mechanical stress, 128
media, 45
mediation, 114
medical, 167
medicine, 137, 140, 165
MEK, 90, 211
membranes, 42, 50, 51, 155
mental retardation, 207
mesenchyme, 7, 8
mesentery, 7
mesoderm, 7, 114, 183
mesothelium, 7, 171, 207
messenger RNA, 86, 134, 196
messengers, 78
Metabolic, 50
metabolic changes, 217
metabolic disorder(s), 210
metabolic syndrome, 53
metabolism, 24, 34, 35, 39, 43, 44, 46, 49, 50, 51, 56, 57, 59, 60, 63, 65, 68, 74, 76, 82, 88, 115, 140, 173, 174, 178, 184, 187, 188, 196, 203, 209, 212, 216
metabolites, 39, 43, 49, 60, 80, 106
metabolized, 57, 58
metabolizing, 58, 60
metalloproteinase, 71, 181, 190, 207, 220
metamorphosis, 144, 202
metastasis, 24
metformin, 134
methanol, 191
methylation, 153, 154, 198
MHC, 148
mice, 7, 8, 37, 42, 43, 52, 53, 58, 60, 64, 68, 80, 84, 85, 86, 92, 93, 109, 117, 125, 130, 133, 141, 149, 152, 162, 177, 178, 188, 190, 191, 192, 193, 205, 209, 224, 225, 226, 228
microcirculation, 97, 119, 191
microorganisms, 147
microscope, 35, 120, 189, 199
microscopy, 4, 13, 17, 20, 21, 30, 35, 91, 105, 113, 119, 120, 144, 156, 201, 202, 205, 208
microsomes, 42, 60, 210, 212
migration, 17, 22, 24, 47, 76, 83, 85, 87, 94, 100, 107, 108, 114, 129, 158, 199, 207, 212, 227
mineralocorticoid, 66, 70, 171
misconception period, 4
mitochondria, 137
mitogen(s), 29, 78, 90, 91, 106, 107, 123, 136, 157, 178, 208
mitosis, 153
MMP(s), 24, 79, 86, 87, 94, 96, 106, 132, 133, 135, 136, 139, 206, 213, 224
MMP-2, 79, 94, 96, 132, 133, 135, 139, 206, 213, 224
model system, 144, 228
models, 80, 93, 131, 133, 135, 140, 179, 181, 184, 209
modifications, 45, 47, 112, 142, 153
mole, 162
molecular weight, 93, 169
molecules, 1, 14, 22, 24, 31, 32, 48, 49, 73, 76, 81, 99, 108, 123, 124, 128, 132, 148, 149, 151
monoclonal antibody, 48
monolayer, 73, 74, 221
morbidity, 130, 141, 155
morphogenesis, 35, 61, 158, 159, 186, 219
morphology, vii, 5, 18, 19, 24, 25, 26, 27, 28, 87, 88, 90, 100, 104, 110, 112, 113, 115, 215, 216
morphometric, 114, 136
mortality, 46, 121, 122, 130
mortality rate, 121, 122
MR, 66, 70, 72
mRNA(s), 41, 46, 48, 57, 68, 69, 70, 71, 76, 77, 81, 84, 91, 96, 107, 108, 109, 123,

125, 131, 133, 134, 136, 138, 141, 143, 151, 154, 194, 196, 222
mucosa, 105, 114
multicellular organisms, 153
mutation(s), 55, 77, 153, 172
myocyte, 91, 224
myofibroblasts, vii, 8, 43, 47, 82, 91, 103, 109, 111, 124, 125, 126, 127, 129, 138, 154, 170, 191, 192, 193, 197, 210, 215, 220, 222
myoglobin, 93
myosin, 109, 221

N

NAD, 142
NADH, 142
natural killer cell, 3, 148
necrosis, 13, 44, 102, 141, 149, 219
nerve, 3, 78, 95, 101, 103, 104, 205, 221
nerve fibers, 95, 101
nerve growth factor, 101, 205, 221
nervous system, 6, 99, 103
neuropeptides, 104
neurotransmitter(s), 78, 103, 104
neutral, 73, 139
NH2, 136
nicotinamide, 157, 201
nitric oxide, 94, 192
nitrogen, 79
nodules, 122, 123
non-structural protein, 140
norepinephrine, 97, 103
Northern blot, 57, 72
NPC, 5, 33, 63, 104, 158, 159
nuclear receptors, 36, 66, 67, 72, 207
nuclei, 110
nucleotides, 31
nucleus, 18, 60, 61, 69, 86
null, 52, 58, 64
nutritional status, 173

O

obesity, 39, 52, 53, 54, 177, 192, 227
obstruction, 109
old age, 117
omission, 131
optical microscopy, 88
organ(s), vii, 3, 9, 40, 41, 55, 62, 63, 65, 85, 93, 103, 105, 106, 112, 113, 122, 123, 125, 129, 130, 131, 147, 151, 155, 161, 162, 165, 190, 195, 203, 208, 218, 223, 224
organelle(s), 17, 37, 42, 73, 110, 183
organism, 81, 144, 153
organize, 129
oxidation, 49, 50, 58, 59, 65, 141, 142
oxidative stress, 48, 70, 76, 79, 140, 141, 191
oxygen, 96, 97, 140

P

pancreas, vii, 3, 106, 107, 114, 165, 170, 219, 222
pancreatic cancer, 107, 108, 199, 203
pancreatic fibrosis, 105, 106, 107, 108, 186, 200, 205
pancreatitis, 105, 106, 107, 108, 186, 200, 225
parallel, 9, 78
parenchyma, 98, 99, 102, 110, 122, 128, 131, 217
parenchymal cell(s), vii, 1, 2, 5, 16, 40, 70, 71, 187, 194, 197, 213, 216, 217
pathogenesis, 1, 48, 53, 54, 96, 97, 112, 137, 141, 145, 186, 193
pathogens, 81, 149, 151
pathophysiological, 75
pathophysiology, 151, 209
pathways, 47, 70, 82, 108, 126, 132, 134, 137, 142, 147, 151, 170, 172, 177, 191, 197, 205, 206
PBMC, 150
PCBs, 162, 179, 189

PCR, 72
pepsin, 83
peptide(s), 76, 85, 89, 108, 148, 152, 184
perfusion, 33, 34, 96, 109
pericytes, 5, 100, 111, 192
peripheral blood, 150, 209
peripheral blood mononuclear cell, 150
permeability, 31
permission, 161
peroxynitrite, 79
PGE, 78
phagocyte, 2, 99
phagocytic cells, 80, 81, 107, 224
phagocytosis, 79, 80, 87, 147, 148, 218
pharmacokinetics, 158
phenobarbitone, 157
phenotype(s), 23, 41, 43, 45, 47, 52, 55, 64, 75, 76, 79, 85, 87, 88, 89, 90, 92, 94, 96, 97, 103, 106, 115, 125, 126, 127, 128, 129, 130, 136, 138, 141, 157, 170, 178, 181, 182, 187, 188, 198, 199, 213, 214, 221
phosphate, 89, 156, 187, 195, 215
phosphoenolpyruvate, 53
phospholipids, 39, 48, 57
phosphorylation, 22, 27, 29, 30, 68, 71, 77, 78, 85, 152, 194
photobleaching, 74, 221
physical structure, 87
Physiological, 174
physiology, 177
PI3K, 91, 123
pigs, 3
pioglitazone, 67, 68, 142, 195
plasma levels, 81, 218
plasma membrane, 17, 51, 55, 75
plasminogen, 69, 86, 133, 202
plasticity, 125
platelets, 85
platform, 73, 182
playing, 71, 113
plexus, 56, 60
point mutation, 52
polar, 9, 12, 13, 14, 16, 49, 60, 161, 162, 163, 211, 218, 225
polarity, 24, 149, 157
polyacrylamide, 82, 92, 93
polymerase, 93
polymerase chain reaction, 93
polypeptide(s), 15, 84, 92, 208
polysaccharides, 87
polystyrene, 19, 21, 22, 26, 27, 87, 88, 156, 158
polyunsaturated fat, 142, 221
pools, 47, 51, 52
population, 91, 96, 121, 127, 130, 131, 157
portal hypertension, 97
portal vein, 33, 34, 38, 62, 127, 144, 151
post-transcriptional regulation, 201
precipitation, 83
precursor cells, 127, 128
predators, 16, 162, 163, 216
preparation, 33, 158
primary cells, 91
primate, 177
priming, 147
progenitor cells, 134, 158
progesterone, 66, 70, 178, 191, 227
prognosis, 122
proline, 83
promoter, 46, 64, 68, 133, 154, 171, 224, 227
pronunciation, 5
propagation, 31
prostaglandins, 78, 103
proteasome, 138
protection, 48, 148
protein family, 50, 222
protein kinase C, 22, 95
protein kinases, 107
protein synthesis, 102, 110, 125, 134, 214, 215
proteinase, 48, 70, 136, 181
protein-protein interactions, 56, 57, 58, 61
proteoglycans, 24, 25, 84, 101, 123
proteolysis, 85, 139, 228
proteome, 83, 92
proto-oncogene, 172
prototype, 52
purification, 33, 34, 35, 188, 193

purity, 13
pylorus, 9

Q

quantification, 222

R

radicals, 79, 80
RANTES, 97
RE, 40, 72, 75
reactions, 56, 88
reading, 69
reality, 180
reasoning, 158
receptors, 8, 13, 24, 36, 40, 47, 49, 60, 66, 73, 77, 78, 81, 84, 85, 90, 93, 96, 97, 103, 108, 110, 136, 138, 141, 149, 172, 176, 177, 180, 181, 186, 191, 200, 202, 208, 211, 212, 220, 224, 227
recognition, 15, 28, 30, 126, 149, 151, 180, 219
recombination, 43
recovery, 103, 120, 131, 138, 139, 143, 204
regenerate, 8
regeneration, vii, 9, 107, 119, 120, 126, 192, 197, 199, 222
regression, 54, 132, 134, 188
relaxation, 97, 192
repair, 96, 109, 128, 175, 179, 190, 193
repressor, 150, 154
reproduction, 49
reproductive organs, 56
RES, 223, 226
researchers, 4, 33, 81, 130, 165
residues, 28, 85
resistance, 53, 54, 94, 95, 96, 139, 211, 226
resolution, 124, 126, 131, 136, 137, 138, 139, 143, 181, 190, 191
response, 8, 19, 26, 42, 46, 61, 69, 76, 77, 78, 81, 84, 85, 88, 91, 96, 97, 98, 100, 103, 114, 122, 123, 128, 131, 135, 136, 142, 148, 149, 150, 151, 156, 157, 158, 181, 200, 205, 221, 227
responsiveness, 77, 84, 148, 178, 201
restoration, 115, 131, 157
reticulum, 15, 51, 74, 82, 135
retina, 36, 213
rhodopsin, 36, 221
risk, 44, 54
RNA, 68, 84, 133, 139
rodents, 81, 119
root, 126
rosiglitazone, 53, 67
rubber, 95

S

salts, 159
SARA, 86
saturated fatty acids, 47
saturation, 57
scar tissue, 123
schistosomiasis, 127
secrete, 3, 26, 34, 40, 41, 79, 82, 99, 105, 106, 108, 111, 112, 147, 179, 207, 215
secretion, 41, 44, 51, 54, 67, 76, 79, 96, 97, 101, 108, 110, 111, 112, 140, 150, 152, 214
selectivity, 49
sensitivity, 53
sensitization, 152
septum, 3, 7, 8
serine, 22, 29, 85, 86, 93, 107
serum, 42, 50, 53, 54, 64, 69, 70, 71, 85, 110, 134, 139, 144, 157, 172, 174, 177, 183, 203, 204, 216, 219
serum albumin, 204
sex, 173
sham, 45
sham-operated animals, 45
shape, 1, 4, 6, 19, 23, 25, 26, 99, 101, 104, 157, 221
shock, 15
shortage, 47, 155
siblings, 52
sieve plate, 100

signal transduction, viii, 17, 22, 27, 29, 30, 85, 95, 133, 150, 177, 190, 194
signaling pathway, 29, 91, 93, 95, 151, 196, 197
signalling, 53, 80, 81, 134
signals, 23, 24, 29, 128, 152, 191, 197, 207, 227
signs, 19, 79, 151, 162
silver, 4, 11, 35, 220
siRNA, 80, 139, 154, 214
skeletal muscle, 51, 59
skin, 60, 114, 170, 187
small intestine, 56, 59, 70, 74
smooth muscle, 8, 13, 95, 126, 127, 220, 222
smooth muscle cells, 8, 95, 126, 127, 220
SNAP, 79
solution, 61
species, 28, 56, 60, 71, 104, 127, 140, 151, 170
spectroscopy, 15, 169
speculation, 122
spelling, 5
spindle, 18, 27
spleen, 51, 105, 161, 162
spontaneous recovery, 131, 139, 144
Sprague-Dawley rats, 198
stability, 123, 157, 158
standardization, 1, 4, 6
stars, 225
state(s), 45, 49, 56, 90, 92, 134, 154, 212
Stellate cell(s) (SC), vii, 2, 181, 216, 224
stem cells, 98, 210, 220
stenosis, 186
steroids, 71
stimulation, 61, 78, 84, 85, 94, 101, 102, 170, 171, 221
stimulus, 90, 95
stress, 15, 19, 26, 29, 70, 79, 88, 137, 141
stroma, 123
stromal cells, 180
structural changes, 122
structure, vii, 3, 7, 19, 23, 25, 27, 28, 31, 66, 73, 82, 87, 88, 89, 122, 153, 154, 156, 158, 159, 175, 180, 182, 189, 193, 194, 199, 214, 216, 217, 223, 224, 225, 226
subcutaneous injection, 113
substitution, 47
substrate, 56, 57, 58, 59, 60, 74, 95
Sudan, 163
sulfate, 24, 26, 83, 87, 184
supplementation, 45, 107, 195
suppression, 68, 78, 134, 172, 217
surface area, 100
surface layer, 172
survival, 26, 49, 139, 140, 143, 162
susceptibility, 47, 138
suspensions, 33
Sweden, 161
sympathetic nervous system, 103
syncytium, 31
syndrome, 55, 58
systolic blood pressure, 53

T

T cell, 128, 137, 147, 148, 193, 225
T lymphocytes, 148
target, viii, 49, 51, 52, 60, 70, 72, 82, 85, 130, 133, 137, 138, 172, 181, 218, 229
T-cell receptor, 148
techniques, vii, 18, 85, 167
technology, 155
TEM, 28, 31, 100, 105, 114, 117, 129
testis, 51, 105, 204
testosterone, 72, 204
textbook, 165
therapeutic agents, 137
therapeutic approaches, 131
therapeutic targets, 92, 123
therapy, viii, 85, 131, 132, 138, 141, 165
thiazolidinediones, 183
third dimension, 178
threonine, 22, 29, 85
thrombin, 70, 76, 136, 197
thymus, 105
thyroid, 51, 66, 177, 218, 219, 225
TIMP, 71, 86, 90, 96, 131, 132, 133, 135, 213

TIMP-1, 71, 90, 131, 132, 133, 135, 213
TIR, 151
TLR, 149, 150, 151, 152
TLR2, 150, 151, 152
TLR4, 149, 150, 151, 152, 215
TLR9, 151
TNF, 68, 84, 90, 106, 135, 142, 150, 152, 222
TNF-α, 222
toxic waste, 159
toxicity, 46, 162, 211
toxicology, 158
toxin, 135
trachea, 105
trade, 157
trade-off, 157
trafficking, 17, 148
trainees, 6
transcription, 9, 36, 47, 49, 61, 69, 70, 75, 77, 90, 91, 93, 133, 140, 169, 172, 186, 210, 218, 224
transcription factors, 47, 49, 90, 91, 93, 186
transcripts, 41, 47, 133, 185
transducer, 102
transduction, 194, 208, 212
transfection, 177
transferrin, 148, 156, 157
transformation, 32, 44, 50, 60, 92, 180
transforming growth factor, 176, 190, 200, 201, 205, 225
translation, 69, 159
translocation, 74, 78, 80, 172
transmission, 28, 73
transplantation, 130, 155, 158
transport, 34, 35, 40, 49, 51, 60, 61, 64, 65, 75, 88, 102, 112, 113, 114, 144, 155, 161, 172, 174, 179, 189, 190, 192, 195, 199, 218, 219
treatment, viii, 22, 23, 41, 44, 46, 47, 65, 68, 76, 83, 84, 86, 89, 92, 94, 105, 106, 107, 123, 124, 130, 132, 133, 134, 136, 137, 141, 144, 154, 171, 181, 200
trichostatin A, 212
triglycerides, 67, 111
trypsin, 111
tumor(s), 19, 102, 107, 108, 114, 138, 183, 203
tumor growth, 107
tumor necrosis factor, 102, 138, 183
tumorigenesis, 24, 35, 61
turnover, 58, 207
type 2 diabetes, 39, 52, 53, 54, 177, 208, 226, 227
tyrosine, 22, 29, 77, 78, 90, 194, 222

U

ultrastructure, 31, 156
underlying mechanisms, 136
uniform, 44
United States, 121, 142, 209
urinary bladder, 105, 227
urokinase, 156, 202
uterus, 60, 105

V

vasculature, 95
vasopressin, 76
VCAM, 150
vector, 39
vegetables, 112
vein, 98, 126, 127
vertebrate evolution, viii, 9
vertebrates, viii, 9, 52, 56, 100, 105, 113, 144, 179, 218, 224
vessels, 103, 127, 129
video microscopy, 20
video-recording, 19, 23, 89
viruses, 122
vision, 49, 52, 64
vitamin C, 89, 156
vitamin D, 66, 70, 183, 200
vitamin K, 71
vitamins, 31
VLA, 179, 220

W

Western blot, 41, 72, 93
Western countries, 140
withdrawal, 134
Wnt signaling, 93, 191
workers, 6
worldwide, 121, 130, 142
wound healing, 96, 122, 123, 131, 151, 154, 198

X

X chromosome, 196

Y

yield, 62, 144, 174

Z

zinc, 141, 200